Lecture Notes in Artificial Intelligence 6747

Edited by R. Goebel, J. Siekmann, and W. Wahlster

Subseries of Lecture Notes in Computer Science

Mor Peleg
Nada Lavrač
Carlo Combi (Eds.)

Artificial Intelligence in Medicine

13th Conference on Artificial Intelligence
in Medicine, AIME 2011
Bled, Slovenia, July 2-6, 2011
Proceedings

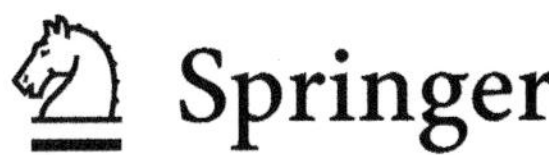

Series Editors

Randy Goebel, University of Alberta, Edmonton, Canada
Jörg Siekmann, University of Saarland, Saarbrücken, Germany
Wolfgang Wahlster, DFKI and University of Saarland, Saarbrücken, Germany

Volume Editors

Mor Peleg
University of Haifa
Department of Information Systems
Haifa 31905, Israel
E-mail: morpeleg@is.haifa.ac.il

Nada Lavrač
Jožef Stefan Institute
Department of Knowledge Technologies
1000 Ljubljana, Slovenia
E-mail: nada.lavrac@ijs.si

Carlo Combi
University of Verona
Department of Computer Science
37134 Verona, Italy
E-mail: carlo.combi@univr.it

ISSN 0302-9743
e-ISSN 1611-3349
ISBN 978-3-642-22217-7
e-ISBN 978-3-642-22218-4
DOI 10.1007/978-3-642-22218-4
Springer Heidelberg Dordrecht London New York

Library of Congress Control Number: 2011930409
CR Subject Classification (1998): I.2, J.3, H.2.8, H.3-4, C.2

LNCS Sublibrary: SL 7 – Artificial Intelligence

Typesetting: Camera-ready by author, data conversion by Scientific Publishing Services, Chennai, India

Printed on acid-free paper

Springer is part of Springer Science+Business Media (www.springer.com)

Preface

The European Society for Artificial Intelligence in Medicine (AIME) was established in 1986 following a very successful workshop held in Pavia, Italy, the previous year. The principal aims of AIME are to foster fundamental and applied research in the application of artificial intelligence (AI) techniques to medical care and medical research, and to provide a forum at biennial conferences for discussing any progress made. For this reason the main activity of the society was the organization of a series of biennial conferences, held in Marseilles, France (1987), London, UK (1989), Maastricht, The Netherlands (1991), Munich, Germany (1993), Pavia, Italy (1995), Grenoble, France (1997), Aalborg, Denmark (1999), Cascais, Portugal (2001), Protaras, Cyprus (2003), Aberdeen, UK (2005), Amsterdam, The Netherlands (2007), and Verona, Italy (2009). This volume contains the proceedings of AIME 2011, the 13th Conference on Artificial Intelligence in Medicine, held in Bled, Slovenia, July 2–6, 2011.

The AIME 2011 goals were to present and consolidate the international state of the art of AI in biomedical research from the perspectives of theory, methodology, and application. The conference included two invited lectures, full and short papers, a special session on "Applications of AI Methods," tutorials, workshops, and a doctoral consortium. In the conference announcement, authors were solicited to submit original contributions regarding the development of theory, techniques, and applications of AI in biomedicine, including the exploitation of AI approaches to molecular medicine and biomedical informatics and to healthcare organizational aspects. Authors of papers addressing theory were requested to describe the properties of novel AI methodologies potentially useful for solving biomedical problems. Authors of papers addressing techniques and methodologies were asked to describe the development or the extension of AI methods and their implementation, and to discuss the assumptions and limitations of the proposed methods and their novelty with respect to the state of the art. Authors of papers addressing systems were asked to describe the requirements, design, and implementation of new AI-inspired tools and systems, and discuss their applicability in the medical field. Finally, authors of application papers were asked to present the implementation of AI systems to solve significant medical problems, to provide sufficient information to allow the evaluation of the practical benefits of such systems, and to discuss the lessons learned.

AIME 2011 received 113 abstract submissions, 92 thereof were submitted as complete papers. Submissions came from 29 different countries, including 8 outside Europe. These numbers confirm the high relevance of AIME in attracting the interest of research groups around the globe. Fifteen of the papers (10 long and 5 short) were submitted to the special session on AI Applications. The papers for the special session went through a separate review process conducted by AIME Board Members Ameen Abu-Hanna and Steen Andreassen, who selected six long papers for inclusion in the special session and also provided recommendations for some papers that were submitted to the special session but were more appropriate for the main session. All other papers, as well as the two most promising papers from the special session that were not selected for inclusion, were carefully peer-reviewed by experts from the Program Committee with the support of additional reviewers. Each submission was reviewed by two to four reviewers, with most submissions reviewed by three reviewers. The reviewers judged the quality and originality of the submitted papers, together with their relevance to the AIME conference. Seven criteria were taken into consideration in judging submissions: the reviewers' overall recommendation, the appropriateness, the technical correctness, the quality of presentation, the originality, the reviewers' detailed comments, and the reviewers' confidence in the subject area.

In four 2–3-hour Skype-based virtual meetings held during March 25–31, 2011, and in several short discussions in subsequent days, a small committee consisting of the AIME 2011 Scientific Chair, Mor Peleg, the AIME 2011 Organizing Committee Chair, Nada Lavrač, and the AIME Chairman of the Board, Carlo Combi made the final decisions regarding the AIME 2011 scientific program.

As a result, 18 long papers (with an acceptance rate of about 26%) and 20 short papers were accepted. Each long paper was presented in a 25-minute oral presentation during the conference. Each short paper was presented in a 5-minute presentation and with a poster. The papers were organized according to their topics in the following main themes: (1) Knowledge-Based Systems; (2) Data Mining; (3) Special Session on AI Applications; (4) Probabilistic Modeling and Reasoning; (5) Terminologies and Ontologies; (6) Temporal Reasoning and Temporal Data Mining; (7) Therapy Planning, Scheduling, and Guideline-Based Care; (8) Natural Language Processing.

AIME 2011 had the privilege of hosting two invited speakers: Manfred Reichert, from the University of Ulm, Germany, and Andrey Rzhetsky, from the University of Chicago, Illinois, USA. Manfred Reichert gave a talk on "What BPM Technology Can Do for Healthcare Process Support," and Andrey Rzhetsky on "Understanding Etiology of Complex Neurodevelopmental Disorders: Two Approaches."

Continuing a tradition started at AIME 2005, a doctoral consortium, organized by Carlo Combi, was held again this year and included a tutorial given by Carlo Combi and Riccardo Bellazzi on how to structure different types of research papers. A scientific panel chaired by Carlo Combi and consisting of Ameen Abu-Hanna, Steen Andreassen, Riccardo Bellazzi, Michel Dojat, Werner Horn, Elpida Keravnou, Peter Lucas, Silvia Miksch, Niels Peek, Silvana Quaglini, Yuval Shahar, and Blaz Zupan discussed the contents of the students' doctoral theses.

Two half-day tutorials were also held one day before the start of the conference: "Introduction to Clinical Data-Mining Methods" given by John H. Holmes and "Personalized Healthcare Information Access" given by Shlomo Berkovsky and Jill Freyne.

Continuing the tradition started at AIME 2009, a significant number of full-day workshops were organized following the AIME 2011 main conference: the workshop entitled "Probabilistic Problem Solving in Biomedicine," chaired by Arjen Hommersom and Peter Lucas; the workshop entitled "KR4HC 2011, Third Knowledge Representation for Health-Care: Data, Processes and Guidelines," chaired by Silvia Miksch, David Riaño and Annette ten Teije; the workshop entitled "IDAMAP (Intelligent Data Analysis in Biomedicine and Pharmacology)" (special topic: Intelligent Data Analysis for Quality and Safety in Healthcare) chaired by Niels Peek, John Holmes, Allan Tucker, and Riccardo Bellazzi; the "Louhi Workshop—Text and Data Mining of Health Documents," chaired by Øystein Nytrø; and "Learning from Medical Data Streams" chaired by Pedro Pereira Rodrigues, Mykola Pechenizkiy, João Gama, and Mohamed Medhat Gaber.

We would like to thank everyone who contributed to AIME 2011. First of all we thank the authors of the papers submitted and the members of the Program Committee together with the additional reviewers. Thanks are also due to the invited speakers as well as to the organizers of the workshops and the tutorials and doctoral consortium. The free EasyChair conference Web system (http://www.easychair.org/) was an important tool supporting us in the management of submissions, reviews, selection of accepted papers, and preparation of the overall material for the final proceedings. We are grateful to the Slovene National Research Agency (ARRS), the Office of Naval Research Global (ONRG) and the Pascal European Network of Excellence (PASCAL2) for their generous financial support. We are also grateful to the collaborators of the Department of Knowledge Technologies of Jožef Stefan Institute, Ljubljana, Slovenia, acting in the local organization team, for their help in organizing the conference. The local team was co-chaired by Tina Anžič, who did a tremendous amount of work which resulted in the smooth running of the conference as a whole. Finally, we thank the Springer team for helping us in the final preparation of this LNCS book.

April 2011

Mor Peleg
Nada Lavrač
Carlo Combi

Organization

Scientific Chair

Mor Peleg

Program Committee

Raza Abidi, Canada
Ameen Abu-Hanna, The Netherlands
(Applications Session Co-chair)
Klaus-Peter Adlassnig, Austria
Steen Andreassen, Denmark
(Applications Session Co-chair)
Pedro Barahona, Portugal
Riccardo Bellazzi, Italy
Petr Berka, Czech Republic
Isabelle Bichindaritz, USA
Elizabeth Borycki, Canada
Aziz Boxwala, USA
Carlo Combi, Italy
(Doctoral Consortium Chair)
Michel Dojat, France
Henrik Eriksson, Sweden
Catherine Garbay, France
Adela Grando, UK
Femida Gwadry-Sridhar, Canada
Peter Haddawy, Macau
Arie Hasman, The Netherlands
Reinhold Haux, Germany
John Holmes, USA
Werner Horn, Austria
Jim Hunter, UK
Hidde de Jong, France
Elpida Keravnou, Cyprus
Pedro Larranaga, Spain
Nada Lavrac, Slovenia (Local Chair)
Johan van der Lei, The Netherlands
Xiaohui Liu, UK
Peter Lucas, The Netherlands
Roque Marin, Spain
Michael Marschollek, Germany
Carolyn McGregor, Canada
Paola Mello, Italy
Gloria Menegaz, Italy
Silvia Miksch, Austria
Stefania Montani, Italy
Mark Musen, USA
Barbara Oliboni, Italy
Niels Peek, The Netherlands
Mor Peleg, Israel (Scientific Chair)
Christian Popow, Austria
Silvana Quaglini, Italy
Alan Rector, UK
Stephen Rees, Denmark
Daniel Rubin, USA
Lucia Sacchi, Italy
Rainer Schmidt, Germany
Brigitte Seroussi, France
Yuval Shahar, Israel
Basilio Sierra, Spain
Costas Spyropoulos, Greece
Paolo Terenziani, Italy
Samson Tu, USA
Allan Tucker, UK
Frans Voorbraak, The Netherlands
Dongwen Wang, USA
Blaz Zupan, Slovenia
Pierre Zweigenbaum, France

Organizing Committee

Tina Anzic (Co-chair)
Damjan Demsar
Matjaz Jursic
Janes Kranjc
Nada Lavrač (Chair)
Dragana Miljkovic
Vid Podpecan
Borut Sluban
Anze Vavpetic

Additional Reviewers

Raphael Bahati
Alessio Bottrighi
Jacques Bouaud
Manuel Campos
Federico Chesani
Matteo Gabetta
Perry Groot
Francisco Guil-Reyes
Maarten van der Heijden
Arjen Hommersom
Jose M. Juarez
Katharina Kaiser
Hameedullah Kazi
Giorgio Leonardi
Mar Marcos
Caterina Marinagi
Andrès Mendez
Dragana Miljkovic
Marco Montali
Giulia Paggetti
Jose Palma
Sergios Petridis
Francesca Pizzorni Ferrarese
Phattanapon Rhienmora
Andreas Seyfang
Nigam Shah
Davide Sottara
Paolo Torroni
Marina Velikova

Doctoral Consortium

Chair: Carlo Combi, Italy

Workshops

Probabilistic Problem Solving in Biomedicine

Co-chairs: Arjen Hommersom (Radboud University Nijmegen, The Netherlands) and Peter Lucas (Radboud University Nijmegen, The Netherlands)

KR4HC 2011, Third Knowledge Representation for Health-Care: Data, Processes and Guidelines

Co-chairs: Silvia Miksch (Vienna University of Technology, Austria), David Riaño (Universitat Rovira i Virgili, Spain), and Annette ten Teije (Vrije Universiteit Amsterdam, The Netherlands)

IDAMAP 2011, Intelligent Data Analysis in Biomedicine and Pharmacology Special Topic: Intelligent Data Analysis for Quality and Safety in Healthcare

Co-chairs: Niels Peek (University of Amsterdam, The Netherlands), John Holmes (University of Pennsylvania School of Medicine, USA), Allan Tucker (Brunel University, London, UK), Riccardo Bellazzi (University of Pavia, Italy)

Louhi Workshop – Text and Data Mining of Health Documents

Chair: Øystein Nytrø (Norwegian University of Science and Technology, Norway)

Learning from Medical Data Streams

Co-chairs: Pedro Pereira Rodrigues (University of Porto, Portugal), Mykola Pechenizkiy (Eindhoven University of Technology, The Netherlands), João Gama (University of Porto, Portugal), and Mohamed Medhat Gaber (University of Portsmouth, UK)

Tutorials

Introduction to Clinical Data-Mining Methods

John H. Holmes (University of Pennsylvania School of Medicine, USA)

Personalized Healthcare Information Access

Shlomo Berkovsky (CSIRO ICT Centre, Australia) and Jill Freyne (CSIRO ICT Centre, Australia)

Table of Contents

Invited Talks

1. Knowledge-Based Systems

2. Data Mining

3. Special Session on AI Applications

4. Probabilistic Modeling and Reasoning

5. Terminologies and Ontologies

6. Temporal Reasoning and Temporal Data Mining

7. Therapy Planning, Scheduling and Guideline-Based Care

8. Natural Language Processing

Understanding Etiology of Complex Neurodevelopmental Disorders: Two Approaches

Andrey Rzhetsky

Depts. of Medicine and Human Genetics, Computation Institute and Institute of Genomics and Systems Biology, University of Chicago, Chicago, Illinois, USA
arzhetsk@medicine.bsd.uchicago.edu

Abstract. Complex human phenotypes, such as autism, schizophrenia, and anxiety, undoubtedly partially overlap in genomic variations that predispose to or protect against these maladies. (Genetic overlap of complex phenotypes has gained increasing experimental support and is no longer just an ungrounded scientific hypothesis.) Furthermore, as yet largely unknown shared environmental factors likely tend to trigger the manifestation of more than one phenotype. Although it may seem overly ambitious to target multiple phenotypes jointly, we believe we can obtain much more information from existing data and gain new insights into individual phenotypes by modeling phenotypes jointly. My talk sketches two distinct computational approaches to this problem.

Keywords: computational approaches for modeling joint phenotypes, neurodevelopmental disorders.

M. Peleg, N. Lavrač, and C. Combi (Eds.): AIME 2011, LNAI 6747, p. 1, 2011.

What BPM Technology Can Do for Healthcare Process Support

Manfred Reichert

Institute of Databases and Information Systems, Ulm University, Germany
manfred.reichert@uni-ulm.de

Abstract. Healthcare organizations are facing the challenge of delivering personalized services to their patients in a cost-effective and efficient manner. This, in turn, requires advanced IT support for healthcare processes covering both organizational procedures and knowledge-intensive, dynamic treatment processes. Nowadays, required agility is often hindered by a lack of flexibility in hospital information systems. To overcome this inflexibility a new generation of information systems, denoted as process-aware information systems (PAISs), has emerged. In contrast to data- and function-centered information systems, a PAIS separates process logic from application code and thus provides an additional architectural layer. However, the introduction of process-aware hospital information systems must neither result in rigidity nor restrict staff members in their daily work. This keynote presentation reflects on recent developments from the business process management (BPM) domain, which enable process adaptation, process flexibility, and process evolution. These key features will be illustrated along existing BPM frameworks. Altogether, emerging BPM methods, concepts and technologies will contribute to further enhance IT support for healthcare processes.

1 Introduction

Business process support has been a major driver for enterprise information systems for a long time. Its overall goal is to overcome the drawbacks of functional over-specialization and lack of process control. Technology response to this business demand was met with a suite of technologies ranging from office automation tools to workflow systems to business process management technology.

Just as database management systems provide a means of abstracting application logic from physical data aspects, workflow management systems separate coordinative process logic from application code [1, 2]. Although workflow technology has delivered a great deal of productivity improvements in industry, it has been mainly designed for the support of pre-specified and repetitive business processes requiring a basic level of coordination between human performers and required application services. More recently *business process management* (BPM) has been used as broader term to reflect the fact that business processes may or may not involve human participants, cross organizational boundaries, and require a high degree of flexibility [3, 4].

M. Peleg, N. Lavrač, and C. Combi (Eds.): AIME 2011, LNAI 6747, pp. 2–13, 2011.

Currently, there is a widespread interest in BPM technologies in a variety of domains, especially in the light of emerging software paradigms surrounding service-oriented computing and its application to dynamic service orchestration and choreography. In this context, the notion of PAIS (*Process Aware Information System*) provides a guiding framework to understand and deliberate on the above developments [5]. As fundamental characteristic, a PAIS provides the basic means to separate process logic from application code. Furthermore, it has to cover all phases of the process lifecycle; i.e., process design, process implementation, process configuration, process enactment, process monitoring and diagnosis, and process evolution [6]. At *build-time* the process logic has to be explicitly defined based on the constructs provided by a *process modeling language*. In this context, a variety of *workflow patterns* (e.g., control and data patterns, resource patterns, time patterns) have been suggested enabling the comparison and evaluation of existing modeling languages and tools [7–10]. Other works, in turn, target at improved process model quality and understandability [11–13]. At *run-time* a PAIS executes the processes according to the defined logic (i.e., process model) and orchestrates required application services and other resources. Examples of PAIS-enabling technologies include *process management systems* like ADEPT2 [14], AristaFlow [15], and YAWL [16] as well as *case handling frameworks* like FLOWer [4] and PHILHarmonic Flows [17].

In spite of several success stories on the uptake of PAISs in industry and the growing process-orientation of enterprises, BPM technologies have not had the widespread adoption in the healthcare domain yet [18]. A major reason for this has been the rigidity enforced by first generation workflow management systems, which inhibits the ability of a hospital to respond to process changes and exceptional situations in an agile way [19]. When efforts are taken to improve and automate the flow of healthcare processes, however, it is extremely important not to restrict physicians and nurses. Early attempts to change the function-oriented views of patient processes have been unsuccessful whenever rigidity came with them. Variations in the course of a disease or a treatment process are deeply inherent to medicine, and the unforeseen event is to some degree a "normal" phenomenon. Therefore, healthcare process support craves for advanced BPM technologies enabling *flexible*, *adaptive* and *evolutionary* processes in large scale.

For many years the BPM community has recognized that a PAIS needs to be able to cope with real-world exceptions, uncertainty, and evolving processes [20]. To address respective needs a variety of process support paradigms like *adaptive processes*, *case handling*, and *constraint-based processes* have been suggested and been applied in practice. Basically, these paradigms allow for coordinated process support (involving human actors) and application service orchestration on the one hand, while enabling process flexibility, process adaptation, and process evolution on the other hand. For example, *adaptive PAISs* allow dynamically changing the process model of an ongoing process instance during run-time [21], while constraint-based paradigms enable loosely specified process models, which can be dynamically refined at the process instance level obeying pre-defined constraints [22]. Taking these technological developments from the BPM area, new perspectives for the realization of flexible, *process-aware hospital information systems* emerge.

This keynote presentation elaborates on advanced BPM methods, concepts and technologies developed during the last decade. Emphasis is put on key features enabling process flexibility, process adaptation, and process evolution. Based on them advanced PAIS can be realized being able to flexibly cope with real-world exceptions, uncertainty, and change. Respective methods, concepts and technologies will foster the development of a new generation of process-aware healthcare information systems.

Section 2 draws a realistic picture of the environment in which a process-aware hospital information systems must run. Section 3 discusses core contributions from the BPM domain enabling flexible and dynamic process support. Finally, the paper concludes with a short summary and outlook in Section 4.

2 Hospital Working Environment

This section motivates the need for healthcare process support and discusses the conditions under which a process-aware hospital information system must operate [18, 19].

Generally, in hospitals, the work of physicians and nurses is burdened by numerous organizational as well as medical tasks. Medical procedures must be planned and prepared, appointments be made, and results be obtained and evaluated. Usually, in the diagnostic and treatment process of a particular patient various, organizationally more or less separate units are involved. For a patient treated in a department of internal medicine or surgery, for example, tests and procedures at the laboratory and the radiology department may become necessary. In addition, specimen or the patients themselves have to be transported, physicians from other units may need to come and see the patient, and reports have to be written, sent, and evaluated. Thus, the cooperation between organizational units as well as the medical staff is a vital task with repetitive, but nevertheless non-trivial character. Processes of different complexity and duration can be identified. One can find short organizational procedures like order entry and result reporting for radiology, but also complex and long-running (even cyclic) treatment processes like chemotherapy for in- and out-patients.

Physicians have to decide which interventions are necessary or not - under the perspective of costs and invasiveness - or which are even dangerous because of possible side-effects or interactions. Many procedures need preparatory measures of various, sometimes considerable complexity. Before a surgery can take place, for example, a patient has to undergo numerous preliminary examinations, each of them requiring additional preparations. While some of them are known in advance, others may have to be scheduled dynamically, depending on the individual patient and her state of health. All tasks may have to be performed in certain orders, sometimes with a certain time distance between them. After an injection with contrast medium was given to a patient, for example, some other tests cannot be performed within a certain period of time. Usually, physicians have to coordinate the tasks related to their patients manually, taking into account all the dependencies existing between them. Changing a schedule is not trivial and requires time-consuming communication. For some procedures, physicians from various departments have to work together; i.e., coherent series of appointments have to be arranged and for each step actual and adequate information has to be provided. Typically, each unit involved in the treatment process concentrates on the function it has to perform. Thus, the process is subdivided into partial, function- and organization-oriented views, and optimization usually stops at the border of the department. For all these reasons many problems result:

- Patients have to wait, because resources (e.g., physicians, rooms or technical equipment) are not available.
- Medical procedures may become impossible to perform, if information is missing, preparations have been omitted, or a preceding procedure has been postponed, canceled or requires latency time. Depending procedures may then have to be re-scheduled as well resulting in numerous phone-calls and time losses.
- If any results are missing but urgently needed, tests or procedures may have to be performed repeatedly.

Because of this, from the patient as well as from the hospital perspective unpleasant and undesired effects occur: Hospital stays can be longer than necessary and the costs or even the invasiveness of the patient treatment may increase. In critical situations, missing information may lead to late or even wrong decisions. Investigations have shown that medical personnel is aware of these problems and that computer systems helping to make appointments and providing the necessary information would be highly welcome by nurses and physicians. In an increasing way it is being understood that correlation between medicine, organization and information is high, and that current organizational structures and hospital information systems offer sub-optimal support. This is even more the case for hospital-wide and cross-hospital processes and for health care networks.

The roles of physicians and nurses complicate the problem. They are responsible for many patients and they have to provide an optimal treatment process for each of them. Medical tasks are critical to patient care and even minor errors may have disastrous consequences. The working situation is further burdened by frequent context switches. Physicians often work at various sites of a hospital in different roles. In many cases unforeseen events and emergency situations occur, patient status changes, or information necessary to react is missing (up to: "where is my patient?"). In addition, the physician is confronted with a massive load of data to be structured, intellectually processed, and put into relation to the problems of the individual patient. Typically, physicians tend to make mistakes (e.g., wrong decisions, omissive errors) under this data overload.

From the perspective of a patient, a concentration on his treatment process is highly desirable. Similarly, medical staff members wish to treat and help patients and not to spend their time on organizational tasks. From the perspective of health care providers, the huge potential of the improvement of healthcare processes has been identified: length of stay, number of procedures, and number of complications could be reduced. Hence there is a growing interest in process orientation and quality management. Medical and organizational processes are being analyzed, and the role of medical guidelines describing diagnostic and treatment steps for given diagnoses is emphasized [23–25].

3 IT Support for Healthcare Processes

3.1 Flexibility Demands of Healthcare Processes

Obviously, the IT support for healthcare processes must not introduce rigidity or restrict medical staff members in their daily work. Generally, physicians and nurses must be free to react and are trained to do so. In an emergency case, for example, physicians may collect information about a patient by phone and proceed with the treatment process, without waiting for the electronic report to be written. Furthermore, medical procedures may have to be aborted if the patient's health state gets worse or the provider finds out that a prerequisite is not met. Such deviations from the pre-planned process are frequent and form a key part of process flexibility in hospitals. Any computer-based system which is used to assist physicians and nurses in their daily work, therefore, must allow them to gain complete initiative whenever needed. In particular, process-aware hospital information systems must be easy to handle, self-explaining, and - most important - their use in exceptional situations must be not more cumbersome and time-consuming than simply handling the exception by a telephone call to the right person. Otherwise the PAIS will not be accepted by hospital staff.

In summary, process-aware hospital information system must be able to cope with exceptions, uncertainty, and evolving processes.

3.2 Pre-specified vs. Loosely Specified Process Models

In the predominant process support paradigm, PAISs require the *a priori* specification of all process details. The resulting pre-specified process models are then used as schema for process execution. Typically, such a *pre-specified process model* defines all activities to be executed, their control flow and data flow dependencies, organizational entities performing the activities, the data objects manipulated by them, and the application services invoked during their execution. In this context, a variety of *modeling patterns* has been suggested [7–10], which can be used as building blocks for creating process models and which allow adding some build-in-flexibility to these models (i.e., *flexibility-by-design*).

However, IT support for healthcare processes demands a more agile approach recognizing the fact that in dynamic environments pre-specified processes are outdated fast and thus require closer interweaving of modeling and execution. Consequently, any PAIS relying on pre-specified process models not only needs to be able to adequately cope with real-world exceptions [26], to adapt the execution of single process instances (i.e., business cases) on-the-fly [27], to efficiently deal with uncertainty [20], and to cope with variability [28], but must also support the evolution of business processes over time, e.g., due to changing regulations or organizational changes [29, 30]. Respective features are provided by adaptive PAISs [21, 27] that have emerged in the BPM area during the last years.

In addition to pre-specified processes, which provide a reliable schema for process execution and thus are well suited for automating repetitive and rather predictable processes, existing approaches also allow process designers to only provide a *loosely specified process model* [31, 32] which can then be refined by end-users during run-time taking predefined *constraints* into account (e.g., mutual exclusion of two activities or activity orders to be obeyed).

In practice, there also exist processes that can neither be adequately captured in pre-specified models nor in constraint-based ones. In particular, it has been recognized that knowledge-intensive processes (e.g., treatment processes) cannot always be "straight-jacketed" into activities. Prescribing an activity-centric process model for them would lead to a "contradiction between the way processes can be modeled and the preferred work practice" [33]. As shown in the context of the PHILharmonicFlows project a major reason for this deficiency stems from the unsatisfactory integration of processes and data in existing activity-centric PAISs [34, 35]. To remedy this deficiency, [36] analyzed various processes from different domains which are not adequately supported by existing PAIS. As a major insight it was found out that in many cases process support requires *object-awareness*. In particular, process support has to consider *object behavior* as well as *object interactions*, and should therefore be based on two levels of granularity. Besides this, object-awareness requires *data-driven process execution* and integrated access to processes and data. PHILharmonicFlows has identified basic properties of object-aware processes as well as fundamental requirements for their operational support. The developed PHILharmonicFlows framework [17] addresses these requirements and enables *object-aware process management* in a comprehensive manner distinguishing between micro and macro processes. For example, a *micro process* may coordinate the processing of a particular medical order, whereas a *macro process* may comprise all micro processes related to a particular entity (e.g., patient) as well as their coordination dependencies.

3.3 Dealing with Exceptions, Uncertainty and Evolving Processes

For more than a decade the BPM community has recognized that PAISs need to provide different kinds of build- and run-time flexibility [20]. Consequently, a variety of techniques have been developed ranging from fully pre-specified processes with certain built-in flexibility to ad-hoc adaptations of pre-specified processes during their execution to loosely specified processes (that have to be concretized during run-time). Generally, existing approaches can be characterized along three fundamental dimensions, namely IT support for adaptation, flexibility, and evolution:

- **Adaptation** represents the ability of the implemented processes to cope with exceptional circumstances [27]. On the one hand, existing PAISs like

YAWL [16] provide support for the handling of expected exceptions, which can be anticipated and thus be pre-specified in the process model. Complementaty to this, adaptive PAISs like ADEPT2 [37] enable the handling of unanticipated exceptions, e.g., through structural ad-hoc adaptations of single process instances (e.g., by adding, deleting or moving process activities during run-time). Thereby, users are assisted in defining ad-hoc adaptations and in reusing knowledge gathered in similar problem context in the past [6, 38]. Clearly, dynamic process adaptations necessitate a comprehensive framework ensuring correctness and robustness of the PAIS. The ADEPT2 framework, for example, provides sophisticated methods, concepts and tools for achieving these goals. In particular, ADEPT2 enables instance-specific changes of a pre-specified model in a controlled, correct and secure manner [27, 39]. This, in turn, can be considered as fundamental driver enabling flexible and dynamic processes in complex application environments. Note that when providing support for ad-hoc adaptations users are no longer forced to bypass the PAIS when unplanned exceptions occur. Instead, single processes instances can be dynamically adapted to the real-world situation if required. Finally, deviations from the pre-specified model are documented in respective change logs [40].

- **Flexibility** represents the ability of a process to execute on the basis of a loosely or partially specified model which is completed at run-time and may be unique to each process instance [31, 32]. Due to the high number of choices, not all of which can be anticipated and hence be pre-specified in a process model, frameworks like DECLARE [31] and Alaska [41] allow defining process models in a more relaxed manner; the model can be defined in a way that allows individual instances to determine their own (unique) processes. In particular, declarative approaches allow for loosely specified process models by following a constraint-based approach. While pre-specified process models define exactly how the overall task has to be accomplished, constraint-based process models focus on what should be done by describing the set of activities that may be performed as well as the constraints prohibiting undesired process behavior. Therefore, constraint-based approaches provide more build-in flexibility when compared to completely pre-specified process models. Potential advantages include the absence of over-specification and the provision of more maneuvering room for end-users. Generally, loosely specified models raise a number of challenges including the flexible configuration of process models at design time or their constraint-based definition during runtime. Due to the high number of run-time choices, in addition, more sophisticated user support (e.g., recommender systems) becomes necessary when compared to PAIS relying on fully pre-specified models. Finally, the integration of pre-specified and constraint-based processes constitutes an emerging area which is particularly important for the healthcare domain. In particular, well established criteria are needed to be able to decide which approach to take in which scenario and how to combine the two paradigms in the best possible way.

- **Evolution** represents the ability of a process implemented in a PAIS to change when the business process evolves, e.g., due to legal changes or process optimizations [30, 42]. The assumption is that the processes have pre-specified models, and a change causes these models to be modified. The biggest challenge then is the handling of the potentially large number of long-running process instances, which were initiated based on the old model but are required to comply with the new specification from now on. Approaches like WASA2, ADEPT2 and WIDE allow process engineers to migrate such process instances to the new model version, while ensuring PAIS robustness and process consistency (see [43, 44]). Moreover, pre-specified process models often have to be changed to cope with model design errors, technical problems or poor model quality. In the latter context process model refactorings have been suggested to foster internal process model quality and to ensure maintainability of the PAIS over time [11, 45].

3.4 Dynamic Processes and Process Learning

In practice, there often exists a significant gap between what is prescribed in a model and what actually happens. Generally, a PAIS records the actual execution behavior of a collection of process instances in an *execution log*. Furthermore, adaptive PAISs document deviations from pre-specified models in *change logs*. In this context *process mining* strives to deliver a concise assessment of the organizational reality by mining these logs of dynamic processes [46]. *Process discovery* algorithms, for example, analyze execution logs and derive process models from them reflecting the actual process behavior best. *Conformance testing*, in turn, analyzes and measures discrepancies between the original model of a process and the actual execution of its instances (as recorded in execution logs). Finally, *log-based verification* checks the execution log for conformance with desired or undesired properties; e.g., process instance compliance with corporate guidelines or global regulations. Furthermore, *change mining* not only considers execution logs of process instances, but additionally analyzes the structural changes applied during the execution of process instances; i.e., they allow visualizing and analyzing dynamic deviations from pre-specified processes [47]. Finally, *process variants mining* [48, 49] allows discovering an optimal *reference process model* being "close" to a given collection of process variants; e.g., process instances derived from the same model, but structurally differing due to ad-hoc changes applied to them.

4 Summary and Outlook

When targeting IT support for healthcare processes it is important to distinguish the patient-specific medical treatment processes from the organizational procedures (e.g. order handling and result reporting) that generally coordinate the cooperation between staff members and organizational units within a hospital [18]. While the former are knowledge-intensive and highly dynamic processes, the latter constitute repetitive processes that capture the organizational knowledge necessary to coordinate daily tasks among staff members and between organizational units (e.g., wards and medical departments). Basically, BPM provides methods, concepts and tools for supporting both categories of processes. In particular, the described technological developments will allow providing the required process dynamics and flexibility, and thus foster the realization of a new generation of process-aware hospital information systems.

Still there is a gap between technology-driven approaches developed by the BPM community and methodological-based approaches suggested in the medical informatics field (e.g., clinical guideline support). Besides there still exists a number of challenges to be tackled in order to provide support for both organizational procedures and complex patient treatment processes. Amongst others these challenges include the process-oriented integration of heterogeneous systems, the embedding of IT process support into routine work practice, the learning from past process executions, the evolution of process knowledge over time, the real-time tracking of healthcare processes, and the coordination of interrelated processes (e.g., corresponding to the same patient). These issues are unlikely to be solved in near future, but indicate that interdisciplinary research is needed to further enhance IT support for healthcare processes.

References

1. Reijers, H.A., van der Aalst, W.M.P.: The effectiveness of workflow management systems: Predictions and lessons learned. Int'l Journal of Inf. Mgmt., 457–471 (2005)
2. Mutschler, B., Weber, B., Reichert, M.: Workflow management versus case handling - results from a controlled software experiment. In: Avanzi, R.M., Keliher, L., Sica, F. (eds.) SAC 2008. LNCS, vol. 5381, pp. 82–89. Springer, Heidelberg (2009)
3. Weske, M.: Business Process Management: Concepts, Methods, Technology. Springer, Heidelberg (2007)
4. Weber, B., Mutschler, B., Reichert, M.: Investigating the effort of using business process management technology: Results from a controlled experiment. Science of Computer Programming 75, 292–310 (2010)
5. Dumas, M., ter Hofstede, A.H.M., van der Aalst, W.M.P. (eds.): Process Aware Information Systems. Wiley Publishing, Chichester (2005)
6. Weber, B., Reichert, M., Wild, W., Rinderle-Ma, S.: Providing integrated life cycle support in process-aware information systems. Int'l J of Cooperative Information Systems 18, 115–165 (2009)
7. Lanz, A., Weber, B., Reichert, M.: Workflow time patterns for process-aware information systems. In: Bider, I., Halpin, T., Krogstie, J., Nurcan, S., Proper, E., Schmidt, R., Ukor, R. (eds.) BPMDS 2010 and EMMSAD 2010. LNBIP, vol. 50, pp. 94–107. Springer, Heidelberg (2010)
8. Russell, N., ter Hofstede, A., van der Aalst, W., Mulyar, N.: Workflow control-flow patterns: A revised view. Technical Report BPM-06-22, BPMcenter.org (2006)
9. Russell, N., van der Aalst, W.M.P., ter Hofstede, A.H.M.: Exception handling patterns in process-aware information systems. In: Martinez, F.H., Pohl, K. (eds.) CAiSE 2006. LNCS, vol. 4001, pp. 288–302. Springer, Heidelberg (2006)

10. Weber, B., Rinderle, S., Reichert, M.: Change patterns and change support features in process-aware information systems. In: Krogstie, J., Opdahl, A.L., Sindre, G. (eds.) CAiSE 2007 and WES 2007. LNCS, vol. 4495, pp. 574–588. Springer, Heidelberg (2007)
11. Weber, B., Reichert, M., Reijers, H., Mendling, J.: Refactoring large process model repositories. Computers and Industry (2011)
12. Reijers, H., Mendling, J.: Modularity in process models: Review and effects. In: Dumas, M., Reichert, M., Shan, M.-C. (eds.) BPM 2008. LNCS, vol. 5240, pp. 20–35. Springer, Heidelberg (2008)
13. Mendling, J., Reijers, H.A., van der Aalst, W.M.P.: Seven process modeling guidelines (7PMG). Information and Software Technology 52, 127–136 (2009)
14. Reichert, M., Rinderle, S., Kreher, U., Dadam, P.: Adaptive process management with ADEPT2. In: Proc. ICDE 2005, pp. 1113–1114 (2005)
15. Reichert, M., et al.: Enabling Poka-Yoke workflows with the AristaFlow BPM Suite. In: Proc. BPM 2009 Demonstration Track. CEUR Workshop Proceedings, vol. 489 (2009)
16. ter Hofstede, A.H.M., van der Aalst, W.M.P., Adams, M., Russell, N.: Modern Business Process Automation: YAWL and Its Support Environment. Springer, Heidelberg (2009)
17. Künzle, V., Reichert, M.: PHILharmonicFlows: towards a framework for object-aware process management. Journal of Software Maintenance and Evolution: Research and Practice (2011)
18. Lenz, R., Reichert, M.: IT support for healthcare processes - premises, challenges, perspectives. Data and Knowledge Engineering 61, 39–58 (2007)
19. Dadam, P., Reichert, M., Kuhn, K.: Clinical workflows - the killer application for process-oriented information systems? In: Proc. BIS 2000, pp. 36–59 (2000)
20. Weber, B., Sadiq, S., Reichert, M.: Beyond rigidity - dynamic process lifecycle support: A survey on dynamic changes in process-aware information systems. Computer Science - Research and Development 23, 47–65 (2009)
21. Reichert, M., Rinderle-Ma, S., Dadam, P.: Flexibility in process-aware information systems. In: Jensen, K., van der Aalst, W.M.P. (eds.) Transactions on Petri Nets and Other Models of Concurrency II. LNCS, vol. 5460, pp. 115–135. Springer, Heidelberg (2009)
22. Weber, B., Reijers, H.A., Zugal, S., Wild, W.: The declarative approach to business process execution: An empirical test. In: van Eck, P., Gordijn, J., Wieringa, R. (eds.) CAiSE 2009. LNCS, vol. 5565, pp. 470–485. Springer, Heidelberg (2009)
23. Lenz, R., Blaser, R., Beyer, M., Heger, O., Biber, C., Baumlein, M., Schnabel, M.: IT support for clinical pathways–lessons learned. Intl. J. Med. Inform. 76, 397–402 (2007)
24. Peleg, M., Tu, S.W.: Design patterns for clinical guidelines. Intl. J. Med. Inform. 47, 1–24 (2009)
25. Peleg, M., Keren, S., Denekamp, Y.: Mapping computerized clinical guidelines to electronic medical records: Knowledge-data ontological mapper (KDOM). J. Biomed. Inform. 41, 180–201 (2008)
26. Reichert, M., Dadam, P., Bauer, T.: Dealing with forward and backward jumps in workflow management systems. Software and System Modeling 1, 37–58 (2003)
27. Reichert, M., Dadam, P.: ADEPT_{flex} – supporting dynamic changes of workflows without losing control. Journal of Intelligent Inf. Sys. 10, 93–129 (1998)
28. Hallerbach, A., Bauer, T., Reichert, M.: Capturing variability in business process models: The Provop approach. Journal of Software Maintenance and Evolution: Research and Practice 22, 519–546 (2010)

29. Reichert, M., Rinderle, S., Dadam, P.: On the common support of workflow type and instance changes under correctness constraints. In: Chung, S., Schmidt, D.C. (eds.) CoopIS 2003, DOA 2003, and ODBASE 2003. LNCS, vol. 2888, pp. 407–425. Springer, Heidelberg (2003)
30. Rinderle, S., Reichert, M., Dadam, P.: Flexible support of team processes by adaptive workflow systems. Distributed and Parallel Databases 16, 91–116 (2004)
31. Pesic, M.: Constraint-Based Workflow Management Systems: Shifting Control to Users. PhD thesis, Eindhoven University of Technology (2008)
32. Sadiq, S., Sadiq, W., Orlowska, M.: A framework for constraint specification and validation in flexible workflows. Information Systems 30, 349–378 (2005)
33. Sadiq, S., Orlowska, M.: On capturing exceptions in workflow process models. In: Proc. BIS 2000 (2000)
34. Künzle, V., Reichert, M.: Integrating users in object-aware process management systems: Issues and challenges. In: Rinderle-Ma, S., Sadiq, S., Leymann, F. (eds.) BPM 2009. LNBIP, vol. 43, pp. 29–41. Springer, Heidelberg (2010)
35. Künzle, V., Reichert, M.: Towards object-aware process management systems: Issues, challenges, benefits. In: Halpin, T., Krogstie, J., Nurcan, S., Proper, E., Schmidt, R., Soffer, P., Ukor, R. (eds.) Enterprise, Business-Process and Information Systems Modeling. LNBIP, vol. 29, pp. 197–210. Springer, Heidelberg (2009)
36. Künzle, V., Weber, B., Reichert, M.: Object-aware business processes: Fundamental requirements and their support in existing approaches. Int'l Journal of Information System Modeling and Design 2, 19–46 (2011)
37. Dadam, P., Reichert, M.: The ADEPT project: A decade of research and development for robust and flexible process support - challenges and achievements. Computer Science - Research and Development 23, 81–97 (2009)
38. Rinderle, S., Weber, B., Reichert, M., Wild, W.: Integrating process learning and process evolution – A semantics based approach. In: van der Aalst, W.M.P., Benatallah, B., Casati, F., Curbera, F. (eds.) BPM 2005. LNCS, vol. 3649, pp. 252–267. Springer, Heidelberg (2005)
39. Weber, B., Reichert, M., Wild, W., Rinderle, S.: Balancing flexibility and security in adaptive process management systems. In: Proc. CoopIS 2005, pp. 59–76 (2005)
40. Rinderle, S., Reichert, M., Jurisch, M., Kreher, U.: On representing, purging, and utilizing change logs in process management systems. In: Dustdar, S., Fiadeiro, J.L., Sheth, A.P. (eds.) BPM 2006. LNCS, vol. 4102, pp. 241–256. Springer, Heidelberg (2006)
41. Weber, B., Pinggera, J., Zugal, S., Wild, W.: Alaska simulator toolset for conducting controlled experiments on process flexibility. In: Soffer, P., Proper, E. (eds.) CAiSE Forum 2010. LNBIP, vol. 72, pp. 205–221. Springer, Heidelberg (2011)
42. Casati, F., Ceri, S., Pernici, B., Pozzi, G.: Workflow evolution. Data and Knowledge Engineering 24, 211–238 (1998)
43. Rinderle, S., Reichert, M., Dadam, P.: Evaluation of correctness criteria for dynamic workflow changes. In: van der Aalst, W.M.P., ter Hofstede, A.H.M., Weske, M. (eds.) BPM 2003. LNCS, vol. 2678, pp. 41–57. Springer, Heidelberg (2003)
44. Rinderle, S., Reichert, M., Dadam, P.: Correctness criteria for dynamic changes in workflow systems – a survey. Data and Knowledge Engineering 50, 9–34 (2004)
45. Weber, B., Reichert, M.: Refactoring process models in large process repositories. In: Bellahsène, Z., Léonard, M. (eds.) CAiSE 2008. LNCS, vol. 5074, pp. 124–139. Springer, Heidelberg (2008)

46. Van der Aalst, W., Reijers, H., Weijters, A., van Dongen, B., de Medeiros, A.A., Song, M., Verbeek, H.: Business process mining: An industrial application. Information Systems 32, 713–732 (2007)
47. Günther, C., Rinderle, S., Reichert, M., van der Aalst, W.: Change mining in adaptive process management systems. In: Proc. CoopIS 2006, pp. 309–326 (2006)
48. Li, C., Reichert, M., Wombacher, A.: Discovering reference models by mining process variants using a heuristic approach. In: Dayal, U., Eder, J., Koehler, J., Reijers, H.A. (eds.) BPM 2009. LNCS, vol. 5701, pp. 344–362. Springer, Heidelberg (2009)
49. Li, C., Reichert, M., Wombacher, A.: The MinAdept clustering approach for discovering reference process models out of process variants. Int'l Journal of Coop. Inf. Sys. 19, 159–203 (2010)

Elicitation of Neurological Knowledge with ABML

Vida Groznik[1], Matej Guid[1], Aleksander Sadikov[1], Martin Možina[1], Dejan Georgiev[2], Veronika Kragelj[3], Samo Ribarič[3], Zvezdan Pirtošek[2], and Ivan Bratko[1]

[1] Artificial Intelligence Laboratory, Faculty of Computer and Information Science, University of Ljubljana, Slovenia
[2] Department of Neurology, University Medical Centre Ljubljana, Slovenia
[3] Faculty of Medicine, University of Ljubljana, Slovenia

Abstract. The paper describes the process of knowledge elicitation for a neurological decision support system. To alleviate the difficult problem of knowledge elicitation from data and domain experts, we used a recently developed technique called ABML (Argument Based Machine Learning). The paper demonstrates ABML's advantage in combining machine learning and expert knowledge. ABML guides the expert to explain critical special cases which cannot be handled automatically by machine learning. This very efficiently reduces the expert's workload, and combines it with automatically learned knowledge. We developed a decision support system to help the neurologists differentiate between three types of tremors: Parkinsonian, essential, and mixed tremor (co-morbidity). The system is intended to act as a second opinion for the neurologists, and most importantly to help them reduce the number of patients in the "gray area" that require a very costly further examination (DaTSCAN).

1 Introduction and Motivation

Essential tremor (ET) is one of the most prevalent movement disorders. [2] It is characterized by postural and kinetic tremor with a frequency between 6 and 12 Hz. ET usually starts in one hand and then spreads to the neck and vocal cords, giving the characteristic clinical picture of the disease. Parkinsonian tremor (PT), on the other hand, is a resting tremor classically described as "pill rolling" tremor with a frequency between 4 and 6 Hz. It is one of the major signs of Parkinson's disease (PD), which also includes bradykinesia, rigidity and postural instability. Although distinct clinical entities, ET is very often misdiagnosed as PT. [10] Co-existence of both disorders is also possible [9], additionally complicating the differential diagnosis of tremors.

Digitalized spiralography is a quantitative method of tremor assessment [5], based on spiral drawing on a digital tablet. In addition to precise measurement of tremor frequency, spiralography describes tremors with additional parameters — these, together with physical neurological examination, offer new means to differentiate between numerous types of tremors [4,5], including ET and PT.

M. Peleg, N. Lavrač, and C. Combi (Eds.): AIME 2011, LNAI 6747, pp. 14–23, 2011.

The use of spiralography for diagnostic purposes is a relatively recent idea, and only a few centers in the world are currently using it, among them Columbia University Medical Center and University Clinical Centre Ljubljana.

The paper describes the process of building a decision support system (DSS) for diagnosing and differentiating between aforementioned three types of tremors, namely ET, PT, and mixed tremor (MT; both ET and PT at the same time). It mainly focuses on the task of knowledge acquisition as this is usually the most challenging part of the project. The motivation for the DSS is as follows. Although several sets of guidelines for diagnosing both ET and PT do exist [3,8], none of them enjoys general consensus in the community. Furthermore, none of these guidelines takes into account additional information from spiralography. Our DSS combines all sources of knowledge, experts' background knowledge, machine-generated knowledge, and spiralography data in an attempt to improve prediction accuracy. However, at the same time and even more importantly, our DSS uses a very comprehensible model, making it very suitable for explaining its decisions and could be used as a teaching tool as well.

Apart from improved data acquisition and storage, the main expected benefits of our DSS are twofold. By acting as a second opinion, mostly for difficult cases, the combined diagnostic accuracy is expected to increase, reducing the need for patients to undergo (a) an invasive, and (b) very expensive further examination (DaTSCAN). This will also save both patients' and doctors' time.

The knowledge acquisition process was based on Argument Based Machine Learning (ABML) [7]. ABML seamlessly combines the domain expert's knowledge with machine-induced knowledge, and is very suitable for the task of knowledge elicitation as it involves the expert in a very natural dialogue-like way [6]. The expert is not required to give general knowledge of the domain (which can be hard), but is only asked to explain concrete examples which the machine cannot correctly classify on its own. The process usually results in improved accuracy and comprehensibility. [7] Such focused knowledge elicitation also saves a lot of expert time.

The organization of the paper is as follows. The next chapter details the domain, data, and experimental setup. Chapters 3 and 4 describe ABML and the process of knowledge elicitation, respectively. We present and discuss the results in Chapter 5, and give some conclusions and plans for further work at the end.

2 Domain Description and Experimental Setup

Our data set consists of 67 patients diagnosed and treated at the Department of Neurology, University Medical Centre Ljubljana. The patients were diagnosed by a physician with either ET, PT or MT which represent possible class values for our classification task.

The patients are described using 70 attributes. They were reduced to 45 attributes during the preprocessing of the data. The excluded attributes contained mostly unknown values and were as such irrelevant for building the model. About a half of these attributes were derived from the patient's history data and the neurological examination, the other half includes data from spiralography.

The class distribution is: 32 patients diagnosed with ET, 17 patients with PT and 18 patients with MT. These were divided into a learning set with 47 cases and a test set with 20 cases preserving stratified class distribution. Such testing set-up was necessary as ABML does not enable easy cross-validation.

During the ABML process some of the attributes were replaced by new ones containing the expert's knowledge of the domain. This usually meant combining two or more attributes.

3 Argument Based Machine Learning (ABML)

Argument Based Machine Learning (ABML)[7] is machine learning extended with concepts from argumentation. In ABML, arguments are used as means for experts to elicit some of their knowledge through explanations of the learning examples. The experts need to focus on one specific case at the time only and provide knowledge that seems relevant for this case. We will use the ABCN2 [7] method, an argument based extension of the well-known CN2 method [1], that learns a set of unordered probabilistic rules from examples with attached arguments, also called *argumented examples.*[1]

The problem domain described in this paper contains a class variable with three values: ET, PT, and MT. Since the MT class contains patients with essential tremor and Parkinsonian tremor, a rule learning method will have difficulties distinguishing between ET and MT (and likewise between PT and MT). To avert this difficulty, we decided to translate our three-class problem into two two-class problems. In the first, ET and MT are combined in EMT (*essential mixed*) class. The common property of the patients in the EMT class is that they all contain some signs of essential tremor. The rules for EMT would therefore contain in their conditions the attributes that are indicating essential tremor and are not indicating Parkinsonian tremor.

In the learning problem with EMT and PT, we learn a set of rules for EMT class only, as learning rules for PT class would be hard for the same reasons as mentioned above. The second problem is analogous to the first one, where PT and MT are combined into PMT (*Parkinsonian mixed*) class. The results of learning in the second problem is a set of rules for PMT class.

Rules are a way to represent knowledge, however to provide classifications, we need a mechanism to enable reasoning about new cases. We developed a technique that can infer a classification in one of three possible classes from rules for EMT and PMT classes. Let example e be covered by rules R_{EMT} for EMT and rules R_{PMT} for PMT. Let $P(e = EMT)$ be the predicted class probability of the best rule (with highest predicted class probability) from R_{EMT} and $P(e = PMT)$ the predicted class probability of the best rule from R_{PMT}. If

[1] Reader can find more about ABML and ABCN2 in [7] and at its website `www.ailab.si/martin/abml`.

R_{EMT} is empty, $P(e = EMT) = 0$. Then, our method will predict the following probabilities for the three classes:

$$P(e = ET) = 1 - P(e = PMT)$$
$$P(e = PT) = 1 - P(e = EMT)$$
$$P(e = MT) = P(e = EMT) + P(e = PMT) - 1,$$

where $P(e = ET)$, $P(e = PT)$, $P(e = MT)$ correspond to predicted probabilities of ET, PT, and MT classes, respectively. Example e is classified as the class with the highest predicted probability.

3.1 Interactions between Expert and ABCN2

As asking experts to give arguments to the whole learning set is not feasible, we use the following loop to pick out the *critical examples* that should be explained by the expert.

1. Learn a hypothesis with ABCN2 using given data.
2. Find the most critical example and present it to the expert. If a critical example can not be found, stop the procedure.
3. Expert explains the example; the explanation is encoded in arguments and attached to the learning example.
4. Return to step 1.

To finalize the procedure, we need to answer the following two questions: a) how do we select critical examples? and b) how can we achieve to get all necessary information for the chosen example?

Identifying critical examples. A critical example is an example the current hypothesis can not explain well. As our method gives probabilistic class predictions, we will first identify the "most problematic" example, with highest probabilistic error. To estimate the probabilistic error we used a k-fold cross-validation repeated n times (e.g. $n = 4, k = 5$), so that each example is tested n times. The critical example is thus selected according to the following two rules.

1. If the problematic example is from MT, it becomes the critical example.
2. If the problematic example is from the ET (or PT) class, the method will seek out which of the rules predicting PMT (or EMT) is the culprit for example's misclassification. As the problematic rule is likely to be bad, since it covers our problematic example, the critical example will become an example from PT or MT class (or ET or MT) covered by the problematic rule. Then, the expert will be asked to explain what are the reasons that this patient was diagnosed with Parkinsonian disease (or essential tremor). Explaining this example should replace the problematic rule with a better one for the PMT (or EMT) class, which hopefully will not cover the problematic example.

Are expert's arguments good or should they be improved? Here we describe in details the third (3) step of the above algorithm:

Step 1: Explaining critical example. If the example is from the MT class, the expert can be asked to explain its Parkinsonian and essential signs (which happens when the problematic example is from MT) or to explain only one of the diseases. In other two cases (ET or PT), the experts always explains only signs relevant to the example's class. The expert then articulates a set of reasons confirming the example's class value. The provided argument should contain a minimal number of reasons to avoid overspecified arguments.

Step 2: Adding arguments to example. The argument is given in natural language and need to be translated into domain description language (attributes). If argument mentions concepts currently not present in the domain, these concepts need to be included in the domain (as new attributes) before the argument can be added to the example.

Step 3: Discovering counter examples. Counter examples are used to spot if an argument is sufficient to successfully explain the critical example or not. If not, ABCN2 will select a counter example. A counter example has the opposite class of the critical example, however covered by the rule induced from the given arguments.

Step 4: Improving arguments with counter examples. The experts needs to revise his initial argument with respect to the counter example.

Step 5: Return to step 3 if counter example found.

4 Knowledge Elicitation with ABML

4.1 Argumentation of Examples from Class ET/PT

At the start of the process, only original attributes were used and no arguments have been given yet. Example E.2 (ET - classified as ET in the data set) was the first critical example selected by our algorithm. The expert was asked to describe which features of E.2 are in favor of ET. He selected the following features: resting tremor, rigidity, and bradykinesia, and chose bradykinesia (represented with two attributes in the data set, one for the left side and one for the right side) to be the most influential one of the three features. The expert used his domain knowledge to come up with the following answer: "E.2 is ET because there is no bradykinesia, either on the left nor on the right side." Based on his general knowledge about the domain he also explained that the side (left or right) does not play any particular role for differentiating between ET and PT.

The expert's explanation served the knowledge engineer to induce new attribute ANY.NONZERO.BRADYKINESIA with possible values *true* (bradykinesia is present on the left side *or* on the right side) and *false* (bradykinesia was not indicated on either side). At the same time the original two attributes were excluded from the domain – it is their combination (reflected in the expert's argument) that provides relevant information according to the expert.

Based on the expert's explanation, argument "ANY.NONZERO.BRADYKINESIA is *false*" was added as the argument for ET to the critical example E.2. No counter examples were found by the method and thus the first iteration was concluded. New rules were induced before entering the next iteration. One of the notable changes was that the following rule occurred:

IF ANY.NONZERO.BRADYKINESIA = *false* THEN *class* = EMT; [20,0]

The rule covers 20 learning examples, and all of them are from class ET.

4.2 Argumentation of Examples from Class MT

In the previously described iteration the critical example E.2 was classified as purely ET by the neurologist. In one of the following iterations, however, the critical example E.61 was classified as both PT and ET. In such a case, the expert is asked to describe which features are in favor of ET *and* which features are in favor of PT. The expert explained that the presence of postural tremor speaks in favor of ET, while the presence of rigidity speaks in favor of PT. Again he relied on his general knowledge to advocate that keeping separate attributes for both the left and the right side does not have any impact on deciding between ET and PT, and suggested one attribute for each feature instead.

Attributes ANY.NONZERO.POSTURAL.TREMOR and ANY.NONZERO.RIGIDITY were introduced into the domain instead of the original ones that describe features postural tremor and rigidity. The former was used as an argument for ET and the latter was used as an argument for PT — both of these arguments were added to the critical example E.61. While no counter examples were found for the expert's argument in favor of ET, the method selected E.45 (ET) as counter example for his argument in favor of PT.

The expert was now asked to compare the critical example E.61 with counter example E.45, and to explain what is the most important feature in favor of PT that applies for E.61 and it does *not* apply for E.45. According to the expert's judgement, it was the presence of harmonics in E.45 (or their absence in E.61), which are typical for ET. The following attribute that was added into the domain earlier, ANY.HARMONICS, with possible values of *true* and *false* was added to the previous argument. However, the method then found another counter example, E.30 (ET). The expert explained that the tremor in E.30 did not have symmetrical onset, as opposed to the one in the critical example. The argument was further extended using the attribute SIM.TREMOR.ONSET and added to the critical example E.61. No new counter examples were found and this particular iteration was therefore concluded.

4.3 Improving on the Arguments

There are three possible ways for the expert's arguments to be improved: (1) by the expert, with the help of counter examples selected by the method, (2) by the method alone, and (3) by the expert, upon the observation of induced rules. The first option was covered in the previous subsection. In the sequel, the latter two options are described.

In the first iteration (as described in 4.1), the expert's arguments proved to be sufficient for the method to induce rules with clear distributions. Sometimes, however, the method automatically finds additional restrictions to improve the expert's argument. Such was the case in one of the following iterations, where the following argument occurred: "ANY.NONZERO.RESTING.TREMOR IS *true* AND ANY.HARMONICS IS *false* AND SIM.TREMOR.ONSET IS *false*." The following rule that also occurs in the final model was induced with help of this argument:

IF ANY.NONZERO.RESTING.TREMOR = *true* AND ANY.HARMONICS = *false*
AND SIM.TREMOR.ONSET = *false* **AND any.Spiro.ET.no.other** = ***false***
THEN class = PMT; [0,14]

The method automatically improved on the expert's argument by adding an additional restriction in the above rule. The attribute ANY.SPIRO.ET.NO.OTHER was introduced by the expert in one of the previous iterations. It's meaning is the following: if qualitative assessment of the spiral in any of the eight observations (attributes) in the original data is essential, and none of them is Parkinsonian (or any other), then the value of ANY.SPIRO.ET.NO.OTHER is *true*, otherwise it is *false*. The above rule covers 14 examples (all of them from class ET) and was particularly praised by the expert – one of the reasons for this being that it effectively combines clinical data with the results of spiralography.

The third possibility occurred only once in the ABML knowledge elicitation process presented in this paper. Upon the final examination of the rules the expert approved all the obtained rules but the following one:

IF ANY.NONZERO.POSTURAL.TREMOR = *true* AND SIM.BRADYKINESIA = *true*
THEN class = EMT; [23,0]

Although the rule covers 23 examples (out of 47) and has a clear distribution, the expert found the attribute SIM.BRADYKINESIA meaningless. This was automatically induced part of the rule from the expert's argument to the example E.61, as described in 4.2. Based on the expert's explanation this argument was now extended to "ANY.NONZERO.POSTURAL.TREMOR is *true* **and any.Nonzero.Bradykinesia** = ***false***." Such changes should not by any circumstances be made *after* examining results on the testing data, and it is particularly important that the expert relies on his common knowledge of the domain when doing this. The following rule was induced from the expert's argument:

IF ANY.NONZERO.POSTURAL.TREMOR = *true*
AND ANY.NONZERO.BRADYKINESIA = *false*
THEN class = EMT; [16,0]

Although the rule has notably worse coverage, the expert found it consistent with his domain knowledge. The expert approved all the rules in the final model and thus the iterative process was concluded.

Table 1. Results before (in brackets) and after knowledge elicitation

	ABCN2 (CN2)	Naive Bayes	Class. Trees	kNN
CA	0.80 (0.60)	0.75 (0.70)	0.50 (0.50)	0.60 (0.55)
AUC	0.86 (0.89)	0.83 (0.84)	0.62 (0.62)	0.76 (0.84)

5 Results and Discussion

5.1 Quantitative Comparison

Table 1 presents the results of applying different machine learning techniques. The numbers represent classification accuracy on the test set after performing knowledge elicitation with ABML, while the numbers in brackets show the accuracy on the initial data set with 45 attributes. Although the newly constructed features improve the accuracy, the small number of available cases limits us from drawing any firm conclusions regarding accuracy at this moment.

The net time investment of the domain expert was slightly more than 20 hours. The knowledge engineers spent approximately 150 hours total.

5.2 Qualitative Comparison of the Initial and the Final Model

The following is a qualitative assessment of the models by the expert. There were 12 rules in the starting model. Seven of them used the duration of the disease or age at disease onset as important attributes in the decision making. Disease duration and age of disease onset are not very informative attributes. Although epidemiological data show that the average age at onset is 40 years for ET and 60 years for PT, both disorders can start at any age. The same is true for disease duration, which obviously directly depends on the age at disease onset. In addition, three other rules used just a single attribute to diagnose a certain tremor type, which, although sensible, is not enough to determine the tremor type. The remaining two rules used sensible combination of attributes. Let us take a closer look at rule #5:

IF AGE $>$ 68.0 AND AGE $\leq$ 76.0 THEN *class* = EMT; [15,0]

This rule is obviously illogical, stating that the essential tremor is defined by age at disease onset. The average age of ET onset as mentioned before is 40 years, although ET can start at any age. In addition, there are no defined criteria for minimal and maximal age at ET onset. Another example is rule #11:

IF RIGIDITY.UPPER.EXTREMITIES.RIGHT $>$ 0.0
AND AGE $\leq$ 83.0 AND DISEASE.DURATION $\leq$ 20.0
THEN *class* = PMT; [0,14]

The first part states correctly that if the rigidity is greater at least in one upper extremity, this is a sign of PT. The other two conditions are completely incorrect. There is no upper limit for the age at disease onset for either PT or ET. Also illogical is the last condition, as both disorders can last more than 20 years or as short as 1 month for example.

There were 13 rules at the end of the process, all correct and completely different from the starting rules. Seven of them were strong, so one could diagnose PT or ET with great probability just relying on a single rule. The other rules were less reliable, yet still logical. For example, rule #2:

IF ANY.HARMONICS = *yes* THEN *class* = EMT; [10,0]

states that if there are harmonic frequencies in the tremor frequency spectra, then the tremor is essential. It is known that the appearance of harmonic frequencies is very specific for ET. Another similar example is rule #11:

IF ANY.NONZERO.BRADYKINESIA = *true*
AND ANY.NONZERO.RIGIDITY.UPPER.EXTREMITIES = *true*
AND ANY.NONZERO.TREMOR.RESTING = *true*
THEN *class* = PMT; [0,15]

stating that if a patient has a resting tremor, bradykinesia, and rigidity, the tremor is Parkinsonian. This rule, namely the combination of a resting tremor, bradykinesia and rigidity actually clinically defines PT. Rule #9 is from the second, less reliable group:

IF FREE.RIGHT.VELOCITY.TIME = *parkinson* AND TREMOR.NECK ≤ 0.0
THEN *class* = PMT; [0,15]

where PT is defined by absence of head tremor and Parkinsonian type-velocity changes over time of the tremor movements. Head tremor is a specific marker of ET, which combined with a Parkinsonian type of velocity-time changes increases the probability of correctly classifying a tremor as being Parkinsonian.

5.3 Misclassification Analysis

As can be seen from subsection 5.1 our final model misclassified four cases. We asked our domain expert to examine these four cases and the rules responsible for their classification.

After precise evaluation, the expert actually agreed with two of the computer's classifications as he overlooked some of the details at the time of diagnosis. Therefore the class of these two cases should actually be modified.

Moreover, the expert changed the class of another case. In this case he did not agree with the computer's evaluation, but the rules nevertheless helped the expert to spot the earlier mistake. The remaining case revealed that we lack learning examples to induce better rules for covering these cases. In one case only a single rule from the model triggered and classified MT as PT. In the second case our model misclassified MT as PT. From the medical point of view this error was minor in comparison to the first case. The misclassification occurred as none of the rules for ET in the model were appropriate for this case.

If we were to use the correct class for the two test cases reevaluated by the expert, the CA of the final model would raise to 90% and the CA of the initial model would drop to 55%. Nevertheless, the number of test cases available is too small to rely on these results. As more patients will be enrolled in the study, we will be able to better assess the prediction accuracies of the models.

6 Conclusions and Further Work

The paper detailed some aspects of building a decision support system for diagnosing and differentiating between three types of tremors. Our DSS also takes into account the information from spiralography, potentially improving classification accuracy. Although the accuracy of the system improved over the initial model (using unaided machine learning) on our test set, the small number of available cases prevents us from drawing any serious conclusions at this moment. However, new patients will constantly be enrolled into the study. This will enable us to precisely quantify the accuracy of the system in the long run.

An even more important aspect from our point of view, is the comprehensibility of the final model. It was judged very positively by the experts. Since the DSS is able to comprehensibly support its suggestions, it might also be a valuable teaching tool. This is another direction for further work.

We have also measured the net time involvement of the expert in building a knowledge base for the system. We believe ABML saves a significant amount of expert's time, and the expert agreed that the process itself felt very natural and stimulating. However, it is very difficult to make a fair comparison with other methods, and we resolved to just stating the net times measured.

References

1. Clark, P., Boswell, R.: Rule induction with CN2: Some recent improvements. In: Kodratoff, Y. (ed.) EWSL 1991. LNCS, vol. 482. Springer, Heidelberg (1991)
2. Deuschl, G., Wenzelburger, R., Loeffler, K., Raethjan, J., Stolze, H.: Essential tremor and cerebellar dysfunction: Clinical and kinematic analysis of intention tremor. Brain 123(8), 1568–1580 (2000)
3. Hughes, A., Daniel, S., Kilford, L., Lees, A.: Accuracy of clinical diagnosis of idiopathic Parkinson's disease: a clinico-pathological study of 100 cases. Journal of Neurology, Neurosurgery, and Psychiatry 55(3), 181–184 (1992)
4. Kraus, P., Hoffmann, A.: Spiralometry: Computerized assessment of tremor amplitude on the basis of spiral drawing. Movement Disorders 25(13), 2164–2170 (2010)
5. Miotto, G.A.A., Andrade, A.O., Soares, A.B.: Measurement of tremor using digitalized tablets. In: Fiftht Conferencia de Estudos em Engenharia Eletrica, CEEL (2007)
6. Možina, M., Guid, M., Krivec, J., Sadikov, A., Bratko, I.: Fighting knowledge acquisition bottleneck with argument based machine learning. In: The 18th European Conference on Artificial Intelligence (ECAI), Patras, Greece (2008)
7. Možina, M., Žabkar, J., Bratko, I.: Argument based machine learning. Artificial Intelligence 171(10/15), 922–937 (2007)
8. Pahwa, R., Lyons, K.E.: Essential tremor: Differential diagnosis and current therapy. American Journal of Medicine 115, 134–142 (2003)
9. Quinn, N., Schneider, S., Schwingenschuh, P., Bhatia, K.: Tremor: Some controversial aspects. Movement Disorders (in print)
10. Thanvi, B., Lo, N., Robinson, T.: Essential tremor — the most common movement disorder in older people. Age and Ageing 35(4), 344–349 (2006)

Intelligent Configuration of Social Support Networks Around Depressed Persons

Azizi A. Aziz, Michel C.A. Klein, and Jan Treur

Agent Systems Research Group, Department of Artificial Intelligence
Vrije Universiteit Amsterdam, De Boelelaan 1081, 1081 HV Amsterdam, The Netherlands
{mraaziz,michel.klein,treur}@few.vu.nl

Abstract. Helping someone who is depressed can be very important to the depressed person. A number of supportive family members or friends can often make a big difference. This paper addresses how a social support network can be formed, taking the needs of the support recipient and the possibilities of the potential support providers into account. To do so, dynamic models about the preferences and needs of both support providers and support recipients are exploited. The outcome of this is used as input for a configuration process of a support network. In a case study, it is show how such an intelligently formed network results in a reduced long term stress level.

Keywords: Agent-Based Modeling, Configuration, Cognitive Models, Social Support Networks, Unipolar Depression.

1 Introduction

Stress is an ever present aspect of life. Long term exposure to stress, often leads to depression [7]. A depression is a mood disorder characterized by a depressed mood, a lack of interest in activities normally enjoyed, fatigue, feelings of worthlessness and guilt, difficulty concentrating and thoughts of death and suicide [4]. If a person experiences the majority of these symptoms for longer than a two-week period they may be diagnosed with major depressive disorder. There has been much recent emphasis on the role of social support network to overcome stress [1, 4]. Social support network refers to the provision of psychological and material resources from the social network, intended to enhance an individual's ability to cope with stress [1]. Essentially, it involves interpersonal transactions or exchanges of resources between at least two persons intended to improve the well-being of the support recipient. From this view, it can promote health through a stress buffering process, by eliminating or reducing effects from stressors.

In this paper it is addressed how a social support network can be formed, taking the needs of the support recipient and the possibilities of the potential support providers into account. This approach can provide a basis for an intelligent application that dynamically suggests support networks based on information available in social network software. The contribution of this paper is twofold. First, an extension of an existing model on preferences for types of social support from the perspective of the recipient (the patient) is presented. The extension describes the process of responding to a request of a specific type from the perspective of the support provider: the social

M. Peleg, N. Lavrač, and C. Combi (Eds.): AIME 2011, LNAI 6747, pp. 24–34, 2011.

network member that might provide support (Section 2). Second, an approach to use this extended model is proposed for the automated selection of a subset of the patient's social network members that together will provide optimal support (Section 3). In Sections 4 and 5 a fictitious case study is described that illustrates this process. Finally, Section 6 concludes the paper.

2 Dynamic Model of Support Receipt and Provision Process

In this section the support provision and receiving process will be discussed, and a computational model for these processes is presented.

2.1 Important Concepts in Support Receipt and Provision

Before the introduction of the formal model, first the factors will be discussed of the process of giving and receiving support that are important according to the literature. Published studies on this process have usually focused on the perspective of the recipient, provider, and relationship [5]. One of the salient factors to ensure support can be provided is the request for support. Requests for support may be expressed either *directly* or *indirectly*. Direct request strategies differ from indirect strategies primarily with regard to two inextricably fused aspects; namely, their communicative clearness and their demand characteristics [10]. In this case, personality plays a central role to determine either direct or indirect request is expressed, for example; individuals' with neuroticism to express their request emotional support request through unpleasant emotions gestures. Another important component related to the support recipient factors is the requested support (*need of support*). Support recipients must recognize the need for support and be willing to accept assistance. This factor is influenced by peoples' perceptions of their expectations of others (*perceived the availability of support*) [14].

Types of support needed are highly related with recipients' social tie preference. For example, one reason why individuals may opt for a weak tie support members (e.g: colleague) is that weak ties often provide access to diverse points of information (*informational support*) [10]. In additional to this, researchers have found that health concerns are often difficult topics for people to discuss, especially with interacting with the close tie members. However, other types of support such as *instrumental, emotional* and *companionship* are highly related to the strong tie (close friends, family) preference [6]. Another important factor to allow social support is the provider's willingness to help. If the willingness is high, then one is more likely to provide support and vice versa [6, 11]. Provider's willingness is related to the personality attributes and *altruistic* behaviour. The *agreeableness* and highly altruistic individuals contribute to a higher willingness level to help compare those who are not.

2.2 Formal Specifications of Support Recipient and Provision Process

The characteristics of the proposed (extension of the) model are heavily inspired by the research discussed in the previous section on support receipt and provision process. In Figure 1, the states that are depicted in grey represent states that have been modeled in the previous work. The same holds for the dashed lines. Readers interested in these relationships are directed to [2, 3]. In the formalization, all nodes are designed in a way to have values ranging from 0 (low) to 1 (high). To represent these relationships in agent terms, each variable will be coupled with an agent's name (*a* or *b*) and a time variable *t*. When using the agent variable *a*, this refers to the agent's support receipt, and *b* to the agent's support provision.

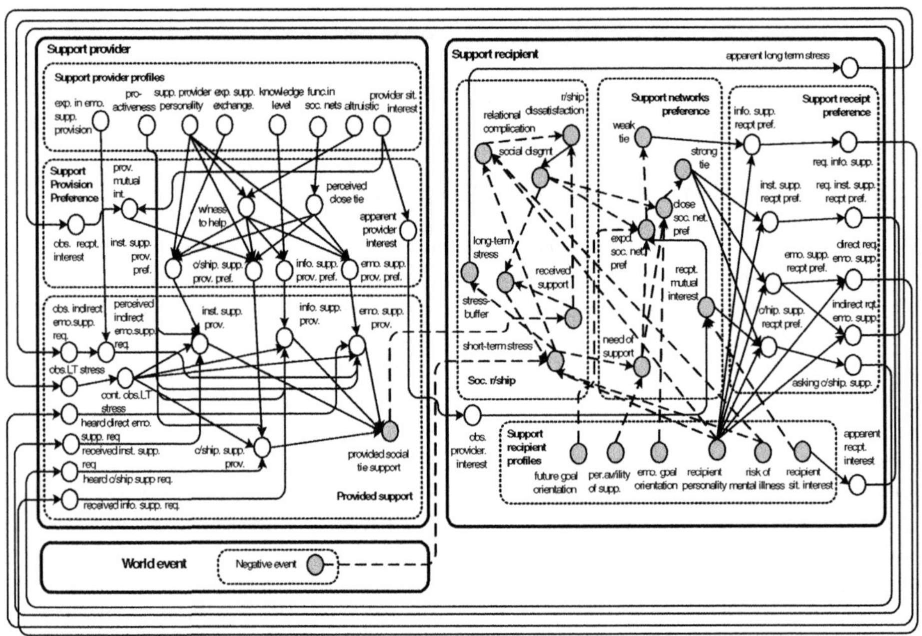

Fig. 1. Global Relationships of Variables Involved in the Support Receipt and Provision Process

Long Term Stress, and Social Disengagement: In the model, the world events are generated by simulating potential effects throughout *t* time. Short-term stress (*StS*) refers to the combination of negative events, risk in mental illness (vulnerability), and neurotic personality. Related to this, accumulation series of *StS* will develop the long term stress (*LtS*). Relational dissatisfaction (*RdS*) is determined by relational complication when no support is given. Social disengagement (*SdG*) is primarily contributed the accumulation exposure towards relational dissatisfaction.

$$LtS_a(t+\Delta t) = LtS_a(t) + \eta_L.[Pos(StS_a(t) - LtS_a(t)).(1 - LtS_a(t)) - Pos(-(StS_a(t) - LtS_a(t)).StS_a(t))].\Delta t \quad (1)$$

$$SdG_a(t+\Delta t) = SdG_a(t) + \psi_S.(1-SdG_a(t).[(RdS_a(t)-SdG_a(t))].SdG_a(t).\Delta t \quad (2)$$

Need of Support, Recipient Mutual Interest: Combination of short term stress (*StS*) and perceived the availability of support (*PvS*) triggers the need of support. Recipient mutual interest (*RmT*) is determined by number of similar interest between provider (*OpI*) and recipient (*RsI*) interest related to *n* activities.

$$NoS_a(t) = StS_a(t).PvS_a(t) \quad (3)$$

$$RmT_a(t) = \sum sim(RsI_a(t), OpI_a(t))/\ n \quad (4)$$

Support Preference (Informational, Instrumental, Emotional, Companionship): Informational support preference (*FrP*) is expressed by combining weak tie preference (*WsP*) and conscientiousness personality (*RcS*). While, combination of strong tie preference (*SsP*) with extraversion (*ReV*) generates instrumental support preference (*NrP*), and neurotic personality generates emotional support preference (*ErP*). The value of companionship support preference (*CrP*) depends by strong tie preference in combination of with the risk in mental illness (*RmI*), and extraversion personality.

$$FrP_a(t) = WsP_a(t).RcS_a(t) \quad (5)$$
$$NrP_a(t) = SsP_a(t).ReV_a(t) \quad (6)$$
$$ErP_a(t) = SsP_a(t).RnU_a(t) \quad (7)$$
$$CrP_a(t) = [\psi_c.RmI_a(t) + (1-\psi_c).ReV_a(t)].SsP_a \quad (8)$$

Provider Mutual Interest, Willingness to Help: Provider mutual interest (*PmT*) is calculated using a similar concept as in recipient mutual interest. Willingness to help (*WsH*) is modelled by instantaneous relations of agreeableness (*PaG*) and altruistic (*AiC*) personality.

$$PmT_b(t) = \sum sim(OrI_b(t), PsI_b(t))/\ n \quad (9)$$
$$WsH_b(t) = \Omega_w.PaG_b(t) + (1-\Omega_b).AiC_b(t) \quad (10)$$

Support Provision Preference (Informational, Instrumental, Emotional, Companionship): All support provision preferences require willingness to help (*WsH*) in the model, and with its additional attributes. For example, informational provision preference (*FsF*) needs a knowledge level about the problem (*KwL*). While, instrumental provision (*IsF*) is calculated using the combination of agreeableness (*PaG*), perceived close tie (*PcT*), and experience in supportive exchange (*EsE*). Emotional support provision (*EsF*) depends on perceived close tie, and agreeableness. Finally, companionship support provision (*CsF*) requires provider mutual interest, perceived close tie, and extraversion personality (*PeV*).

$$FsF_b(t) = \tau_f.WsH_b(t) + (1-\tau_f).KwL_b(t) \quad (11)$$
$$IsF_b(t) = [\varphi_I.PaG_b(t) + (1-\varphi_I).EsE_b(t)].WsH_b(t).PcT_b(t) \quad (12)$$
$$EsF_b(t) = [\lambda_e.PcT_b(t) + (1-\lambda_e).PaG_b(t)].WsH_b(t) \quad (13)$$
$$CsF_b(t) = [\gamma_c.PmT_b(t) + (1-\gamma_c).PcT_b(t)].PeV_b(t).WsH_b(t) \quad (14)$$

Provided Support: In general, specific supports (informational (*IfP*), emotional (*EsP*), instrumental (*InP*), and (*CsP*)) can be measured by combining some proportion of proactive effort (*PaC*), and an active observation of long term stress (*AoS*) with particular support preference attributes and support requests (informational (*RfR*),direct emotional (*DeR*), indirect emotional (*PiE*), instrumental (*RnR*), and companionship (*HcR*) support requests). These support requests are combined to model accumulated suppot (*ApS*), and later, provided support (*PsS*).

$$IfP_b(t) = PaC_b(t).AoS_b(t) + (1-PaC_b(t)).FsF_b(t).RfR_b(t) \quad (15)$$
$$EsP_b(t) = PaC_b(t).AoS_b(t) + (1-PaC_b(t)).\ [\rho_e.DeR_b(t) + (1-\rho_e).PiE_b(t)].EsF_b(t) \quad (16)$$
$$InP_b(t) = PaC_b(t).AoS_b(t) + (1-PaC_b(t)).IsF_b(t).RnR_b(t) \quad (17)$$
$$CsP_b(t) = PaC_b(t).AoS_b(t) + (1-PaC_b(t)).HcR_b(t).EsF_b(t) \quad (18)$$
$$AoS_b(t+\Delta t) = AoS_b(t) + \lambda_a.[Pos(AlS_b(t)- AoS_b(t)).(1-AoS_b(t))- (-\ Pos(AlS_b(t) - AoS_b(t))).AoS_b(t)].\Delta t \quad (19)$$

$$PsS_b(t+\Delta t) = PsS_b(t) + \beta_p.[Pos(f(ApS_b(t))\text{-} PsS_b(t)).(1\text{-}PsS_b(t))–(\text{-}Pos(f(ApS_b(t))\text{-} PsS_b(t))).PsS_b(t)].\Delta t \quad (20)$$

where, $f(ApS_b(t))$ is a logistic unit function, $2.(1/(1+\eta.e^{-\alpha(ApS_b(t))})\text{-}0.5)$, and $ApS_b(t) = IfP_b(t)+ EsP_b(t)+ InP_b(t)+ CsP_b(t)$

The operator Pos for the positive part is defined by Pos(x) = $(x + |x|)/2$, or, alternatively; Pos$(x) = x$ if $x\geq 0$ and 0 else. For the similarity function, $sim(.)$ is defined by $sim(x,y) = 1$ if $x=y$ or otherwise 0.

3 Configuring Social Support Networks

In order to achieve an intelligent assignment of people to a social support network, an approach has been followed in which the dynamic domain model for support receipt-provision process is used as basis for a configuration process. The description of how a domain model can be used to support a person is sometimes called a *support model.* Based on the required support, this support model selects people from an individual's social network and assigns them to the social support network.

3.1 Concepts in the Configuration Approach

Configuration is an application area in Artificial Intelligence that deals with the formation of complex solutions from a set of simpler components. It has been developed in a number of domains, such as manufacturing, medical therapy, industrial plans, personalized marketing ordering, and electronics design [8, 13, 15]. Technically, configuration is the process of creating a technical system from a predefined set of potential objects / components. It begins with broad specifications, and end with in depth specifications of what components are needed and how they are to be arranged [13]. The outcome of such a process has to fulfil a set of given constraints and requirements. Requirements differ from constraints in that constraints must not be violated (*logical consistency*), while requirements must be fulfilled (*logical consequence*) [15]. The configuration itself is performed in an incremental approach, where each step represents a configuration result and possibly includes testing, or simulating with constraint techniques. In general, there are two types of configuration methods namely; 1) *representation-oriented*, and 2) *task-oriented* [15]. The main objective of representation-oriented view is to find the right representation for expressing the structure of the problem domain, while in task-oriented, it focuses to identify the sub-problems to be solved [8]. Several configuration methods such rule-based configuration, dynamic constraint satisfaction problem, and resource-based configuration fall under the group of representation oriented methods. Meanwhile, case based reasoning and hierarchical method can be grouped under task-oriented methods. A detailed discussion on these methods is beyond the scope of this article. Readers interested in those methods will find [13, 15] useful.

3.2 Interaction between Domain and Support Model

There are two fundamental steps in the design of a support model for support provision task assignment. The first is that information about human's states and profiles is fed into a dynamic model of social receipt and provision, which will result in requirements and constraints about the support network. In the second step this will be used to select social support members within the observed social networks. More importantly, this support model will assign support provision task among selected members in line with their resources and preferences. Figure 2 depicts interactions between support model and dynamics model.

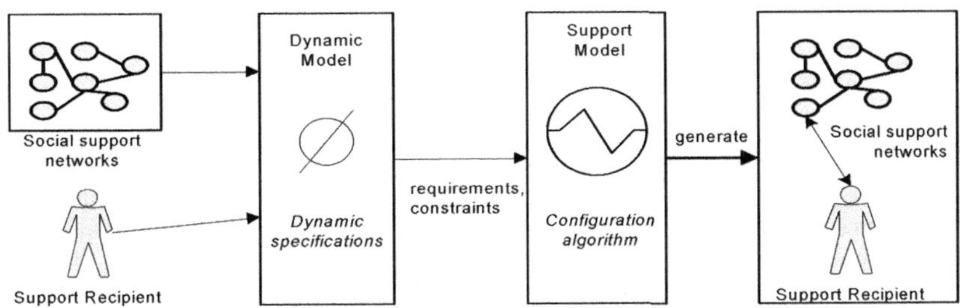

Fig. 2. Interaction between support and dynamic models

As can be seen in Figure 2, important information of all members in social networks and a potential support recipient will be fed into the dynamic model. Within the dynamic model, instantaneous and temporal relationships will compute both support receipt and provision preferences. Moreover, within the dynamic model, information about support recipient's well-being, such as long-term stress can be monitored. This is crucial as it is a vital indicator when to activate the support model.

In this paper, a resource-based configuration approach is used. This approach assumes that all individual components can be viewed as providing a resource needed in the system. The aim of the configuration model is to select the correct set of support providers based on their ability and the type of support they can provide. The structure of relationships between requested and provided support are not expressed in terms of individual or one-to-one matching, but in terms of their preferences. Therefore, it is possible to describe members providing multiple types of supports and utilizing these preferences. For example, a requirement for a support of 0.3 (on the scale between 0 and 1) can be satisfied by using three support providers with 0.1 amount each.

3.3 A Configuration Algorithm to Assign Support Members

In this paper, the configuration process utilizes support recipient information (from the agent's model) to select support members that available for support provision. The crucial information (*requirements*) needed for a configure process are; 1) tie's preferences, 2) long-term stress, 3) support receipt preferences, 4) function in social networks, and 5) support provision preferences. Using this information with a set of configuration rules, an algorithm to generate a set of social support members to provide support is developed (see Algorithm 1 for details). At the start of this algorithm, a set of constraints, like preference number of providers, percentage of assigned supports, and a level of acceptance burden must be initialized first.

Algorithm 1. Steps in the Configuration Process

Input: task assignment, number of support provider, acceptable support provider's burden level, and configuration requirements.
Output: A set of selected support providers
Process: Repeat steps S1-S10 until one of the stopping criteria is satisfied.
S1: Check support receipt long term stress and need of help to start the process.
S2: Input task assignment, number of support provider, and acceptable burden level. Stop if no more task assignment or number of support provider can be assigned
S3: Determine the support network preferences,
weak_ tie_ preference (%) = (WsP / (WsP + SsP)).100.
strong_ tie_ preference (%) = (SsP / (WsP + SsP)).100.
S4: Evaluate support receipt preference (requested support).
S5: Assign support provision according to required preferences and tasks equally. Member with a high support provision will be chosen first, and so forth. If the task assigned or tie preference > the number of support provider, repeat S2.
S6: Assign support providers corresponding to their support provision preferences.
S7: Always assign emotional and companionship support to members in close tie networks if such support resources are still available. Otherwise assign it to another member within weak tie group.
S8: Compute the ratio of provided support over requested support.
overall_provided_support(%)=Σ(provided_support)/Σ(requested_*support).100*
S9: Evaluate support provider burden. If it exceeds the acceptable burden, repeat S2.
burden_provider (%) = Σ(provided_support)/Σ(support_preference).100
S10: Evaluate assigned support. If assigned support ≥ requested support then construct the list contains the assigned members to provide support, else repeat S2.

Information such as a function in social networks can be used to choose the right support provider. If any individual experiences a heighten long term stress level but do not have any support network preferences, then the agent will have its own autonomy to select suitable individuals for support provision purposes. The expected result from this algorithm is the assignment of social provision tasks for support members in social support networks. Figure 3 summarizes the outcome of this process.

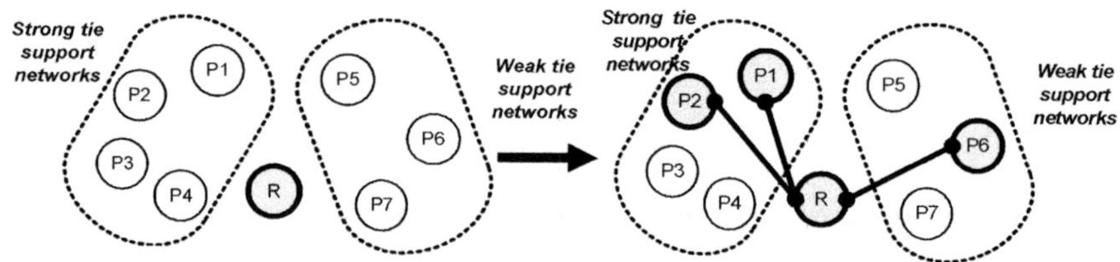

Fig. 3. Social Support Assignment within Social Support Networks

From Figure 3, consider this example; *R* requires social support from his/her support networks (*P1, P2,..., P6*). To assign support provision task, the support model will extract important information from the domain model, and perform a configuration process. Based on several pre-determined requirements and constraints, the support model will generate a list contains potential members to provide support. Potential support providers will be selected either from a strong tie network, or a weak tie network, or both networks (in above example, it was from both networks, *P1* and *P2* from the strong tie support networks, and *P6* from the weak tie support networks).

4 Case Study

In this section, a simple case study to show the results of support model is presented. The proposed model has been implemented in visual programming platform by constructing several scenarios to generate simulation traces. For the sake of brevity, only two types of support request and provision will be discussed.

4.1 Support Assignment

In this case study, eleven different fictional persons are studied under several parameters and attributes for social support receipt and provision. Consider this example: *"Piet experiences stress and seeks for help. From his personality and preferences, he needs more informational support (0.7) than companionship support (0.3). What is more, he prefers members from a weak tie network (0.7) to a strong tie network (0.2). Within his social support networks, he has four members in a strong tie and six members in a weak tie network."* From these members, the support provision availability is the following (*tie network, informational support, companionship support*); **Kees** (*strong, 0.3,0.4*), **Peter** (*strong, 0.1,0.5*), **Anke** (*strong, 0.5,0.5*), **Frieda** (*strong, 0.2, 0.4*), **Jasper** (*weak, 0.5,0.1*), **Bert** (*weak, 0.3, 0.2*), **Johan** (*weak, 0.2, 0.1*), **Sara** (*weak, 0.6,0.2*), **Vincent** (*weak, 0.1, 0.2*), and **Kim** (*weak, 0.2, 0.1*). In this case, three individuals were assigned to provide help. Note that this information is generated from the dynamic model of support receipt and provision process.

Using a support tie preference, he prefers 78 % from support members in a weak tie (≈ 2 members), and 22 % from a strong tie (≈ 1 member). Furthermore, 50 % of provision tasks have been assigned to both members in a weak tie and 100 % for a member in a strong tie. As for the accepted burden level, each individual should not exceed more than 60 % of his/her ability. Based on available information, the algorithm generates this result (see Table 1).

Table 1. Selected Support Provision Members

Name (strong tie)	Info.	C/ship	Name (weak tie)	Info.	C/ship
Kees	-	-	Jasper	0.25	-
Peter	-	-	Bert	-	-
Anke	0.15	0.3	Vincent	-	-
Frieda	-	-	Sara	0.30	-
			Johan	-	-
			Kim	-	-
Provided support *(%)*	**21 %**	**100 %**		**79 %**	

From this, support burden is calculated; where Anke will contribute 45 % of her total ability to support, follow by Jasper (42 %), and Sara (38%). If any of these figures exceed the accepted burden level, a new support distribution will be asked. If necessary, the algorithm will select another member to provide support. In this case,

Anke will provide 30 % of her preference in informational support, and 60 % in companionship support. Both Jasper and Sara will provide 50 % of their ability to provide informational support to Piet.

4.1 Simulation Results

To analyse the configuration results from our case study, the model presented in Section 2 is used to determine the effect of different variants of support networks. Three conditions have been simulated; namely 1) no support is assigned, 2) random support assignment, and 3) configured support assignment. In the first condition, no support is assigned to help support recipient. As for the second condition, three support members were selected randomly (random numbers were generated to select support members). For the last condition, support members were selected from the list generated by a proposed configuration algorithm. During this simulation, a person (support recipient) has been exposed to an extreme of stressors, to represent the prolonged stressors throughout a life time. The outcomes from these conditions are measured using the individual's long-term stress, and social disengagement levels. These results show selection the right support members have a substantial impact on the course of the long-term stress on support recipient.

For simplicity, the current simulations used the following parameters settings: t_{max}=1000 (to represent a monitoring activity up to 42 days), Δt=0.3, flexibility rates = 0.3, and regulatory rates = 0.5. These settings were obtained from previous systematic experiments to determine the most suitable parameters values in the model. For all cases, if the long term stress is equal or greater than 0.5, it describes the support recipient is experiencing stress condition. These experimental results will be discussed in detail below.

Results #1: No Support Provided. During this simulation, a person receives no support from its social network. The person experiences very negative events throughout the simulation time. Since the person needs help, but no support has been provided, then a person is unable with the incoming stressors. This results in an increase of the long-term stress. In case the person is more vulnerably towards stress, the long-term stress increases more quickly and therefore it takes more time for the person to recover. For this case, Figure 4(a) shows the effect on social disengagement where it represents a potential risk to isolate from any social interactions. This condition is one of the precursors to develop a depression if no support is given in future [11]. Similar findings can be found in [9, 10].

Results #2: Random Support Assignment. The analysis of random support assignment helps to understand the effect of support provision assignment without a proper strategy. Figure 4 (b) depicts the effect from this support. As it can be seen in Figure 5, this result provides evidence that by randomly selecting support members is not the best choice if there are many possible variants in support requests and provider's preferences. Although, apparently the long-term stress is decreasing slightly, is not enough to guarantee a person to recover from the incoming stressors. In addition to this, there is a possibility to have a support provider with no support provision preference that matches with the support needed. Thus, a person will have least a chance to recover. On the other hand, if a support provider with the right support

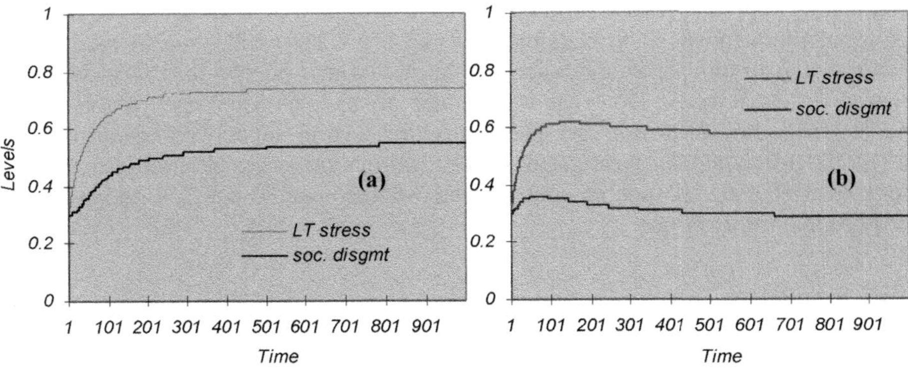

Fig. 4. Person with (a) No Support and (b) Random Support Provision

preference was chosen, there is a risk that it might burden the provider [5, 7]. Having this in motion will hamper the effectiveness of support receipt and provision process.

Results #3: Configured Support Assignment. In this scenario, a person receives support from suggested support members by the configuration approach. Figure 5 shows a more consistent and gradual decrease in a long-term stress level, compared to the random support assignment. For this scenario, it can be seen that the social disengagement is decreasing, and potentially to show that a person is accepting social support and improving the social interaction within a social support network. This condition occurs almost within the majority of individuals when they received the right support by their support members [4, 10, 11].

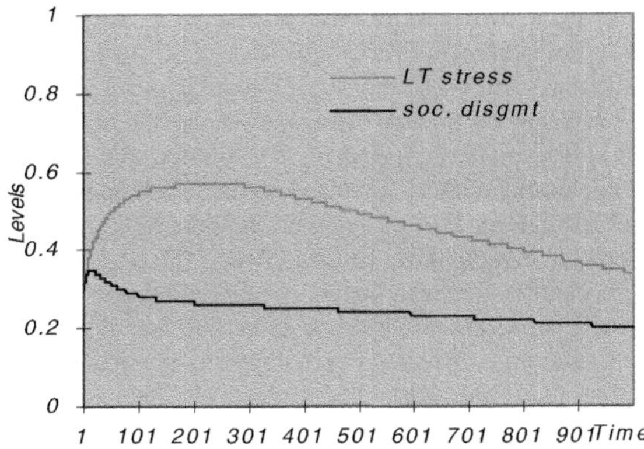

Fig. 5. Person with Configured Support Provision

5 Conclusion

The case study illustrates that the dynamic model about support provision and receipt together with a configuration algorithm can be used to intelligently form a social support network around persons experiencing stress. The simulations suggest that such an assignment results in a lower long term stress level and a reduced level of social disengagement. Ultimately, this might help people in preventing depression or recovering from a depression. Social networks have always been important in stress reduction, but since social network software (e.g. Facebook, MySpace) has become enormously popular in recent times, it starts to become realistic to think about automating support network formation. Much information about social relations and personal characteristics are available nowadays. For the application of the dynamic models used in this paper, more specific information is needed than what is usually shared via social media. However, it is not unrealistic to envision applications that ask people for such information for specifically this goal of support provision. In future research, it should be investigated which information is essential for an effective formation of a social support network and whether people are able and willing to provide that information.

References

1. Adelman, M.B., Parks, M.R., Albrecht, T.L.: Beyond close relationships: support in weak ties. In: Albrecht, T.L., Adelman, M.B. (eds.) Communicating Social Support, pp. 126–147 (1987)
2. Aziz, A., Treur, J.: Modelling Dynamics of Social Support Networks for Mutual Support in Coping with Stress. In: Nguyen, N.T., Katarzyniak, R.P., Janiak, A. (eds.) New Challenges in Computational Collective Intelligence. SCI, vol. 244, pp. 167–179. Springer, Heidelberg (2009)
3. Aziz, A.A., Klein, M.C.A., Treur, J.: An Agent Model for a Human's Social Support Network Tie Preference during Unipolar Depression. In: Proceedings of the 9th International Conference on Intelligent Agent Technology (IAT 2009), pp. 301–306. IEEE Computer Society Press, Los Alamitos (2009)
4. Bolger, N., Zuckerman, A., Kessler, R.C.: Invisible support and adjustment to stress. Journal of Personality and Social Psychology 79(6), 953–961 (2000)
5. Burleson, B.R.: Emotional Support Skills. In: Handbook of Communication and Social Interaction Skills, pp. 551–594 (2003)
6. Cohen, S.: Social Relationships and Health. American Psychologist 59, 676–684 (2004)
7. Etzion, D.: Moderating Effect of Social Support on the Stress-Burnout Relationship. Journal of Applied Psychology 69, 615–622 (1984)
8. Fohn, S.M., Liau, J.S., Greef, A.R., Young, R.E., O'Grady, P.J.: Configuring Computer Systems through Constraint-Based Modelling and Interactive Constraint Satisfaction. Computer in Industry 27, 3–21 (1995)
9. Goldsmith, D.J.: Communicating Social Support, pp. 25–33. Cambridge University Press, Cambridge (2004)
10. Haines, V.A., Hurlbert, J.S., Beggs, J.J.: Exploring the Determinants of Support Provision: Provider Characteristics, Personal Networks, Community Contexts, and Support Following Life Events. J. Health and Social Behaviour 37, 252–264 (1996)
11. Helgeson, V.S.: Social Support and Quality of Life. Supplement: Multidisciplinary Perspectives on Health-Related Quality of Life, vol. 12, pp. 25–31 (2003)
12. Stice, E., Ragan, E.J., Randall, P.: Prospective Relations between Social Support and Depression: Differential Direction of Effects for Parent and Peer Support? Journal of Abnormal Psychology 113(1), 155–159 (2004)
13. Stumptner, M.: An Overview of Knowledge-Based Configuration. AI Communications 10, 111–125 (1997)
14. Tausig, M., Michello, J.: Seeking Social Support. Basic and Applied Social Psychology 9(1), 1–12 (1988)
15. Yang, D., Dong, M., Miao, R.: Development of a Product Configuration System with an Ontology-based Approach. J. Computer-Aided Design 40, 863–878 (2008)

Argumentation-Logic for Explaining Anomalous Patient Responses to Treatments

Maria Adela Grando[1], Laura Moss[2,3,4], David Glasspool[1], Derek Sleeman[2,3], Malcolm Sim[2], Charlotte Gilhooly[2], and John Kinsella[2]

[1] School of Informatics, University of Edinburgh, UK
{mgrando,dglasspo}@inf.ed.ac.uk
[2] Academic Unit of Anaesthesia, Pain, and Critical Care Medicine, School of Medicine, University of Glasgow, UK
laura.moss@glasgow.ac.uk
[3] Department of Computing Science, University of Aberdeen, UK
[4] Department of Clinical Physics, University of Glasgow, UK

Abstract. The EIRA system has proved to be successful in the detection of anomalous patient responses to treatments in the Intensive Care Unit (ICU). One weakness of EIRA is the lack of mechanisms to describe to the clinicians, rationales behind the anomalous detections. In this paper, we extend EIRA by providing it with an argumentation-based justification system that formalizes and communicates to the clinicians the reasons why a patient response is anomalous. The implemented justification system uses human-like argumentation techniques and is based on real dialogues between ICU clinicians.

Keywords: knowledge-based expert systems, explanation, argumentation logic, ontology, intensive care unit.

1 Introduction

EIRA (Explaining, Inferencing, and Reasoning about Anomalies) [1] helps users detect anomalous patient responses to treatment in the Intensive Care Unit (ICU) domain and provides decision support for clinicians by generating explanations for the anomalies. EIRA is based on complex algorithms that reflect the problem solving methods used by ICU clinicians in detecting and resolving anomalies. While EIRA has proved to be very accurate [2], it lacks a justification system that could make explicit, in a user-friendly way, the complex rationality behind the algorithms; such an extension would allow the system to be updated more easily with new knowledge; this is an important weakness that needs to be addressed.

In this work we abstracted EIRA's algorithms for a specific domain to use a more flexible reasoning process based on logical argumentation. The first stage of this work involved using the Argumentation Service Platform with Integrated Component (ASPIC) engine (http://aspic.acl.icnet.uk/) to model exchanges of arguments made by ICU clinicians to develop schemes for use in EIRA. The second stage involved the

M. Peleg, N. Lavrač, and C. Combi (Eds.): AIME 2011, LNAI 6747, pp. 35–44, 2011.

implementation of these schemes in EIRA to allow EIRA's reasoning to be exposed to clinicians. A subsequent evaluation showed that most clinicians found the display of the argumentation results to be useful when faced with complex anomalous scenarios.

This paper is organized as follows; section 2 provides background to this work; in section 2.1 EIRA is described; in section 2.2 the use of ASPIC is explored to formalize and evaluate the main arguments given in a dialogue between two clinicians from Glasgow Royal Infirmary's ICU; in section 3 the enhanced version of EIRA is described, detailing the elements from EIRA which are kept (ontologies, algorithms) and those added in order to incorporate the functionality of the ASPIC engine; finally in section 4 we explain our future plans.

2 Background

2.1 EIRA

Anomalous scenarios play a key role in knowledge discovery; Kuhn [3] defines an anomaly as a violation of the "*paradigm-induced expectations that govern normal science*". Anomalies are of interest as they often point to the inadequacy of a currently held theory and require refinement of the related theory; consequently this can provide the impetus for the discovery of further domain knowledge. EIRA [4] helps to detect anomalous patient responses to treatment in the ICU domain and assists clinicians by providing potential explanations for why the anomaly may have occurred. The explanations generated by EIRA can be considered as an anomaly-driven refinement of the clinician's theory. One proposed function of EIRA is that it will be used by ICU clinicians as an 'offline' aid/tutoring tool.

EIRA comprises: a knowledge base consisting of several instantiated OWL ontologies (http://www.w3.org/2004/OWL/) and a Java program implementing strategies extracted from domain experts' protocols. As shown in Figure 1, for each patient, EIRA also has access to data containing physiological parameters, and drug and fluid infusions. When attempting to detect anomalies, EIRA identifies the drugs given to the patient at a particular time point from the patient's data and retrieves the anticipated effects of administering each drug from the ICU ontology. When the anticipated response(s) do not occur, the actual response observed in the data is noted (Figure 2). For example, EIRA's anomaly detection algorithm may determine that:

Patient Data contains: Adrenaline is administered to a patient and this is followed by a decrease in the patient's mean arterial pressure (MAP).
EIRA's Knowledge Base contains: Adrenaline should increase MAP.
EIRA suggests that: A patient has responded anomalously to adrenaline.

To generate context-dependent hypotheses for why the detected anomalies may have occurred, EIRA proceeds with each of the implemented strategies (algorithms) and, if appropriate, explanations are presented to the user (Figure 3).

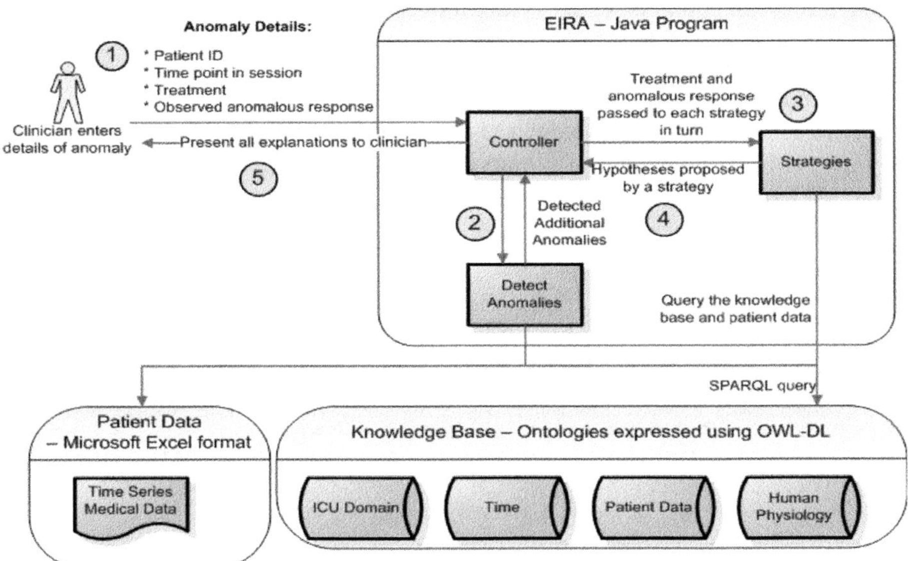

Fig. 1. EIRA system. (1) ICU clinician enters an anomaly into EIRA. (2) EIRA can detect additional anomalies. (3),(4) EIRA's explanations (reinterpretations) are generated by the application of strategies with medical domain knowledge represented in several ontologies. (5) The explanations generated for the anomaly are presented to the ICU clinician.

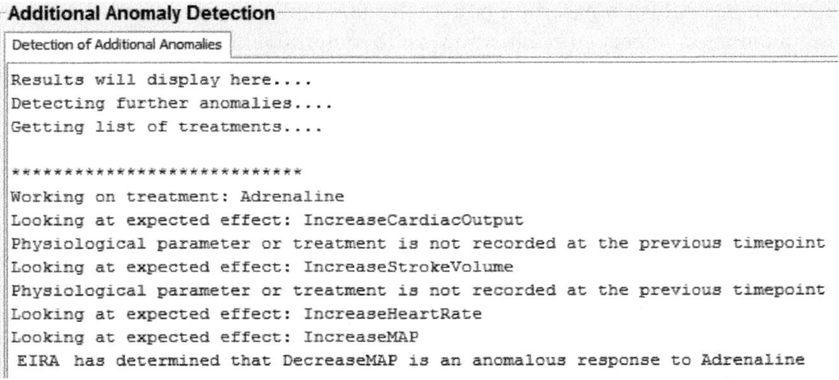

Fig. 2. EIRA's display of detected anomalies

For example, for the above anomaly, EIRA suggests that the patient's high MAP decreased because the patient's condition may have been improving at the same time (i.e. it invokes the Overall Patient Improvement algorithm). To generate this explanation, EIRA examined the patient data to determine whether, over the previous six hours, the majority of the physiological parameters in the patient's dataset showed an improvement.

A current limitation of EIRA is that it does not justify its conclusions; it does not explain *how* it determined that a patient response is anomalous and it does not explain *how* it generated an explanation for why the anomaly occurred. Justification for EIRA's conclusions is important for the clinician's acceptance [5] and to allow the clinician to criticize the knowledge and reasoning processes used by EIRA.

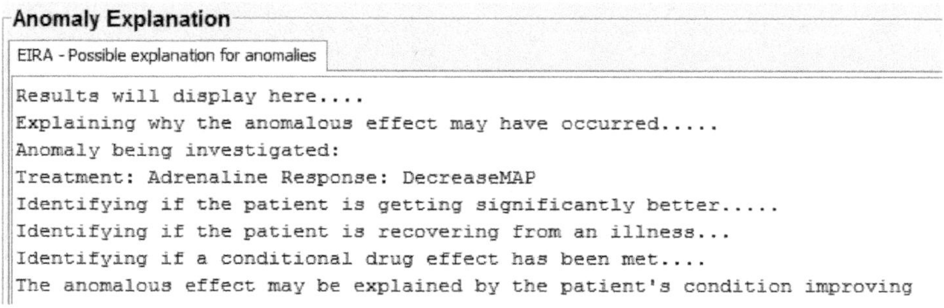

Anomaly Explanation

EIRA - Possible explanation for anomalies

```
Results will display here....
Explaining why the anomalous effect may have occurred.....
Anomaly being investigated:
Treatment: Adrenaline Response: DecreaseMAP
Identifying if the patient is getting significantly better.....
Identifying if the patient is recovering from an illness...
Identifying if a conditional drug effect has been met....
The anomalous effect may be explained by the patient's condition improving
```

Fig. 3. EIRA's display of anomaly explanation

2.1 Using ASPIC in the Intensive Care Unit (ICU) Domain

During the past three decades much research has been done on the enhancement of the justification capabilities of *knowledge-based systems* and decision support systems. In parallel, *argumentation logic* has evolved as a formal framework for modelling human collaborative deliberations, interchanging arguments in favour or against some conclusion based on potentially incomplete or inconsistent information. In argumentation theory the intention is to determine if a particular proposition follows from certain assumptions even if some of these assumptions are disproved by other assumptions. Furthermore, arguments can have relative strengths, which provide a very human-like approach to reasoning.

In this work we propose an enhanced version of EIRA where the process used to construct justifications is a combination of algorithms and ontology-based argumentation reasoning. We retain from EIRA the algorithms that evaluate the patient's physiological measurements and use them to generate factual arguments. But in the enhanced system we have rewritten EIRA's algorithms to detect anomalies that are based on complex medical knowledge into schemes which form reasoning templates that can be used as argument generators. The schemes are expressed in terms of concepts from EIRA's medical ontologies. For instance, consider the scheme: *there is an anomaly if there is a difference between a patient's observed and expected behaviour*. Only at run time is a scheme instantiated to become an argument by using domain information retrieved from EIRA's ontologies and the patient's physiological measurements. For example, using EIRA's algorithms, the following argument can be created from the previous scheme: *the behaviour of the patient is anomalous because an increase in the blood pressure was observed although a decrease was expected*. After the generation of arguments and their interactions, a graph is created showing which are attacked or which are defending themselves from attacks. Based on this evaluation the system can determine if a patient's response to treatment is anomalous.

To investigate whether we could formalize exchanges of arguments in this particular domain (in preparation for enhancing EIRA) an exercise was carried out to model the main arguments exchanged in dialogues from the ICU using a particular argumentation framework. Previously, sessions had been held with ICU clinicians from Glasgow Royal Infirmary to understand how two clinicians, who had disagreed on whether a patient's response to treatment was anomalous, exchanged arguments in order to arrive at a consensus. One particular disagreement consisted of one clinician believing that on the 2nd day of a patient's stay, the patient's cardiac output increased when given noradrenaline (a cardiac drug) and he considered this anomalous; whilst the other clinician believed that although the dose of noradrenaline given to the patient was very high and the patient's cardiac output was high he did not believe the situation was anomalous. During the session the clinicians discussed possible explanations for why the patient's cardiac output increased and if that was anomalous. We have formalized the main arguments exchanged in the session using the ASPIC engine; to do this we have carried out the following tasks:

1. Defined a knowledge base: this contains a knowledge base of facts and a set of rules. Facts are defined as [optional fact name] α.n and rules are of the form [optional rule name] ß <-α_1,..., α_t. n, where ß, α ,α_1,..., α_t are expressed as first order literals and their negations and $0<n\leq 1$ is numeric support for the rule. Facts can have support $0<n\leq 1$, strict rules have support 1.0 and defeasible rules can be assigned support $0<n<1$.

The greater the numeric support, the more confidence there is in the validity of the rule. Here we follow the convention for qualitative support adopted in the Tallis (http://www.cossac.org/tallis) decision support system: (++) for conclusive arguments, (+) for positive support, (-/+) for neutral support, (-) for negative support, and (–) for exclusive support; to do this conclusive arguments are assigned 1, positive support corresponds to 0.7, neutral support is equivalent to 0.5, negative support is assigned 0.3, and exclusive support receives 0. We have assigned qualitative support levels based on our judgment of the level of assertiveness shown in the dialogue transcript by the participating clinicians. In the future, the extended EIRA system could assign support to arguments on the basis of evidence gathered from previously recorded deliberations.

To define our knowledge base we adopted the notion of an anomaly used in EIRA: an anomaly exists if a clinician has an acceptable argument for an expected effect, but there is evidence that the expected effects did not happen (arguments **[a1] [a2],** *defined below*). According to EIRA, when the clinicians administer a drug at time t1 with a known expected effect, then they can confidently expect to see the drug's effect at a time t2 where t2>t1 (**[a3]**). We also added to the knowledge base the facts **[a4][a5]** to state that the observation of no increase in an attribute value is different from an observed increase. From the clinician's dialogue we know that at time t1, patient p has severe sepsis, is vasodilated, and has been administered noradrenaline, as stated by the facts **[a6]** to **[a9]**. It is also stated in the transcript that at time t2, where t2>t1, there is an increase in the patient's cardiac output, expressed in **[a10][a11]** and a highly expected effect of noradrenaline is not to increase the patient's cardiac output (**[a12]**). Finally, in the dialogue the clinicians agree that most probably the noradrenaline is not producing the expected effect for patient p at time t1. Below we formalize in ASPIC the above arguments:

Rules:
[a1] anomaly <- expected(Patient, Attribute, Expected, t2), observed(Patient, Attribute, Observed, t2), different(Expected, Observed) 1.0.
[a2] anomaly <- ~expected(Patient, Attribute, Expected, t2), observed(Patient, Attribute, Observed, t2), ~different(Expected, Observed) 1.0.
[a3] expected(Patient, Attrib, Expect,t2) <- administered(Patient, D, t1), expected_effect(D, Attrib, Expect), greater(t2,t1) 0.7.
Facts:
[a4] different(no_increase, increase) 1.0. [a5] different(increase, no_increase) 1.0.
[a6] patient(p) 1.0. [a7] severe_sepsis(p,t1) 1.0. [a8]vasodilated(p,t1) 1.0.
[a9] administered(p, noradrenaline, t1) 1.0.
[a10] observed(p, cardiac_output, increase, t2) 1.0 [a11] greater(t2,t1) 1.0
[a12] expected_effect(noradrenaline, cardiac_output, no_increase) 0.7

2. *Defined argument interactions*: three different types of attack relations can be defined: rebutting, restricted rebutting, and undercutting. For instance, the literals *~a 0.3* and *a 0.5* are both valid and their associated arguments rebut (or contradict) each other. Similarly, an argument formed from the fact a. and the rule b<- a 0.9. rebuts an argument formed from the fact ~b 0.4. Strict arguments cannot be rebutted. Under restricted rebutting, an argument whose top rule is strict cannot be rebutted by an argument whose top rule is defeasible. Rules can be named and undercut (by a counter argument) by writing a fact or rule whose head is the contradiction of that name; if argument A undercuts (i.e. is a counter argument to) argument B, then A claims that some rule in B is not applicable. For instance, if noradrenaline is not working (i.e. not having the expected effects) then the defeasible argument that we named **a3** could be undercut:
~[a3] <- ~working(p,noradrenaline,t1), expected_effect(noradrenaline, cardiac_output, non_increase) 0.7.

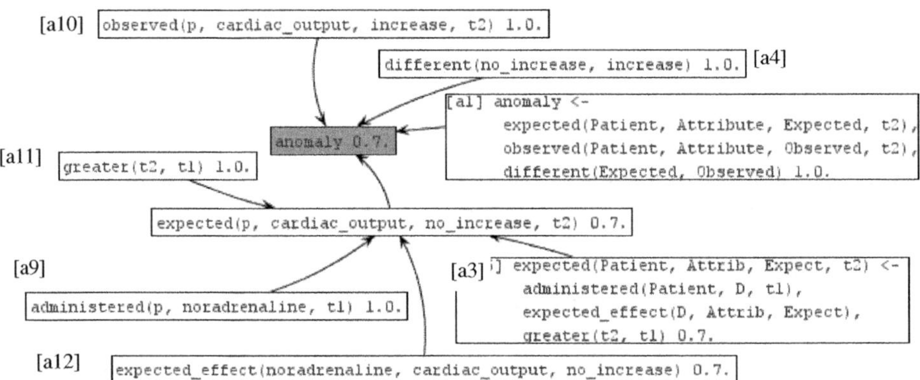

Fig. 4. Argumentation graph returned by the ASPIC engine when the user queries if the patient's response to treatment is anomalous

3. *Evaluated argument status:* based on the interacting arguments and Dung's calculus of opposition [6] the ASPIC engine determines the status of the arguments based on Dung's grounded semantics: if argument A is attacked by some argument B,

then A can be reinstated as an acceptable argument if its attacker B is itself attacked. When the query **anomaly** is introduced, the results of the inferences performed by the ASPIC engine are shown as an argumentation graph (Figure 4). Here we have set the ASPIC engine to use the weakest link valuation, which assigns the support for the main argument as the minimum support over all of its subarguments. In the diagram, arrows represent inference, shaded boxes indicate an undefeated main argument, and non-shaded boxes indicate an unevaluated argument (usually a subargument). As found in the clinicians' dialogue transcript, the ASPIC engine has detected that the patient's increase in cardiac output is anomalous. One explanation, as shown in Figure 4, is that after administering noradrenaline to a patient (according to the known expected effects of the noradrenaline drug in this context) the patient's cardiac output should decrease.

3 The Implemented EIRA Extension

When attempting to detect an anomaly in the ICU domain, EIRA identifies the drugs given to the patient (from the patient dataset) and retrieves the anticipated effects of administering each drug from the ICU domain ontology. The ICU domain ontology contains three types of knowledge: disorders, treatments, and disorder severity scores. The drug class (a subclass of treatment) describes how drugs are used as treatments in the ICU domain. An instance of the drug class (e.g. adrenaline) is related to an instance of the physiological effect class (e.g. Increase in MAP), which is defined in the human physiology ontology, via the 'expectedDrugEffect' property. The human physiology ontology models, at a high level, knowledge regarding organs and organ systems, clinical features, and physiological effects. The 'physiological effects' class represents different types of effects that occur in the human body; two types of effects have been defined: parameter changes and symptoms.

EIRA then analyses the patient data to determine the physiological effect that has occurred after the drug was administered to the patient. To do this, the human physiology ontology is queried to identify which instance of the physiological effect class has been observed in the patient dataset. To establish whether an anomaly has occurred, two instances of the physiological effect class are compared; the first taken from the query of the ICU domain ontology to determine the expected effect of a drug, and the second from the query to determine the observed response in the patient dataset. If the two instances are not equivalent, then an anomaly has occurred. The information about the anomaly (the drug, the expected effect, and the observed effect) is then displayed to the user on EIRA's original GUI (shown in Figure 2).

This simple comparison of ontology instances does not currently allow for a sufficient justification to be produced for *how* EIRA has detected an anomaly. Subsequently, EIRA's evaluation of whether the observed response to a drug is different to the expected response has been replaced by the ASPIC argumentation framework (through ASPIC java libraries). To create an ASPIC knowledge base, schemes have been implemented in EIRA based on the previous modelling of clinician argumentation (described in section 2.2). The schemes were obtained by replacing specific terms in the ASPIC arguments from section 2.2 for terms from the ICU domain ontology and the patient dataset (indicated by [*italics*]). For example in argument **[a9] administered(p, noradrenaline, t1)1.0** we replaced the specific drug noradrenaline for the generic term *[drug]*. Below we provide several examples of schemes introduced in EIRA:

- **[scheme9]administered(p, [*drug*], t1) 1.0.**
- **[scheme10]observed(p, [*observed parameter*], [*observed effect*], t2)1.0.**
- **[scheme12]expected_effect([*drug*],[*expected effect parameter*], [*expected effect*])0.7.**
- **[scheme1]anomaly <- expected(Patient, Physiological_Effect, Expected, t2), observed(Patient, Physiological_Effect, Observed, t2), different(Expected, Observed)1.0.**
- **[scheme2]anomaly <- ~expected(Patient, Physiological_Effect, Expected, t2), observed(Patient, Physiological_Effect, Observed, t2), ~different(Expected, Observed)1.0.**
- **[scheme3] expected(Patient, Attrib, Expect, t2) <- administered(Patient, D, t1), expected_effect(D, Attrib, Expect), greater(t2,t1)0.7**

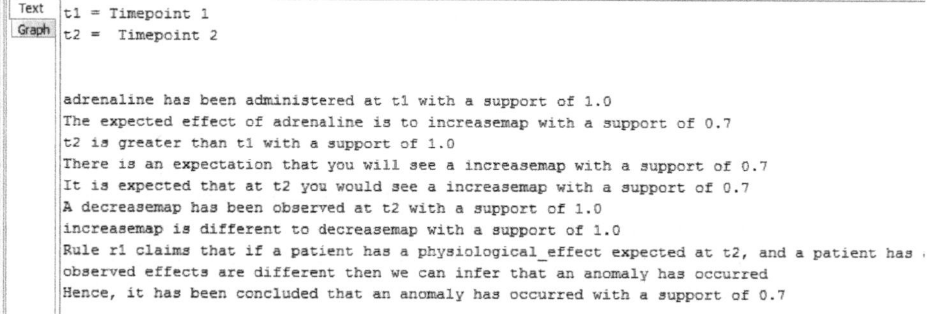

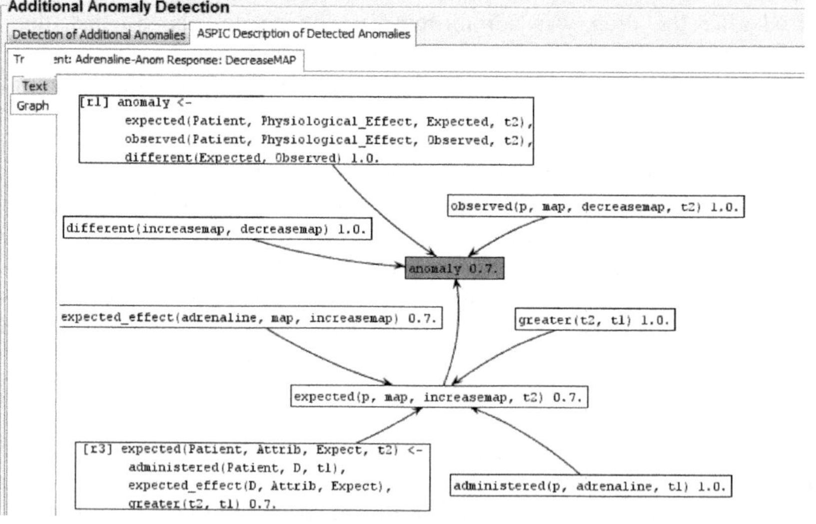

Fig. 5. ASPIC inferences for the detection of an anomaly

Schemes are instantiated (where appropriate) at run time with relevant ontology instances. For example, the scheme **administered(p, [*drug*], t1)1.0.** is instantiated at run time as *administered(patient99, adrenaline, (12/08/2010 3:00:00))1.0.*

For each expected effect of a drug, there are three alternative effects: an increase in a physiological parameter, a decrease in a physiological parameter, or no change in a physiological parameter. Depending on the expected effect (e.g. increase in MAP), the other physiological effects (e.g. decrease in MAP and constant MAP) are determined by further queries of the Human Physiology ontology. Therefore, the following scheme is added to EIRA: **different([*expected effect*],[*different effect*])1.0.**

Once the knowledge base has been completed, the ASPIC argumentation engine determines the state of the arguments and whether an anomaly has occurred. The results are presented to the clinician in the form of an argumentation graph and an equivalent textual representation (Figure 5). The use of schemes allows the methods used to construct the argumentation framework to be separated from the form and content of arguments, as proposed in [7]. As in [8] the content of arguments is generated from queries of a domain ontology used as a reference source.

4 Evaluation and Future Work

In the enhanced EIRA system we have achieved the following: 1) made more explicit EIRA's reasoning by implementing schemes that can be inspected, verified, and easily changed; 2) achieved sound justifications; and 3) allowed defeasible reasoning; that is achieving the detection of anomalies even with contradictory arguments.

For the evaluation of the potential clinical benefit of the enhanced EIRA system we held interviews with 3 specialty registrars (in Anaesthesia, Pain, and Critical Care). It became clear from these discussions that in some scenarios the extra information provided by the ASPIC-generated justification was not required as the clinician clearly understood why an anomaly had been identified; this was why, in general, two of the clinicians preferred EIRA's original presentation of detected anomalies. However, the clinicians suggested that when they were faced with a complex anomaly, or one which they did not agree with, they liked having access to the additional information provided by the argumentation inferences. Subsequently, it is suggested that the ASPIC generated justifications should be considered as an *additional* feature available to the clinicians.

Our future plans are to further extend EIRA to allow interactions with the user in order to discuss the explanations generated by the system. The user should be allowed to introduce at run-time his own arguments supporting/attacking explanations provided by EIRA. In addition, EIRA should be able to instantiate from its library of design-time schemes, new arguments attacking/supporting the user's arguments, adding them to the argumentation graph under construction. The deliberation would finish when neither EIRA nor the user can add a new argument or they both agree on the conclusion. The benefits that this planned extension of EIRA could bring to the ICU are: 1) A well-principled methodology to *create/correct the medical knowledge and strategies* on which the tool is based; 2) A way to *suggest extensions in the data collected by the patient's management system* and subsequently used by EIRA. This process will show if some data is required by the decision process but was not available to EIRA; 3) A tool that could be used to *train junior clinicians* by helping them to understand why the system's solution is better/different from the one they expected; 4) A methodology to *learn the techniques used by clinicians when arguing*.

This work has focussed on the use of anomalies to perform decision support, the development of ASPIC schemes based on ICU clinicians' dialogue, and the implementation of these schemes in a decision support tool to provide an argumentation-based justification for its decision making. From the theoretical point of view this research will allow us to tackle interesting open problems. According to [9] *"Currently there exists no artificial agent or knowledge-based system that possesses both argumentation and explanation capabilities." "Now, can the same knowledge base be used to generate argumentative and explanatory discourse?"*

Acknowledgements. Richard Appleton, Rachel Harrison, and Chris Hawthorne (Academic Unit of Anaesthesia, Pain, and Critical Care, University of Glasgow). Kathryn Henderson and Jennifer McCallum (Glasgow Royal Infirmary). Matthew South (Robotics Research Group, University of Oxford). This work was an extension of the routine audit process in Glasgow Royal Infirmary's ICU; requirements for further Ethical Committee Approval have been waived.

References

1. Moss, L.: Explaining Anomalies: An Approach to Anomaly-Driven Revision of a Theory. PhD Thesis, University of Aberdeen (2010)
2. Moss, L., Sleeman, D., Sim, M., Booth, M., Daniel, M., Donaldson, L., Gilhooly, C., Hughes, M., Kinsella, J.: Ontology-Driven Hypothesis Generation to Explain Anomalous Patient Responses to Treatment. Knowledge Based Systems 23(4), 309–315 (2010)
3. Kuhn, D.: The Structure of Scientific Revolutions. University of Chicago Press, Chicago (1962)
4. Moss, L., Sleeman, D., Booth, M., Daniel, M., Donaldson, L., Gilhooly, C., Hughes, M., Sim, M., Kinsella, J.: Explaining Anomalous Responses to Treatment in the Intensive Care Unit. In: Combi, C., Shahar, Y., Abu-Hanna, A. (eds.) Proc. of the 12th Conf. on AI in Medicine. LNCS, pp. 250–255. Springer, Heidelberg (2009)
5. Gonul, M.S., Onkal, D., Lawrence, M.: The Effects of Structural Characteristics of Explanations on the use of a DSS. Decision Support Systems 42(3), 1481–1493 (2006)
6. Dung, P.M.: On the Acceptability of Arguments and its Fundamental Role in Non Monotonic Reasoning, Logic Programming and N-person Games. J. Artificial Intelligence 77, 321–357 (1995)
7. Gordon, T.F., Walton, D.: Legal Reasoning with Argument Schemes. In: Hafner, C.D. (ed.) Proc. 12th Int. Conf. on Artificial Intelligence and Law, pp. 137–146. ACM Press, New York (2009)
8. Williams, M.H.: Integrating Ontologies and Argumentation for Decision-Making in Breast Cancer. PhD thesis. University College London (2008)
9. Moulin, B., Irandoust, H., Belanger, M., Desbordes, G.: Explanation and Argumentation Capabilities: towards the creation of more persuasive agents. Artificial Intelligence Review 17, 169–222 (2002)

How to Use Symbolic Fusion to Support the Sleep Apnea Syndrome Diagnosis

Adrien Ugon[1,2], Jean-Gabriel Ganascia[1], Carole Philippe[2], Hélène Amiel[2], and Pierre Lévy[2]

[1] Laboratoire d'Informatique de Paris 6, Paris
{adrien.ugon,jean-gabriel.ganascia}@lip6.fr
[2] Hôpital TENON, AP-HP, Paris
{carole.philippe,pierre.levy}@tnn.aphp.fr,
amielhelene@gmail.com
[3] Inserm UMR s 707, paris
[4] UPMC-Paris6, Inserm U707, paris

Abstract. The Sleep Apnea Syndrome is a sleep disorder characterized by frequently repeated respiratory disorders during sleep. It needs the simultaneous recording of many physiological parameters to be diagnosed. The analysis of these curves is a time consuming task made by sleep Physicians. First, they detect some physiological events on each curve and then, they point out links between respiratory events and their consequences. To support the diagnosis, we used symbolic fusion on elementary events, which connects events to their sleep context - sleep-stage and body position - and to the respiratory event responsible of their occurrence. The reference indicator is the Apnea-Hypopnea Index (AHI), defined as the average hourly frequency of arisen of Apneas or Hypopneas while the patient is sleeping. We worked on the polysomnography of 59 patients, that were first completely analyzed by a sleep Physician and then analyzed by our method. We compared the ratio of the AHI got by the automatic analysis and the AHI got by the sleep Physician.

$$\delta = \frac{AHI(automaticanalysis)}{AHI(SleepPhysicianAnalysis)}$$

Globally, we overvalued the count of apneas and hypopneas for the group of patients with $AHI \leq 5$, that are considered as healthy patients. In average, for these patients, $\delta = 2,71$. For patients with mild or moderate Sleep Apnea Syndrome we globally found a similar AHI. In average, for these patients, $\delta = 1,04$. For patients with severe Sleep Apnea Syndrome, we undervalued a little the count of respiratory events. In average, for these patients, $\delta = 0,83$. This leads to the same severity class for most of the patients.

Keywords: symbolic fusion, signal processing, event extraction, Sleep Apnea Syndrome.

M. Peleg, N. Lavrač, and C. Combi (Eds.): AIME 2011, LNAI 6747, pp. 45–54, 2011.

1 Introduction

1.1 The Sleep Apnea Syndrome

The Sleep Apnea Syndrome (SAS) is a sleep disorder characterized by recurrent respiratory events during sleep, causing excessive sleepiness, cognitive deficits [1] and road traffic accidents [2].

By people suffering from SAS, cessations and decreases of the air flow are observed. This has for consequences a poor quality of sleep. Its association with increased cardiovascular [3] and cerebrovascular [4] morbidity is clearly recognized. Young and colleagues estimated that 2% of women and 4% of men of middle age meet the criteria for the clinical syndrome of sleepdisordered breathing [5].

The polysomnography (PSG) is the medical examination used to detect the sleep disorders. It consists of simultaneously recording physiological activity during a night.

The diagnosis consists in two tasks. First are counted and analyzed the number of each respiratory event and their eventual consequences on other physiological parameters; this task is called the *scoring*. The second task of the diagnosis consists in gathering all the events and specific medical information from the medical file and give the conclusion using medical knowledge. In particular is used .the Apnea-Hypopnea Index (AHI) that is the average hourly frequency of occurrence of apnea or hypopnea while the patient is sleeping. Any dependence to a sleep-context, position and/or sleep-stage, is for instance a useful information for the diagnosis and the choice of treatment.

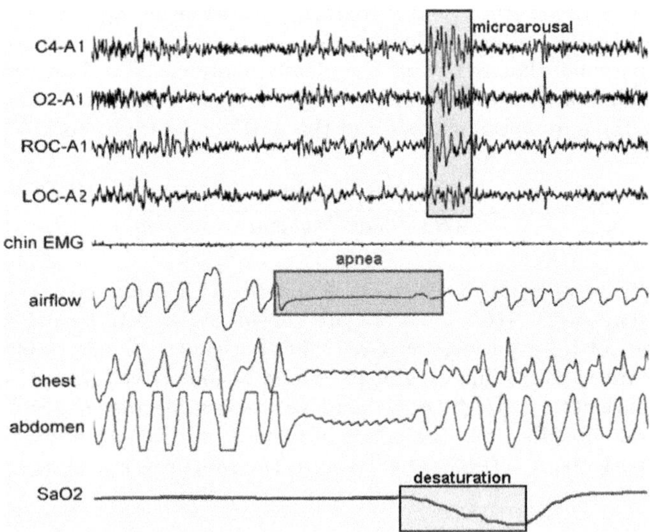

Fig. 1. Polysomnographic Data

The necessary events for the diagnosis are respiratory events - apneas and hypopneas -, *desaturations* and *microarousals*, which are very short awakenings that last between 3 and 10 seconds. The position and the sleep stages need also to be known as a sleep context of arisen of the events. Desaturations are a $\geq 3\%$ decrease of the level of oxygen in the blood (cf figure 1).

1.2 Data Intepretation

In sleep medicine, the American Academy gives the reference rules, terminology and technical specifications for acquisition of physiological parameters and their interpretation. The "AASM Manual for the Scoring of Sleep and Associated Event" [6] specifies the necessary sensors to use to acquire reliable data and the definition of physiological events used as indicators of the disease.

Thus should be recorded during the polysomnography : electroencephalographic (EEG) derivations recording brain activity, electroocculographic (EOG) derivations recording eyes movements, Chin electromyographic (EMG) derivation recording muscle tone, Leg EMG derivations recording legs movements, Airflow, Respiratory Effort, Oxygen blood-saturation (SpO_2), electrocardiographic (ECG) derivation and body position.

It is demonstrated in [7] that there is a tremendous variability among polysomnography technologists and that this variability is mostly reduced with a reliable computer-assisted scoring system (cf [8]).

Respiratory Events

An apnea (cf figure 1) is defined as a drop in the peak air flow excursion by $> 90\%$ of baseline, with an amplitude reduction that lasts at least 10 seconds [6].

The apneas are then classified in obstructive, mixed or central apneas depending of the inspiratory effort during the absence of airflow. In case of presence of continuous or increased effort throughout the entire period, it is classified as an obstructive apnea. If the effort is absent during the whole cessation of airflow, the apnea is considered as central. If there is no effort at the beginning of the period, and then a resumption of inspiratory effort in the second portion of the event, the apnea is classified as a mixed apnea.

There is no consensus on hypopneas definition. There are two used definitions in [6] :

- There is a drop by $\geq 30\%$ of baseline in the nasal pressure signal excursions, during at least 10 seconds and followed by a $\geq 4\%$ desaturation from pre-event baseline or an arousal.
- There is a drop by $\geq 50\%$ of baseline in the nasal pressure signal excursions, during at least 10 seconds and followed by a $\geq 3\%$ desaturation from pre-event baseline or an arousal.

Scoring of Sleep Stages

During a night, sleep is composed of 5 or 6 sleep cycles, that last about 90 minutes. Every cycle is composed itself by sleep stages, that could be considered as the depth of sleep. At the beginning of the cycle, during a few minutes, is the N1 sleep stage. It is followed by the N2 sleep-stage, that constitutes 60% of all sleep; it is called "light sleep". Then, we find the N3 sleep-stage, that is called "deep sleep". At the end of the cycle, we find the REM-sleep (Rapid Eyes Movement-Sleep), this is the sleep-stage where we mostly dream. Each sleep stage is recognizable, by 30-seconds epochs, by the main frequency of EEG waves and the presence of specific patterns. These patterns are too short to be automatically recognized with reliability. Of course, the Physicians also use the knowing of preceding sleep-stage.

Usually, EEG waves are grouped by frequency ranges (cf Table 1).

Table 1. EEG frequency range

frequency range	class label
0-4 Hz	δ
4-7 Hz	θ
8-12 Hz	α
12-30 Hz	β

The whole polysomnographic recording should be analyzed by 30-seconds epochs; Each of them should be associated to a sleep stage. This analysis is called the *scoring*.

1.3 Goal of the Paper

In previous works ([9] and [10]), we showed that sleep-context - Sleep stage and position - allows to have extra information that could directly be used by Sleep Physicians for diagnosis.

Our goal is to automatize the calculation of the AHI. Our add-on is to offer to the doctor the sleep-context of arisen of the respiratory events and their physiological consequences. We use two consecutive steps in that aim. In the first step are extracted the elementary physiological events from the recorded curves. In the second step, we fuse linked events.

The remainder of the paper is organized as follows. Section 2 provides the prior medical knowledge and the symbolic fusion. Later, results are illustrated and described in Section 3. Finally, Method and Results are discussed in Section 4.

2 Method

2.1 Input Data Description

We used 215 polysomnographic recordings as input data, that were each composed of 3 EEG channels - C3-A2, C4-A1 and O1-A2 -, 2 electroocculographic

(EOG) channels (Left and Right), 1 Chin electromyographic (EMG) channel recording the muscle tone, 1 canula recording the nasal respiratory air flow, 2 thoracic and abdominal belts recording thoracic and abdominal movements, that are directly linked to the activity of respiratory muscles, and thus to the respiratory effort and 1 SpO_2 channel, 1 Pulse channel, 1 ECG Channel, 2 legs EMG channels and finally the body-position channel. Sleep Physicians were asked to analyze these 59 polysomnographic recordings and give their conclusion; each patient polysomnography was analyzed by one sleep Physician.

The recordings were made and scored with the EMBLA System® and last each 14 to 15 hours.

From these 215 recordings, we could use the whole dataset for the sleep stages scoring, but only 59 recordings for the complete treatment. Indeed, our method needs all signals to be interpretable. The main problems were unusable format for body position and SpO_2 channel that got loose during the night.

Sleep Physicians were asked to score the sleep stages of these 215 polysomnographic recordings; each polysomnography was analyzed by one sleep Physician.

2.2 Sleep Stage Scoring

Given an epoch, we described the recordings with 24 parameters, 8 for each of the 3 types of sensors - EEG, EOG and EMG -. For EEG and EOG, there are several curves. Thus, each parameter is computed for each different curve. Except for parameter 2, the final parameter is the mean value of the different *temporal* computed parameters. Parameter 2 is a class belonging. The final parameter is the most frequent class. For instance, there are 3 EEG curves. For a given epoch E1, parameter 1 will be computed for each of the 3 recorded curves. Let us call $P1_A$, $P1_B$ and $P1_C$ these 3 *temporal* parameters. The final EEG parameter 1 for this epoch E1 is the mean value of $P1_A$, $P1_B$ and $P1_C$.

signal processing : parameters extraction
The 8 parameters that we used are :

1. The first parameter is the power of the recorded signal. For one given real signal x, its power is defined by :

$$Power(x) = \frac{1}{T} * \sum(x(t)^2)$$

   where x(t) is the amplitude of the signal at t-time and T is the length of the signal (30 seconds in our case)
2. The second parameter is the main frequency Class. Using a Fast Fourier Transform (FFT), coefficients are grouped by frequency classes. Then, to each group is associated the median Fourier coefficient. The second parameter is thus the group identifier with the maximum median coefficient value. For the EEG curves was used the frequency range from table 1; for EOG and Chin EMG curves, frequency range from table 2. EMG and EOG thresholds were defined and adjusted for this study.

Table 2. EOG and EMG frequency ranges

class label	EOG	EMG
δ	0-2 Hz	0-2 Hz
θ	2-3 Hz	2-3 Hz
α	3-20 Hz	3-4 Hz
β	$> 20Hz$	$> 4Hz$

3. The third parameter is the frequency to which is associated the maximum coefficient value in the FFT.
4. The fourth parameter is the most frequent local main frequency class. A FFT is computed on each 1-second window of the treated epoch. There are thus 30 *local* windows for one given epoch. For each window is associated the main frequency class. The fourth parameter of the whole epoch is the most frequent main frequency class found from the 30 studied windows.
5. The fifth parameter is the proportion of 1-second window with β local main frequency class.
6. The sixth parameter is the proportion of 1-second window with α local main frequency class.
7. The seventh parameter is the proportion of 1-second window with θ local main frequency class.
8. The eighth parameter is the proportion of 1-second window with δ local main frequency class.

Classification
The classifier is a binary decision tree. Its parameters were learnt with WEKA on a learning-set, that was constituted of 191.389 epochs, that is the half of the whole dataset, constituted by 215 patients' polysomnographies. Different decision trees of WEKA were tested and REPTree used with Bagging metaclassifier got the best results.

2.3 Symbolic Fusion

The goal of symbolic fusion is to work on symbolic complex objects and to connect them to each other, following predefined rules. (cf [11] and [12]). It is opposed to the numeric fusion that works directly on curves. Objects need to be represented in their complexity. The rules for fusion should be perfectly defined.

In our case, the fusion will be made on physiological events. Represented under the formalism of conceptual graphs, they are fused in order to associate to each respiratory event all its eventual consequential physiological events and its sleep-context of arisen. This allows to enrich the respiratory event.

In that aim, we have to consider, one by one, the complex respiratory events. We consider that an event can be a consequence of a respiratory event if it arises in the 20 seconds after the end of the respiratory event.

At the beginning, we have three lists of events : complex respiratory events, O_2-desaturations and microarousals. Each respiratory event is described by its type, its beginning-time and ending-time. For each of them, we look after a desaturation and/or a microarousal that would arise in the next 20 seconds after the ending-time of the respiratory event. If found, we fuse them, by enriching the complex respiratory event with this new information (cf figure 2).

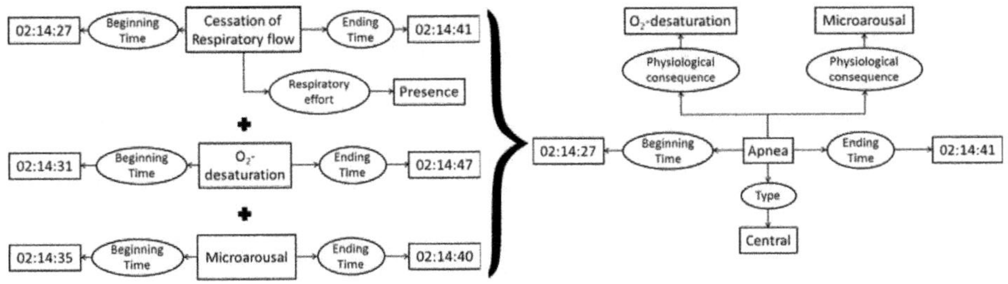

Fig. 2. Example of Data fusion

At the end of this step, each complex respiratory event is described by its type (Obstructive Apnea, Central Apnea, Mixed Apnea or Hypopnea), its beginning-time, its ending-time and its physiological consequences.

3 Results

3.1 Sleep Stages Recognition

First was evaluated the algorithm of recognition of sleep-stages. This evaluation was made on our dataset of 215 patients' polysomnographies. This dataset is constituted 382.778 30-seconds epochs. Globally, 82,21% of the epochs were correctly scored. More in details, were correctly labelled 93,57% of Wakefulness epochs, 65,82% of REM sleep-stage epochs, 25,6% of N1 sleep-stage epochs, 76,38% of N2 sleep-stage epochs, 75,52% of N3 sleep-stage epochs. These results are represented on figure 3.

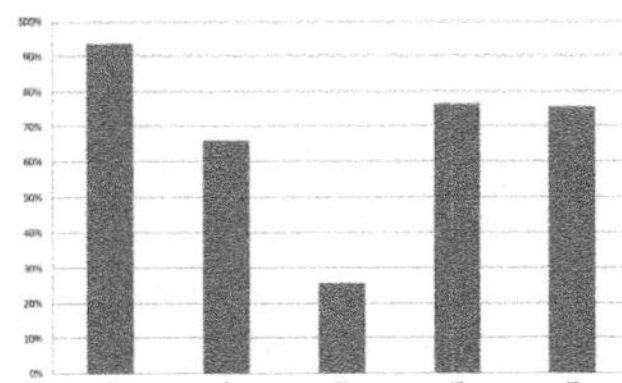

Fig. 3. Detection of sleep stages

Given the fact that the sleep stages scoring of two human polysomnography technologists may coincide from 70% to 90% (cf [14]), our results are satisfying but could probably be improved.

3.2 Symbolic Fusion

The complete method was applied to 59 patients for the evaluation.

The evaluation was made by comparing the AHI got by our method to the one got by the Physician's analysis.

On the figure 4, we compare the AHI got by the Physician (x-axis) and by our automatic analysis (y-axis). We added the median axis, on which should be ideally every point and the different groups of severity of the Sleep Apnea Syndrome

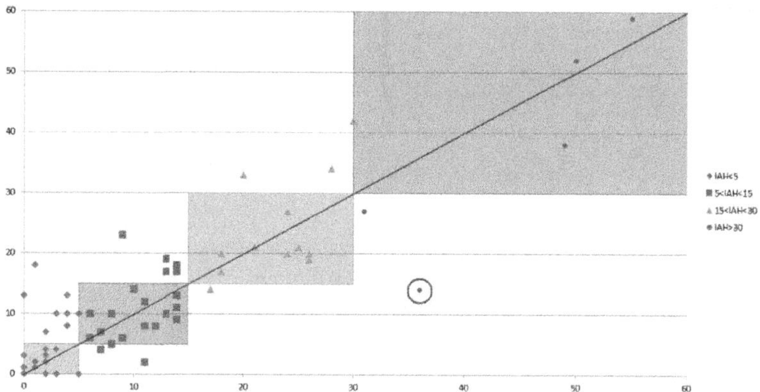

Fig. 4. Comparison of AHI depending on the severity of the Sleep Apnea Syndrome

The AHI got by our method is mostly very close to the one got by the Physician. In our evaluation, there was only one patient (in the red circle on the figures 4) whose results were very different from the Physician's; with our method, we would conclude that this patient has a light Sleep Apnea Syndrome, although the Physician concluded to a severe syndrome. We cannot yet explain this difference of results.

4 Discussion

4.1 Sleep Stages Scoring

Salih Günes et al. presented in [15] a recent study with a sleep stage recognition system using *k*-means clustering based feature weighting. The system works on 129 frequency parameters extracted from EEG signals. The results are similar to ours (cf table 3)

4.2 Symbolic Fusion

The originality of our approach holds on the symbolic fusion. The common approach for medical decision support is to use signal processing or classification

Table 3. Comparison of success rates between Günes et al. and our method

Sleep stage	Günes et al.	**our method**
W	80%	**93,57%**
R	81%	**65,82%**
N1	7,33%	**25,6%**
N2	88,9%	**76,38%**
N3	65,34%	**75,52%**

with numeric entries. This makes the problem very complex. To solve it, the chosen solution is often to reduce the number of entry-signals, typically to work on one single channel. Many research teams try to find one single physiological parameter that could be easily explored and give satisfying and accurate results for a diagnosis of Sleep Apnea Syndrome(cf [16] and [17]). With this approach, they try to elaborate a discriminating numerically-computed parameter. Thus, they often leave aside some information. The symbolic fusion has the advantage of keeping all information.

This evaluation needs to be completed by an evaluation of the quality of the decision made by Physicians using our method, and in particular, the contextual-AHI. This is possible only after a training-step, in which Physicians should use these indexes to get used to their interpretation.

Our method allows to add other consequential physiological events, like legs movement or cardiac events, what will be done in the future.

References

[1] McNicholas Walter, T.: Diagnosis of Obstructive Sleep Apnea in Adults. Proceedings of the American Thoracic Society 5, 154–160 (2008)

[2] George, C.F.P.: Reduction In motor vehicle collisions following treatment of sleep apnoea with nasal. CPAP Thorax 56(7), 508 (2001)

[3] Marin, J.M., Carrizo, S.J., Vicenter, E., Agusti, A.G.: Long term cardiovascular outcomes in men with obstructive sleep apnoea-hypopnea with or without treatment with continuous positive airway pressure: an observational study. Lancet 365(9464), 1046–1053 (2005)

[4] Arzt, M., Young, T., Finn, L., Skatrud, J.B., Bradley, T.D.: Association of sleep-disordered breathing and the occurrence of stroke. AM. J. respir. Crit. Care Med. 172(11), 1447–1451 (2005)

[5] Young, T., Peppard, P.E., Gottlieb, D.J.: Epidemiology of obstructive sleep apnea: a population health perspective. Am. J. Respir. Crit. Care Mer. 165(9), 1217–1239 (2002)

[6] Iber, C., Ancoli-Israel, C.: The AASM Manual for the Scoring of Sleep and Associated Events: Rules, Technology and Technical Specifications Westchester: American Academy of Sleep Medicine

[7] Silber, M.H., Ancoli-Israel, S., Bonnet, M.H., Chokroverty, S., Grigg-Damberger, M.M., Hirshkowitz, M., Kapen, S., Keenan, S.A., Kryger, M.H., Penzel, T., Pressman, M.R., Iber, C.: The Visual Scoring of Sleep in Adults. Journal of Clinical Sleep Medicine 3(2) (2007)

[8] Anderer, P., Moreau, A., Woertz, M., Ross, M., Gruber, G., Parapatics, S., Loretz, E., Heller, E., Schmidt, A., Boeck, M., Moser, D., Kloesch, G., Saletu, B., Saletu-Zyhlarz, G.M., Danker-Hopfe, H., Zeitlhofer, J., Dorffner, G.: Computer-Assisted Sleep Classification according to the Standard of the American Academy of Sleep Medicine: Validation Study of the AASM Version of the Somnolyzer 24 X 7. Neuropsychobiology 62, 250–264 (2010)

[9] Ugon, A., Philippe, C., Pietrasz, S., Ganascia, J.G., Lévy, P.P.: OPTISAS a new method to analyse patients with Sleep Apnea Syndrome. Stud. Health Technol. Inform. 136, 547–552 (2008)

[10] Ugon, A., Philippe, C., Ganascia, J.G., Rakotonanahary, D., Amiel, H., Boire, J.Y., Lévy, P.P.: Evaluating OPTISAS, a visual method to analyse. In: Sleep Apnea Syndromes Conf. Proc. IEEE Eng. Med. Biol. Soc. 2009, pp. 4747–4750 (2009)

[11] Laudy, C., Ganascia, J.-G.: Using Maximal Join for Information Fusion. In: Proceedings of IJCAI (2009)

[12] Laudy, C., Ganascia, J.-G.: Information Fusion Using Conceptual Graphs. In: International Conference on Conceptual Structures (2008) (in proceedings)

[13] Norman, R.G., Pal, I., Stewart, C., Walsleben, J.A., Rapoport, D.M.: Interobserver agreement among sleep scorers from different centers in a large dataset. Sleep 23(7), 901–908 (2000)

[14] Danker-Hopfe, H.E., Kunz, D., Gruber, G., Klo, G., Lorenzo, J.L., Himanen, S.L., Kemp, B., Penzel, T., Röschke, J., Dorn, H., Schlögl, A., Trenker, E., Dorffner, G.: Interrater reliability between scorers from eight European sleep laboratories in subjects with different sleep disorders. J. Sleep Res. 13, 63–69 (2004)

[15] Günes, S., Polat, K., Yosunkaya, S.: Efficient Sleep stage recognition system based on EEG signal using k-means clustering based feature weighting. Expert Systems with Applications 37, 7922–7928 (2010)

[16] Tonelli de Oliveira, A.C., Martinez, D.T., Vasconcelos, L.F., Cadaval Gonalves, S., do Carmo Lenz, M., Costa Fuchs, S., Gus, M., Oliveira de Abreu-Silva, E., Beltrami Moreira, L., Danni Fuchs, F.: Diagnosis of Obstructive Sleep Apnea Syndrome and Its Outcomes With Home. Portable Monitoring Chest 135, 330–336 (2009)

[17] Marcos, J.V., Hornero, R., Álvarez, D., Del Campo, F., Aboy, M.: Automated detection of obstructive sleep apnoea syndrome from oxygen saturation recordings using linear discriminant analysis. Medical and Biological Engineering and Computing 48(9), 895–902

Ontology-Based Generation of Dynamic Feedback on Physical Activity

Wilko Wieringa[3], Harm op den Akker[1,2], Valerie M. Jones[2], Rieks op den Akker[3], and Hermie J. Hermens[1,2]

[1] Roessingh Research and Development
[2] University of Twente, Department of Telemedicine
[3] University of Twente, Department of Human Media Interaction

Abstract. Improving physical activity patterns is an important focus in the treatment of chronic illnesses. We describe a system to monitor activity and provide feedback to help patients reach a healthy daily pattern. The system has shown positive effects in trials on patient groups including COPD and obese patients. We describe the design and implementation of a new feedback generation module which improves interaction with the patient by providing personalised dynamic context-aware feedback. The system uses an ontology of messages to find appropriate feedback using context information to prune irrelevant paths. The system adapts using derived probabilities about user preferences for certain message types. We aim to improve patient compliance and user experience.

1 Introduction

Balancing daily activity is a focus in the treatment of chronic diseases such as Chronic Low Back Pain (CLBP) and Chronic Fatigue Syndrome (CFS) [1], and COPD and obesity. Keeping an active lifestyle, while keeping in mind the limits caused by the disease and the risks of exacerbations, is a major goal in preventing COPD patients from entering a downward spiral of inactivity and disease progression. A popular approach for promoting an active lifestyle is to objectively measure the subject's activity pattern and provide feedback periodically, or at the end of each day. We describe an activity monitoring system which has been trialled on different patient groups including COPD and obese patients. Experience with this system, and reported elsewhere in the literature [2,3] highlights the need for a more sophisticated approach to the delivery of user feedback. Not only the content of the message, but the timing and manner in which it is delivered need to be tuned to the individual and their context. The expression of message content too needs to be varied in order to avoid habituation effects, automatic responses, boredom or irritation. The activity monitoring system consists of a 3D-accelerometer connected via Bluetooth to a PDA. The system logs acceleration every 10 seconds as an integrated value, summed over the three axis of movement. The patient's current activity level is compared to a predefined

M. Peleg, N. Lavrač, and C. Combi (Eds.): AIME 2011, LNAI 6747, pp. 55–59, 2011.

reference, and feedback is given at fixed hourly intervals: "*Encouraging*" to encourage activity, "*Discouraging*" to discourage activity and "*Neutral*" feedback if the patient is doing well.

2 Improving Feedback Message Generation

The objective of the work described here is threefold. First, we aim to bring more variation to the feedback messages presented. Hearing the same messages over and over again reduces the subject's willingness to use the system and comply to the advice given in the feedback [4]. Second, we want to generate messages that are relevant to the subject's current context or environment, e.g. when the weather is good, advise people to go for a walk, when the weather is bad, advise an indoor activity. Third, we want to create a system that can be tuned to the user's personal preferences. If one individual responds better to messages that are given in a commanding tone, the system should adapt to this. In short, the system should be *dynamic*, *context-aware* and *self adapting.*

2.1 Dynamic Message Generation

At the core of the feedback message generation system lies an ontology of feedback messages. Erriquez and Grasso [2] show the viability of this approach over more complex natural language generation methods. Key factors in their approach are scalability and opacity, as for any generated message the reason why that message was generated from the ontology can be deduced. Our OWL2.0[1] ontology contains a set of feedback messages structured in a meaningful way. When the system requests a feedback message, the ontology is traversed, generating a list of possible candidate sentences from which a random selection is made. Initially we generate three message types: "*Neutral*" (when the subject is performing well), "*Encouraging*" (meaning encouraging more activity when the subject is insufficiently active) and "*Discouraging*" (meaning discouraging activity when the subject is too active). We used a threshold of 10% compared to the reference to determine over- or under performing. Each of these *MessageTypes* can be composed of several *MessageComponents*, the top-level entity for all the actual sentences in the ontology. A MessageType currently consists of one *Evaluation* (a message containing factual information on the current activity performance) and either one of *DiscouragingAdvice*, *NeutralAdvice* or *EncouragingAdvice.* An example of a generated EncouragingMessage could be "You have been insufficiently active. [Evaluation] Please go for a walk! [EncouragingAdvice]". We focus here on the advice components as they contain the motivational messages that are of most interest to the physical activity monitoring system. Figure 1 shows part of the message ontology for *EncouragingAdvice*, with the *EncouragingInside* and *Household* entities expanded. The lowest level contains the actual feedback messages (grey circles). At runtime the system traverses this ontology, gathering all the candidate sentences and makes a random

[1] `http://www.w3.org/TR/owl2-overview/`

choice from the message candidates for presentation to the user. This initial version of the system is equivalent to selecting a random message from a list of predefined feedback messages; however, it forms the basis for the next version of our context-aware and self-adapting system, explained in the two following sections.

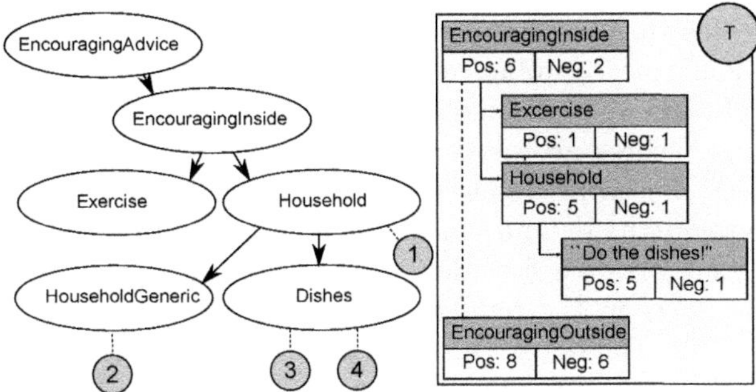

Fig. 1. (Left) Example of the ontology with EncouragingAdvice expanded and individual feedback messages at the leaves. (Right) Compliance database for storing responses (compliance) to feedback messages (see Section 2.3).

2.2 Adding Context-Awareness

Notice in Figure 1 there is a high level split between messages that tell the patient to go outside (*EncouragingOutside*), and those that tell the patient to stay inside (*EncouragingInside*). However a patient should not be sent outside if in a thunderstorm; hence our system is extended to include Boolean functions attached to ontology entities. In this case the *EncouragingOutside* entity has the function `isWeatherGood()` attached, which returns true if the weather at the patient's location can be considered "good". In our Android implementation, this function is implemented by retrieving current location and weather data online and performing a rule-based conversion to Boolean. Similar context functions, using for example location information, could be added to rule out a branch of messages that are only relevant when the patient is at home, or at work. The same schema can also be used to embed user preferences into the selection process for message candidates. If user information, such as dog ownership, is available this can be used to open up branches containing messages related to taking the dog for a walk.

2.3 A Self-adapting Mechanism for Message Selection

Instead of choosing randomly between messages candidates deemed to be relevant given the message ontology and the current contextual state, we can learn from the patient's response to previously given feedback messages. We use the same definition of feedback compliance as [5]; the compliance score "*compares* *the amount of activity performed in the 30 minute interval before the feedback event (Δ_1), with the amount of activity performed in the 30 minute interval after the feedback event (Δ_2)"*. The 30 minute interval was chosen for comparability with earlier work, but this value can be seen as a variable that needs further study. For encouraging messages, the subject complied if $\Delta_1 < \Delta_2$, and for discouraging message the subject complied if $\Delta_1 > \Delta_2$. Thirty minutes after each feedback message, the compliance score (`true` or `false`) is fed back to the system. Notice that we look at the time the subject has seen the feedback message for calculating compliance. The number of times each individual message was judged positively and negatively is stored in a `compliance database`. These compliance scores are used to make an informed decision about which message to select. The winner selection algorithm is explained, using the choice between *EncouragingInside* and *EncouragingOutside* in Figure 1 (right) at some state T as an example. We first define *levelData* as the total amount of data available on the *level* in the ontology of our choice. In this case $levelData = 6 + 2 + 8 + 6 = 22$. Furthermore, we define *localTrue* as the number of positive judgments for each individual entity, and *localData* as its total amount of judgements. Then:

$$entityChance(X) = \frac{localTrue}{localData} \times (1 - \frac{localData}{levelData}) \tag{1}$$

$$entityChance(EncouragingInside) = \frac{6}{8} \times (1 - \frac{8}{22}) = \frac{21}{44} = \frac{147}{308} \tag{2}$$

$$entityChance(EncouragingOutside) = \frac{8}{14} \times (1 - \frac{14}{22}) = \frac{16}{77} = \frac{64}{308} \tag{3}$$

After computing the common denominator for each fraction, we define the weight of each entity as their fraction numerator, and their selection probability as $\frac{entityNumerator}{sumOfNumerators}$ (e.g. the selection probability for EncouragingInside is $\frac{147}{211} \approx 70\%$ and for EncouragingOutside $\frac{64}{211} \approx 30\%$). Next we define a lottery, where a total of $100 \times N$ (where N is the number of entities on the current level) balls are divided among the candidates. First a fixed percentage of 20% of the balls is equally divided amongst all candidates, the rest of the balls are divided according to the weights calculated above. In this case: $EncouragingInside = 20 + 160 \times \frac{147}{211} = 131$ and $EncouragingOutside = 20 + 160 \times \frac{64}{211} = 69$. The algorithm has the following three properties: (1) it selects with a higher probability those candidates which have been judged positively more often than negatively (2) it selects with a higher probability those candidates for which less data is available, and (3) there always remains a small probability that a candidate is selected, regardless of positive/negative ratio. These properties ensure that the algorithm (1) learns to give (types of) feedback messages that the individual prefers more often, (2) gathers enough data on all messages to make informed decisions, and (3) does not fully discard messages that so far have a 100% negative judgment.

2.4 Evaluation

In order to evaluate the properties of the system we ran simulations using fictional personas. We generated 300 feedback messages[2] and determined the patient's compliance to those messages on three personas: "sporty", "random" and "housefather". The sporty persona had a high probability of reacting well to sporting activities, while the "housefather" complied better to household activities. After 300 messages, only 18% of the messages generated for the non-random personas were of a disliked category. This shows that adaptation is taking place, although evaluations with real patients is a crucial next step.

3 Discussion

We have described the design and preliminary testing of a feedback message generation component of an activity monitoring system that has been integrated into our Android based framework. Simulation runs indicate that the self-adapting mechanisms work as intended. The next step is to test the system on real patients. Current work focusses on designing an ontology that can be used in large patient trials; the content of the ontology will be defined based on the literature on activity based feedback and on results of patient questionnaires. The ontology will be structured in a logically and semantically sound way in order to optimize learning and context-awareness. By combining the system described here with our previous work on designing a self-learning algorithm for determining the optimal timing for feedback messages for individual patients [5], these two components of the activity monitoring system form the cornerstone for an intelligent Feedback Coach. The coach will be able to act as a virtual companion for patients who try to change their behaviour and lead a more healthy lifestyle. The generic design approach and focus on personalisation also means that this application is not *limited* to patients suffering from chronic diseases.

References

1. Van Weering, M.G., Vollenbroek-Hutten, M.M., Tönis, T.M., Hermens, H.J.: Daily physical activities in chronic lower back pain patients assessed with accelerometry. European Journal of Pain London England 13, 649–654 (2009)
2. Erriquez, E., Grasso, F.: Generation of Personalised Advisory Messages: an Ontology Based Approach. In: Proceedings of the 21st IEEE International Symposium on Computer-Based Medical Systems (CMBS), Jyvaskyla, Finland, pp. 437–442 (2008)
3. Cortellese, F., Nalin, M., Morandi, A., Sanna, A., Grasso, F.: Personality Diagnosis for Personalized eHealth Services. In: Proceedings of the 2nd International ICST Conference on Electronic Healthcare for the 21st Century, pp. 173–180. Springer, Heidelberg (2009)
4. Bickmore, T.W., Picard, R.W.: Establishing and maintaining long-term human-computer relationships. ACM Transactions on CHI 12, 293–327 (2005)
5. op den Akker, H., Jones, V.M., Hermens, H.J.: Predicting Feedback Compliance in a Teletreatment Application. In: Proceedings of ISABEL 2010, Rome, Italy (2010)

[2] 300 is approximately the number of messages that patients received in one month's time in earlier studies.

A Case Study of Stacked Multi-view Learning in Dementia Research

Rui Li[1], Andreas Hapfelmeier[1], Jana Schmidt[1], Robert Perneczky[2], Alexander Drzezga[3], Alexander Kurz[2], and Stefan Kramer[1]

[1] Institut für Informatik/I12, Technische Universität München, Boltzmannstr. 3, D-85748 Garching b. München, Germany
[2] Klinik u. Poliklinik für Psychiatrie u. Psychotherapie, Technische Universität München, Ismaninger Str. 22, D-81675 München, Germany
[3] Nuklearmedizinische Klinik, Technische Universität München, Ismaninger Str. 22, D-81675 München, Germany
kramer@in.tum.de

Abstract. Classification of different types of dementia commonly involves examination from several perspectives, e.g., medical images, neuropsychological tests, etc. Thus, dementia classification should lend itself to so-called *multi-view learning*. Instead of simply combining several views, we use stacking to make the most of the information from the various views (PET scans, MMSE, CERAD and demographic variables). In the paper, we not only show the performance of stacked multi-view learning on classifying dementia data, we also try to explain the factors contributing to its performance. More specifically, we show that the correlation of views on the base and the meta level should be within certain ranges to facilitate successful stacked multi-view learning.

Keywords: Dementia, Alzheimer's Disease, Machine Learning, Multi-View Learning, Stacking, Canonical Correlation Analysis (CCA).

1 Introduction

Research on Alzheimer's disease (AD), the main cause of dementia, has received broad attention from medical experts, psychiatrists, machine learning and data mining researchers. AD is a progressive, degenerative and incurable disease of the brain that causes severe problems with communication, thinking and memory. According to some study, 4.6 million people are diagnosed worldwide with some type of dementia annually, and the number is expected to exceed 100 million by 2050 [1].

Roughly speaking, the study of AD has focused mainly on the pathological causes and the discrimination from other types of dementia or cognitive impairment. This study is dedicated to distinguishing mild cognitive impairment (MCI) from clinically diagnosable AD. MCI is a transitional phase to AD, which, however, does not necessarily end up in it. Hence, distinguishing MCI from AD is of great medical interest. For this purpose and, generally, diagnosing different

M. Peleg, N. Lavrač, and C. Combi (Eds.): AIME 2011, LNAI 6747, pp. 60–69, 2011.

forms of dementia, imaging techniques like magnetic resonance imaging (MRI) and positron emission tomography (PET) are used routinely. Apart from these techniques, clinical variables (e.g., from neuropsychological tests) are employed to assist in the assessment of cases [12]. As this medical domain naturally offers different perspectives or views on patients (e.g., demographic data, neuropsychological tests, imaging data, ...), it lends itself to the application of methods for so-called *multi-view learning* [11]. In particular, we investigate the use of multi-view stacking, which combines the classifications (into the classes MCI or AD) originating from different views into overall classifications. In the paper, we not only present the results of multi-view stacking along those lines, we also attempt to explain the performance of multi-view stacking in terms of correlations between feature groups and correlations between predictions. Finally, we shed some light on the way the different views are combined by the stacking procedure to come up with the overall classification.

2 Related Work

Data mining methods have been used in many applications in dementia research. A survey of methods used for brain imaging data [10] aimed at finding interesting associations and patterns based on image and other clinical data. In a different study [14], SPECT images were used to classify patients with AD based on a linear programming formulation. Clustering and subgroup discovery were studied to incorporate imaging and non-imaging data, where PET images and clinical variables were combined to correlate disease patterns of the brain with neuropsychological tests [12]. Related work [6] applied stacking to the early diagnosis of AD against normal controls (NC) using event related potentials (ERPs) and showed that it outperformed majority voting.

In data mining, stacking [17] has been used widely, but its underlying mechanisms are still not understood completely. Influential work [15] pointed out two interesting facts: First, multi-response linear regression (MLR) was a suitable meta level learner compared to decision trees, Naïve Bayes and KNN. Second, class probabilities (soft) should be used instead of class predictions (hard). The advantage of using class probabilities instead of class predictions was confirmed in further studies [13]. An interesting study argued that meta level correlation is crucial in stacking [5]. Besides, it was demonstrated that stacking is better than selecting the best classifier from the ensemble by cross validation [3]. More recently, stacked graphical learning was proposed for collective classification, showing that it was not only accurate but efficient as well [8].

3 Stacked Multi-view Learning

In this section, we introduce the proposed approach, which is slightly different from standard stacked generalization. Furthermore, we elaborate on the correlation measure using CCA that aims at providing a quantitative explanation of the results.

Algorithm 1. Stacked Multi-View Learning

Data: $\mathcal{D}_i$, $i = 1...n$, n view training data with true label Y.
Training: divide $\mathcal{D}_i$ into J disjoint sets.
for $i = 1$ *to* n **do**
  for $j = 1$ *to* J **do**
    compute class probabilities z_{ij} of set j trained from remaining $\mathcal{D}_i^{(J-j)}$ using base learner $\mathcal{L}_i$.
  end
  Denote z_i as entire predicted class probabilities of $\mathcal{D}_i$.
end
Let $\mathcal{F} = \{z_1, \cdots, z_i, Y\}$, train meta level model ($\mathcal{M}$) based on $\mathcal{F}$ using MLR.
Test: each $\mathcal{L}_i$ gives a prediction (z_i^*) to a test sample $\mathcal{D}_i^*$ trained from $\mathcal{D}_i$, let $\mathcal{F}^* = \{z_1^*, \cdots, z_i^*\}$ to be classified by $\mathcal{M}$ and result in the final prediction.

3.1 Stacking (Stacked Generalization)

Stacking [17] was proposed to combine different classifiers to improve predictive accuracy. By learning how classifiers correlate with each other, the approach aims at outperforming each individual base classifier [5]. Conventionally, base classifiers (orginating from different base learners) are applied to a *single* dataset, and the predicted labels along with their true labels are concatenated and used as training (test) data at the meta level [17,15]. In this study, stacking is applied in a different manner: we stack the predictions from different *views*, i.e. groups of features, and then perform meta level learning, assigning one base learner and classifier to each view. Each base classifier (from a corresponding view) then produces class probabilities (predictions), which are subsequently used to train the meta level model. Once a test sample is presented, each base classifier gives a prediction, and subsequently their predictions are combined by the meta model.

3.2 Canonical Correlation Analysis (CCA)

CCA is applied to measure the correlation between views. It was proposed to measure the linear association between two sets of variables [7]. Let $X = (x_1, x_2, \cdots, x_p)$, $Y = (y_1, y_2, \cdots, y_q)$, $U = \alpha_1 x_1 + \alpha_2 x_2 + \cdots + \alpha_p x_p = \alpha^T X$ and $V = \beta_1 y_1 + \beta_2 y_2 + \cdots + \beta_q y_q = \beta^T Y$ (U and V are called canonical variates). $\Sigma = \begin{pmatrix} \Sigma_{11} & \Sigma_{12} \\ \Sigma_{21} & \Sigma_{22} \end{pmatrix}$, Σ_{11} (or Σ_{22}) is the covariance matrix within set X (or Y), Σ_{12} is the covariance matrix between sets X and Y and $\Sigma_{12} = \Sigma_{21}^T$. CCA seeks to find α_p and β_q such that the following equation is maximized:

$$\rho(\alpha_p, \beta_q) = \alpha_p^T \Sigma_{12} \beta_q \tag{1}$$

$$\text{subject to} \quad \alpha_p^T \Sigma_{11} \alpha_p = 1, \beta_q^T \Sigma_{22} \beta_q = 1$$

As a result, the canonical correlation coefficient can be computed as the square root of the eigenvalues of matrix $\Sigma_{22}^{-1} \Sigma_{21} \Sigma_{11}^{-1} \Sigma_{12}$ for each canonical variates pair.

The number of coefficients equals to $min = \{p, q\}$ with a statistical significance value ($p < 0.05$), therefore $\mathbb{E}(\rho) = \sum_{i=1}^{min\{p,q\}} \rho_i / min\{p, q\}$ is taken as the overall correlation between two feature subsets. Pairwise CCA is performed among views and an averaged value is calculated as the final correlation.

4 Experiments

4.1 Dementia Data

The dementia dataset was provided by the psychiatry and nuclear medicine departments of Klinikum rechts der Isar of Technische Universität München. It covers 127 patients for which both a PET scan and clinical/demographic data are available. From these patients, 57 patients suffered from AD and 70 from MCI.

PET Imaging Data Processing and Feature Extraction. Prior to their use, PET scans are transformed into feature vectors. The Automated Anatomical Labeling (AAL) brain Atlas [16] was applied to obtain 116 pre-defined brain regions modeling the intensities of the interesting brain regions (e.g., Hippocampus) along with their spatial coordinates. This separation was done on a group of 20 cognitively healthy age-matched persons. To inspect the regions more closely, we applied DBSCAN [4] on the 116 previously identified regions and clustered them into 1894 finer groups[1]. Both intensity and coordinates (x, y, z) of each voxel were taken into account during the clustering. Then the mean intensity of each cluster of the MCI and AD PET scans was extracted. Thus, the PET is, at this point, represented as a feature vector consisting of 1894 intensity values. As 1894 features apparently require too much computational effort, we applied the F-score [2] to select the most informative ten features. However, before creating the final feature vector, PET images have to undergo two pre-processing steps: normalization and smoothing (kernel size [8 8 8] mm), which were achieved by SPM8[2].

Non-Imaging Data. Non-imaging data consist of demographic (e.g., age and gender) and clinical data. Clinical variables cover neuropsychological tests that indicate the patients' social behavior, self-care capability and a person's daily ability concerning memory, language and orientation. The tests include: **Con**sortium to **E**stablish a **R**egistry for **A**lzheimer's **D**isease (CERAD) neuropsychological assessment battery, **M**ini-**M**ental **S**tate **E**xamination (MMSE) and the **C**lock **D**rawing **T**est (CDT). The CDT is added to the demographic data in this

---

[1] Parameter ϵ was analytically set according to the input data and the minimum number of points (minPts) = 6. The parameters were set so as to keep the clusters' size roughly balanced.

[2] Statistical Parametric Mapping, `http://www.fil.ion.ucl.ac.uk/spm/software/spm8/`, 2009.

work to form a more informative view for multi-view stacking. The demographic data, CERAD, MMSE form natural views in dementia data.

To examine the factors contributing to the success and failure of multi-view stacking, we additionally created 50,000 datasets with randomly generated views of the same dimensionality as of the natural views (e.g., $dim(\mathcal{V}_1) = dim(PET)$). From these 50,000 trials, we picked the two datasets with the lowest and the highest correlation among the views for further examination (cf. Table 1).

4.2 Results

We ran three experiments to examine the prediction accuracy of stacking compared to a baseline learner. The baseline is a simple prediction based on the whole dataset without any division into views. KNN is chosen as the base learner, as it is one of the simplest and most fundamental learning schemes.[3] KNN was used as first level predictor in the stacking approach, while multi-response linear regression (MLR) was applied as meta learner, since it was shown to be efficient for this purpose [15]. Table 1 gives the performance of the baseline approach (column 'baseline'), predictions using only one view (columns 'PET' to 'Demo') and the accuracy for stacking ('Stacked'). Each experiment was repeated 50 times with a 10-fold cross validation. Class probabilities are used instead of class labels at the meta level. The K in KNN was set to 9 and the probability for each class (AD and MCI) is calculated via majority voting of the first-level learner: $p(AD) = \frac{|votes_{AD}|}{K}$. Various values ($K$) have been tested and values that are relatively large, e.g., 9, yield equally good results.

Table 1. Comparison of accuracy, mean±std%. Baseline: PET, MMSE, CERAD, CDT and Demographic data are pooled into one table for learning. $\mathcal{V}_i$: randomly created view of dementia data with dimension unchanged. In 'Created Views 1', $\mathcal{V}_2$ was set to contain MMSE, since we wanted to observe if a strong individual view takes effect in multi-view stacking.

Natural Views	Baseline	PET	MMSE	CERAD	Demo	Stacked
KNN	76.3±11.1	69.6±12.4	78.1±10.6	80.1±11.0	61.6±13.4	**83.2**±**10.2** •
Created Views 1	**Baseline**	$\mathcal{V}_1$	$\mathcal{V}_2$	$\mathcal{V}_3$	$\mathcal{V}_4$	**Stacked**
KNN	76.3±11.1	72.9±11.6	78.1±10.6	79.6±11.4	61.4±12.9	**81.2**±**11.0** •
Created Views 2	**Baseline**	$\mathcal{V}_1$	$\mathcal{V}_2$	$\mathcal{V}_3$	$\mathcal{V}_4$	**Stacked**
KNN	76.3±11.1	75.6±11.1	66.1±11.8	82.7±10.3	72.0±11.4	**81.1**±**10.3** •

Table 1 shows that the natural views of dementia data presents the best result for all stackings. Moreover, specific views outperform the baseline approach, but do not exceed the performance of stacking. Remarkably, all stacking approaches

[3] Other learning schemes like decision trees, the SVM, etc. are also possible, but beyond the scope of this paper.

Table 2. Description of three factors of stacked multi-view learning on dementia data

	Base Corr.	Meta Corr.	Std. of Accur.
Natural Views	0.63±0.01	0.28±0.04	13.9±5.45
Created Views 1	0.64±0.01	0.27±0.03	13.5±5.19
Created Views 2	0.95±0.01	0.27±0.03	12.2±4.91

outperform the baseline approach. This shows that stacking on random views also increases performance. As for 'Created Views 2', the result of stacking does not outperform $\mathcal{V}_3$ (82.7%), which may due to the too high base level correlation (0.95, cf. Table 2). Detailed explanation will follow in section A.4.

Although the stacked versions of Table 1 show that stacking is better than a baseline, the underlying mechanisms are not yet completely understood. Three parameters that may influence the performance of stacking are: the feature correlation between base views; the meta correlation, i.e., the correlation between the prediction of the separate views; and the variation of accuracy of separate views. Training data are used for these measures, since training data, in reality, are the only ones that we can gain knowledge from. Table 2 gives the values for the base correlation, meta correlation and the standard deviation of the accuracy of the four views. We claim that the prediction accuracy for stacking improves when the base level correlation is relatively high, e.g., in the range of [0.6-0.9]. We can support this fact by examining the relation of the baseline correlation and the prediction improvement (for a more detailed analysis of these factors see Appendix A, and in particular Fig. 1 in Section A.4). As the dementia dataset has a high baseline correlation, stacking is supposed to work on this data. As noted by other authors [5], meta level correlation can be crucial in stacking, which is also supported by Fig. 1 that shows a likely ideal interval of [0.2-05]. Again, the given dementia dataset witnesses a meta correlation in this range. These findings, to some extent, should help explain the performance of stacked multi-view learning on our dementia dataset.

Table 3. Regressors of multiple linear regression of meta level data. P-value in brackets.

	PET	MMSE	CERAD	Demo
MCI	-0.241 (0.0001)	-0.303 (0.0031)	-0.269 (0.0157)	-0.083 (0.1791)
AD	0.339 (0.0006)	0.084 (0.0493)	0.197 (0.0108)	0.183 (0.2060)

Another property of the views is, of course, their natural meaning. In the following, we will briefly analyze the contributions of the different views on the meta level classification. More specifically, we take a look at the coefficients of the MLR model, which is given as:

$$Y = \alpha \cdot \text{PET(MCI)} + \beta \cdot \text{PET(AD)} + ... + \gamma \cdot \text{Demo(AD)} + \text{const.} \quad (2)$$

As the MLR model encodes the two classes in two separate linear models, the task is to find eight regressors (weights) given the training label and meta level class probability. The resulting eight weights are given in Table 3. Following these results, MMSE and CERAD are strong at predicting MCI, since their weights are high (negative because MCI $= 1 <$ AD $= 2$). Whereas PET is strong at recognizing AD due to its highest value of 0.339. This table shows the interaction of these four views, which does not reveal their individual importance but their power in stacking using MLR as a meta learner.

5 Discussion and Conclusions

The paper investigated the use of multi-view stacking for classifying dementia data, in particular for discriminating between Alzheimer's disease and mild cognitive impairment. While a simple KNN prediction including all features achieved a prediction accuracy of 76.3%, stacking on the natural views achieved an accuracy gain of 6.9%. Analyzing the meta level classifier showed that the predictions of the MMSE and CERAD views are important for MCI classification, while the PET view is crucial for AD. Further evaluations on 14 UCI datasets revealed that the performance can be largely attributed to the medium meta-level correlation of the views and the relatively high base-level correlation of the views. These insights were gained by transforming the UCI datasets into multi-view dataset within different ranges of base and meta correlations. Regression analysis showed that views with a high level of base correlation are likely to perform well in stacking. However, if the base correlation is low, stacking may nevertheless perform well. The same is true for the meta correlation: For medium values the performance is likely to increase, but still, this may happen for smaller and larger values. We can thus, to some extent, explain the good performance of stacking in our application domain. Based on these findings, researchers may therefore consider stacking for data from other medical application domains to improve their prediction accuracy whenever there are natural views in the indicated ranges of correlation.

References

1. ALZ. The prevalence of dementia worldwide, Alzheimer's Disease International (2008), http://www.alz.co.uk/adi/pdf/prevalence.pdf
2. Chen, Y.W., Lin, C.J.: Combining svms with various feature selection strategies. In: Feature Extraction, Foundations and Applications (2006)
3. Džeroski, S., Ženko, B.: Is combining classifiers with stacking better than selecting the best one? Machine Learning 54, 255–273 (2004)
4. Ester, M., Kriegel, H.P., Jörg, S., Xu, X.W.: A density-based algorithm for discovering clusters in large spatial databases with noise. In: Proceedings of the 2nd International Conference on Knowledge Discovery and Data Mining (KDD), pp. 226–231. AAAI Press, Menlo Park (1996)
5. Fan, D.W., Chan, P.K., Stolfo, S.J.: A comparative evaluation of combiner and stacked generalization. In: Proceedings of AAAI 1996 workshop on Integrating Multiple Learned Models, pp. 40–46 (1996)

6. Gandhi, H., Green, D., Kounios, J., Clark, C.M., Polikar, R.: Stacked generalization for early diagnosis of Alzheimer's disease. In: Proceedings of the 28th IEEE EMBS Annual International Conference, pp. 5350–5353 (2006)
7. Hotelling, H.: Relations Between Two Sets of Variates. Biometrika 28, 321–377 (1936)
8. Kou, Z.Z.: Stacked graphical models for efficient inference in markov random fields. In: Proceedings of the 2007 SIAM International Conference on Data Mining (2007)
9. Ling, C.X., Du, J., Zhou, Z.H.: When does co-training work in real data? In: Theeramunkong, T., Kijsirikul, B., Cercone, N., Ho, T.-B. (eds.) PAKDD 2009. LNCS, vol. 5476, pp. 596–603. Springer, Heidelberg (2009), `http://dx.doi.org/10.1007/978-3-642-01307-2_58`
10. Megalooikonomou, V., Ford, J., Shen, L., Makedon, F., Saykin, A.: Data mining in brain imaging. In: Statistical Methods in Medical Research, pp. 359–394 (2000)
11. Rüping, S., Scheffer, T. (eds.): Proceedings of the ICML 2005 Workshop on Learning with Multiple Views (2005)
12. Schmidt, J., Hapfelmeier, A., Mueller, M., Perneczky, R., Kurz, A., Drzezga, A., Kramer, S.: Interpreting PET scans by structured patient data: a data mining case study in dementia research. Knowledge and Information Systems 24(1), 149–170 (2010)
13. Sigletos, G., Paliouras, G.s., Spyropoulos, C.D., Hatzopoulos, M.: Combining information extraction systems using voting and stacked generalization. Journal of Machine Learning Research 6, 1751–1782 (2005)
14. Stoeckel, J., Fung, G.: SVM feature selection for classification of SPECT images of Alzheimer's disease using spatial information. In: Proceedings of the Fifth IEEE International Conference on Data Mining, ICDM 2005, pp. 410–417. IEEE Computer Society, Washington, DC (2005)
15. Ting, K.M., Ian, H.W.: Issues in stacked generalization. Journal of Artificial Intelligence Research 10, 271–289 (1999)
16. Tzourio-Mazoyer, N., Landeau, B., Papathanassiou, D., Crivello, F., Etard, O., Delcroix, N., Mazoyer, B., Joliot, M.: Automated anatomical labeling of activations in SPM using a macroscopic anatomical parcellation of the MNI MRI single-subject brain. NeuroImage 15(1), 273–289 (2002)
17. Wolpert, D.H.: Stacked generalization. Neural Networks 5(2), 241–259 (1992)

A Appendix

A.1 UCI Benchmark Datasets

As it is hard to find standard datasets with naturally defined views, we conducted a study with synthetic views on 14 UCI datasets to empirically study the factors contributing to the performance of stacked multi-view learning.

A.2 UCI Data Subsets Generation

The UCI datasets are single view data, hence we randomly sample features into various subsets[4] (views) to create multiple views. The number of views produced is 4 that is the same as the dementia data. 20 randomly sampled datasets are generated for every dataset, making sure that the generated views are approximately equally sized.

[4] UCI datasets were already split into two disjoint subsets for co-training purposes [9].

Table 4. Accuracy comparison between baseline and stacked 4-view learning averaged over 20 randomly sampled sets (mean±std%). Only the mean is given for Base Corr. etc., as the standard deviation is marginal.

Datasets	KNN	Stacked 4-View	Base Corr.	Meta Corr.	Std of Accur.
hepatitis [he]	56.7±8.62	**62.6±3.92**	0.76	**0.31**	7.11
musk [mu]	71.0±3.60	**85.7±0.62**	0.85	**0.48**	1.67
ionosphere [io]	85.1±2.62	87.1±1.39	0.66	0.17	1.93
sonar [so]	68.3±5.27	**74.8±1.78**	0.82	**0.26**	2.93
ozone [oz]	93.3±7.34	93.1±1.30	0.91	0.58	1.49
spectf [sp]	73.8±63.4	74.5±0.94	0.83	0.30	2.62
parkinson [pa]	81.4±6.79	83.1±2.78	0.83	0.30	2.62
promoters [pr]	76.6±6.09	77.6±3.28	0.93	0.29	9.95
german [ge]	70.7±2.19	50.9±1.27	0.51	0.11	1.19
breast [br]	95.0±1.47	90.2±3.81	0.76	0.12	3.69
chess [ch]	91.5±0.96	81.3±4.56	0.46	0.17	9.26
spambase [sb]	91.0±1.03	87.5±1.47	0.44	0.32	5.52
heart [ht]	81.4±3.51	63.1±7.80	0.56	0.17	7.36
australian [au]	85.1±2.30	69.3±8.04	0.46	0.11	6.65

A.3 UCI Data Results

Three factors are analyzed, and the results shown in Table 4. The comparison with the dementia data is straightforward, because they are all of a 4-view scenario.

A.4 Statistical Significance Study Using Regression Analysis

Table 4 reveals that the meta and base level correlation might be associated with the performance of stacking. For example, 'german', 'breast' and 'chess' present low meta correlation and the stacked results are not satisfying, as opposed to 'hepatitis', and 'musk'.

To measure the linear association between accuracy and the conjectured influential factors, we apply linear regression to determine the corresponding regressor (β) indicating their relation. Let Y = accuracy gain = accuracy (stacking) − accuracy (baseline KNN) be the dependent (target) variable, each of 'base corr.', 'meta corr.' and 'std of accur.' be the independent variable X. The task is to find β given Y and X, assuming equation $Y = \beta \cdot X + \text{const}$. The straight black line in Fig. 1 indicates the fitted linear curve with the slope and p-value shown on top. The gray quadratic curve is fitted using quadratic regression if we envision there is a non-linear relation.

Fig. 1 demonstrates that meta correlation is by far the most important factor in terms of accuracy gain. A medium meta correlation would be suggested if the quadratic curve is regarded as more reasonable. The linear curve claims that accuracy grows as meta correlation increases. As for base correlation, the quadratic curve starts to drop at 0.9. View accuracy variation seems to be unimportant.

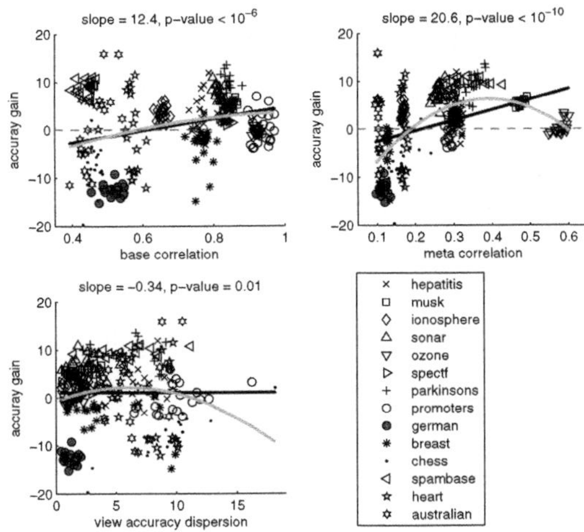

Fig. 1. Regression analysis using all randomly sampled datasets. Each UCI dataset is re-sampled 20 times and each point is a dataset ($20 \times 14 = 280$ in total).

Remarkably, some datasets have high base and meta correlation but perform poorly. Therefore, we do not claim that the higher the correlation of base and meta level, the better the stacking performance, whereas a medium degree might be optimal. It can be easily understood that the meta level learner does not benefit if there is a very high or even perfect correlation. Certainly, there are still exceptional points falling into the optimal range, but behave poorly, which might be due to other reasons, such as the distribution difference between training and test samples, to name only one.

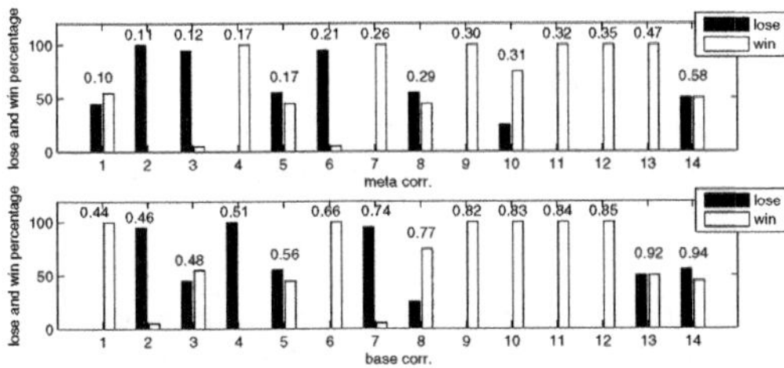

Fig. 2. Percentage of wins (accuracy gain > 0) and losses (accuracy gain < 0) against meta and base level correlation. The correlation is shown on top of the bar.

Statistical Machine Learning for Automatic Assessment of Physical Activity Intensity Using Multi-axial Accelerometry and Heart Rate

Fernando García-García[1,2], Gema García-Sáez[1,2], Paloma Chausa[1,2], Iñaki Martínez-Sarriegui[1,2], Pedro José Benito[3], Enrique J. Gómez[1,2], and M. Elena Hernando[1,2]

[1] Grupo de Bioingeniería y Telemedicina, Universidad Politécnica de Madrid, Spain
{fgarcia,elena}@gbt.tfo.upm.es

[2] Networking Research Center on Bioengineering, Biomaterials and Nanomedicine (CIBER-BBN), Madrid, Spain

[3] Laboratory of Exercise Physiology, Facultad de Ciencias de la Actividad Física y del Deporte (INEF), Universidad Politécnica de Madrid, Spain

Abstract. This work explores the automatic recognition of physical activity intensity patterns from multi-axial accelerometry and heart rate signals. Data collection was carried out in free-living conditions and in three controlled gymnasium circuits, for a total amount of 179.80 h of data divided into: sedentary situations (65.5%), light-to-moderate activity (17.6%) and vigorous exercise (16.9%). The proposed machine learning algorithms comprise the following steps: time-domain feature definition, standardization and PCA projection, unsupervised clustering (by k-means and GMM) and a HMM to account for long-term temporal trends. Performance was evaluated by 30 runs of a 10-fold cross-validation. Both k-means and GMM-based approaches yielded high overall accuracy (86.97% and 85.03%, respectively) and, given the imbalance of the dataset, meritorious F-measures (up to 77.88%) for non-sedentary cases. Classification errors tended to be concentrated around transients, what constrains their practical impact. Hence, we consider our proposal to be suitable for 24 h-based monitoring of physical activity in ambulatory scenarios and a first step towards intensity-specific energy expenditure estimators.

Keywords: physical activity intensity, accelerometry, heart rate, k-means, Gaussian Mixture Models, Hidden Markov Models, F-measure.

1 Introduction

The automatic assessment of physical activity facilitates ambulatory monitoring of lifestyle and may enrich traditional interventions to prevent and/or to manage chronic conditions for which regular exercise is prescribed, like cardiovascular and pulmonary diseases, obesity or diabetes.

M. Peleg, N. Lavrač, and C. Combi (Eds.): AIME 2011, LNAI 6747, pp. 70–79, 2011.

Current gold-standard techniques to measure energy expenditure (EE), i.e. doubly-labeled water and indirect calorimetry, are costly and impractical in free-living conditions.

Thus, a frequent alternative is to use multi-axial accelerometers placed on key locations of the body (hip, wrist, etc.) and to estimate EE by linear regression from acceleration counts and personal characteristics (weight, sex, etc.). However, accelerometry-based techniques are posed to neglect any physical exercise not encompassing movements of the sensor. In addition, the accuracy of such EE estimation formulae has been reported to fluctuate substantially depending –among other factors– on whether the activity under monitoring is or not comparable in terms of type and intensity with the particular set-up used in the experiments to develop and validate the equations (Crouter et al.[1]).

Another common option is to estimate EE from heart rate (HR), since there are physiological evidences for HR exhibiting a linear relationship with oxygen uptake ratios ($\dot{V}O_2$) and energy consumptions in the case of aerobic exercise at intermediate intensity ranges (i.e. around 110–150 bpm[2]). However, such linearity can be adversely affected by a number of other factors –drugs, stress, etc.– and does not hold for anaerobic exercise[3].

Consequently, an increasing number of authors advocate for techniques combining simultaneously accelerometry and HR measurements[2, 4, 5].

On the other hand, after Crouter et al.[1] identified various limitations for the EE regression formulae, different authors have suggested activity-specific EE estimation schemes[6–8], whose first step was to recognize a particular set of activities (e.g. sitting, standing, walking, running, cycling, etc.). Machine learning (ML) techniques have been thoroughly applied in literature to such activity recognition tasks, with noticeable success and a wide range of algorithms, for example: C4.5 trees[8, 9], Naïve Bayes classifiers[8, 9], GMM[10], MLP[11] and SOM[12] neural networks, AdaBoosting[13], etc. Most approaches, like the aforementioned, were based solely on accelerometry; while some others combined it with HR measurements[7, 14].

Conversely, instead of distinguishing among concrete activities from a pre-established set, in this work we will present algorithms to assess physical activity intensity (PAI) from multi-axial accelerometry and HR signals. In current practise and commercial monitoring devices, physical activity is often ranked into intensity levels based simply on 'cut-points' –thresholds– for accelerometer counts and/or HR, either with constant[15] or subject-dependent[16] values. Within the ML literature, some authors defined separate classes for the same exercise performed at different intensities, as in [7, 8]. In this work we will develop a combination of statistical ML techniques to determine PAI in an explicit and activity-independent manner. PAI classes will correspond to standardized intensity range definitions (Ainsworth et al.[17]): rest and sedentary situations, light-to-moderate activity and vigorous exercise.

2 Materials and Methods

2.1 Equipment

ActiTrainer Research accelerometer (ActiGraph, USA) was selected due to its function to record wireless signals from Polar Wearlink heart rate monitors (Polar Electro, Finland). ActiTrainer (51 g, 86×33×15 mm, ±3G dynamic range, 30 Hz sample frequency) registered biaxial acceleration counts $(\mathbf{a}_1, \mathbf{a}_2)$, number of steps –pedometer function– **st** and heart rate **hr**. Measurements were accumulated over 10 s periods –epochs– so that **hr** was physiologically meaningful.

Following manufacturers' guidelines, Polar strap was worn on the chest and ActiTrainer was tightly placed on the hip. Main and secondary axis had vertical and antero-posterior orientation, respectively.

2.2 Experiments and Participants

Two different experiments were conduced.

Exp. 1. aimed to acquire data in free-living conditions. Seven healthy subjects took part: 3 males and 4 females, aged 23–36 and with lifestyles ranging from sedentary to regular athletic training.

Volunteers received instructions on how to wear the sensors and were encouraged to report detailed written descriptions of type, duration and intensity of their physically active periods. They were requested to include: exercise at a self-selected intensity, daily life situations (e.g. sleep, rest, walk, housekeeping, office work, etc.) and the use of transportation (elevator, car, bus, metro).

An heterogeneous set of activities was obtained, including: walking at moderate speeds, dancing, jogging, vigorous endurance running, karate, football, mountain bike, etc. The elimination of periods with ambiguous annotations yielded a total of 149.35 h in 72 sequences. Data were then manually grouped according to Ainsworth et al.'s Compendium[17] into three PAI classes: *(i)* rest and sedentary situations (<3 MET, Metabolic Equivalents), *(ii)* light-to-moderate activity (3–6 MET), and *(iii)* vigorous exercise (>6 MET). See Table 1 for details.

Exp. 2. consisted of a controlled laboratory set-up where physical activity was performed in a gymnasium under researchers' supervision. Three circuit modalities were available, comprising: upper and lower limb exercises in gymnasium machines (e.g. shoulder press), free weight training and a combined weight-aerobic (treadmill running) circuit. Each 64 min session started with a warm-up phase by 5 min of treadmill/elliptical walk and a preliminary circuit lap (7.75 min) with light load. Thereafter, 3 more circuit bouts with high load were performed, each of these bouts separated by 5 min of 'active rests' (i.e. walking)[1].

Nine subjects aged 20–49 years were involved (6 male, 3 female). Three were healthy active males and the remaining 6 individuals suffered overweight

[1] PRONAF Study (Trial registration ClinicalTrials.gov NCT01116856). A complete description of exercises, circuits and protocols can be found in Benito et al.[18].

Table 1. Summary of the collected dataset, divided by experiments and PAI ranges. In *Exp. 2*, 40.9% 'REST' data embraced pre- and post-exercise periods.

	Exp. 1	*Exp. 2*	Total
	149.35 h (83.1%)	30.45 h (16.9%)	179.80 h (100.0%)
REST	105.40 h (70.6%)	12.45 h (40.9%)	117.85 h (65.5%)
LIGHT	26.42 h (17.7%)	5.23 h (17.2%)	31.65 h (17.6%)
VIGOR	17.53 h (11.7%)	12.77 h (41.9%)	30.30 h (16.9%)

($BMI = 28.1 \pm 1.3$ kg $\cdot$ m^{-2}). Informed consent was obtained in all cases. Depending on their availability for the experiment, 5 subjects completed all of the 3 circuits in different days, one subject exercised for 2 sessions and the remaining 3 participants completed only one circuit. In total, 20 sessions were registered. Data were subsequently grouped into the three available PAI ranges, following the same class criteria as for *Exp. 1*.

Combining both experiments, the total amount of time in rest/sedentary situations dominated against the two other PAI classes (see Table 1), what in practice mimics reasonably well realistic data distributions for 24 h-based monitoring scenarios.

2.3 Methodology for Automatic PAI Assessment

2.3.1 Feature Definition. Signals were divided into segments by rectangular non-overlapping windows. Note that the length of such analysis window is an important parameter for our methods, implying a trade-off between: *a)* temporal resolution –short windows necessary–, and *b)* the definition of meaningful features able to capture relevant information about the underlying phenomena –longer windows preferred–. In a preliminary stage, we tested our algorithms for different window lengths, within a range of 0.5–10 min. Evaluating the obtained overall performance in terms of accuracy and temporal resolution, we opted for 2 min windows (12 samples with 10 s epochs).

An extra magnitude, acceleration norm $\|\boldsymbol{a}\| = \sqrt{\mathbf{a}_1^2 + \mathbf{a}_2^2}$, was defined to combine the information from the two axis. Afterwards, statistical descriptives were computed in the time-domain for $\mathbf{a}_1$, $\mathbf{a}_2$, $\|\boldsymbol{a}\|$, **st** and **hr** in each windowed segment; namely: means, standard deviations, medians, maxima, minima and Pearson's correlation coefficients r_{XY} for low-pass filtered versions of the original signals. In total, 35 features were derived.

2.3.2 Dimensionality Reduction. Principal Component Analysis (PCA) was applied to reduce the amount of redundancy present in the data. Given that features are clearly not commensurate (for example: $|r_{XY}| \in [0, 1]$ by definition, while $\|\boldsymbol{a}\|{>}1000$ in many cases), the original feature space was standardized (i.e. subtraction of μ and division by σ in each dimension). This was done to prevent the PCA eigenvectors from being dominated by those features with largest variance, what would have masked much of the relevant information.

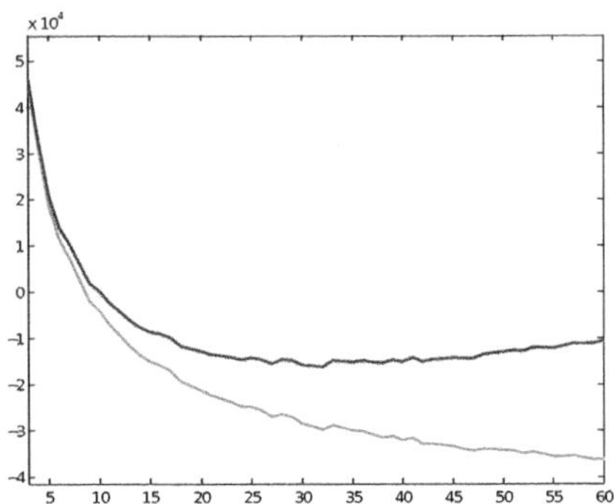

Fig. 1. Average values for Akaike (light line) and Bayes (dark line) information criteria –ordinate– with an increasing number of L mixtures in the GMM –abscissa–

We selected the T=10 eigenvectors with highest eigenvalues λ_i, which explained 81.5% of total variance (79.0% for T=9). After projection onto a new subspace formed by the eigenvectors $\{\boldsymbol{v}_i\}_{i=1}^{T}$, data were again standardized (dividing by $\sqrt{\lambda_i}$) in order to obtain commensurate magnitudes.

2.3.3 Unsupervised Clustering. Two different techniques were compared: k-means clustering and a Gaussian Mixture Model (GMM), the latter option as a particular case of Expectation-Maximization (EM) algorithm where the underlying probability density function is modeled as a mixture (i.e. linear combination) of L Gaussians.

Prior to the automatic learning phase itself, suitable values for parameters k and L had to be chosen. To do so, we assessed the complexity of our 10-dimensional feature space by fitting into the data a GMM with increasing L. For each iteration, average values of Akaike (AIC) and Bayes (BIC) information criteria were computed with a 10-fold cross-validation strategy. Figure 1 depicts an almost monotonically decreasing trend for AIC up to L=60 mixtures, while BIC reached a global minimum for L=32. Since AIC yielded a local minimum for this same number, we accepted L=32 as a reasonable compromise to avoid making the learning process unnecessarily complex. In addition, for k-means we selected k=32 as well, in order to compare both algorithms under equal circumstances (assuming none was favoured by such choice).

2.3.4 Temporal Model. In practise, when individuals exercise, their PAI does not usually fluctuate rapidly; on the contrary, changes tend to be gradual and intensity ranges are often kept almost constant for time periods that broadly exceed the length of our 2 min analysis windows. Consequently, it is common to observe long-term trends with a fixed intensity level; so that PAI for a particular moment shows strong correlation with respect to the PAI at neighbor instants. To benefit from this behaviour, we propose a multi-scale approach from a temporal point of view, where the lower scale corresponds to the span of our analysis window and the higher scale is related to the scope of a Hidden Markov Model (HMM). While extensively used in speech and gesture recognition, different authors have also suggested HMMs to detect physical activities (e.g. falls, sit-to-stand transitions, etc.[19, 20]).

We built a single-layered HMM where: *a)* observations correspond to cluster assignments –which, being 32 possible symbols, lack of intuitive interpretation–, and where *b)* hidden states are assimilated to the targeted PAI classes. During the training phase, emission and transmission matrices (with size 3×32 and 3×3, respectively) were estimated in a supervised manner, i.e. by direct comparison of cluster assignments and PAI labels from the ground truth. During the HMM-based classification stage, the algorithms calculated which sequence of ('hidden') PAI classes most likely originated a given ('observed') sequence of clusters.

2.3.5 Performance Evaluation. While total accuracy is the most common metric for assessing performance in classification tasks, it tends to undervalue achievements on multi-class problems or under notable class imbalance. As both circumstances apply in this work, we opted for using precision and recall metrics instead. For the i-th class:

$$\text{Precision}^{(i)} \equiv \frac{\text{TP}^{(i)}}{\text{TP}^{(i)} + \text{FP}^{(i)}} \qquad \text{Recall}^{(i)} \equiv \frac{\text{TP}^{(i)}}{\text{TP}^{(i)} + \text{FN}^{(i)}} \tag{1}$$

Hence, the harmonic mean between precision and recall (often known as F-measure or F-score) is another convenient metric in our case:

$$\text{F} - \text{measure}^{(i)} \equiv 2\,\frac{\text{Precision}^{(i)} \cdot \text{Recall}^{(i)}}{\text{Precision}^{(i)} + \text{Recall}^{(i)}} \tag{2}$$

Overall classification performance was estimated by 30 independent runs of a 10-fold cross-validation. Full stratification was dismissed because it would remove any temporal coherence. Instead, a partial stratification was implemented: Each of the 92 available sequences was randomly allocated into a fold. Folds were then checked to guarantee that their relative class frequencies were similar to the prior PAI distributions, and to assure that fold sizes were not highly uneven.

3 Results

The dimensionality reduction process showed HR-related features playing prominent roles in the first PCA eigenvectors. Outliers-sensitive features (e.g. maxima, minima) also exhibited a substantial discriminative power, instead of being adversely affected by noise or artifacts.

Table 2 presents a summary of results in terms of total accuracy; as well as precision, recall and F-measure for the three PAI. In general, both k-means and GMM-based algorithms yielded meritorious performance values considering the marked class imbalance in the dataset. k-means outperformed GMM in

Table 2. Classification performance of the proposed algorithms in the whole dataset

	$n = 30$ $\mu \pm \sigma$ [min|max]	**k-means + HMM**	**GMM + HMM**
	Accuracy	86.97 ± 0.67% [85.58%|88.21%]	85.03 ± 0.82% [83.60%|86.96%]
REST	Precision	94.83 ± 0.45% [93.97%|95.73%]	97.11 ± 0.46% [96.11%|98.11%]
	Recall	93.76 ± 0.89% [90.99%|95.01%]	91.08 ± 0.72% [89.42%|93.15%]
	F-Measure	94.29 ± 0.48% [92.99%|94.98%]	94.00 ± 0.45% [93.12%|95.25%]
LIGHT	Precision	73.60 ± 1.99% [69.39%|77.61%]	67.40 ± 3.27% [61.18%|72.32%]
	Recall	63.70 ± 1.49% [60.82%|66.31%]	65.70 ± 1.85% [61.67%|70.33%]
	F-Measure	68.27 ± 1.28% [65.12%|70.97%]	66.48 ± 1.65% [63.45%|69.67%]
VIGOR	Precision	71.89 ± 1.76% [67.39%|74.33%]	64.77 ± 1.57% [60.84%|67.69%]
	Recall	85.01 ± 1.90% [81.13%|88.96%]	81.85 ± 3.61% [75.50%|88.63%]
	F-Measure	77.88 ± 1.26% [75.31%|80.10%]	72.28 ± 1.85% [68.86%|75.47%]

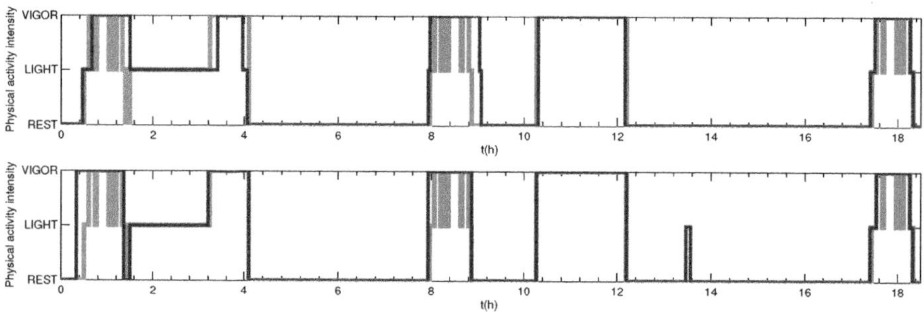

Fig. 2. Top: Example of k-means+HMM classification outputs (dark line, 92.45% accuracy) vs. ground truth (light line) along time. Bottom: GMM+HMM results (dark line, 94.06% accuracy) for the same ground truth sequence as above.

non-sedentary situations (average F-measures: 68.27% and 77.88% for k-means, versus 66.48% and 72.28% for GMM). A two-tailed unpaired t-test found significant differences between methods ($p<0.01$ in all cases, except for F-measure in 'REST', where $p=0.02$).

Figure 2 depicts an example of automatic classification results versus ground truth PAI annotations, obtained for a test subset of data kept apart from the ML training phase. In general, long-term mismatches seldom occur –none in Figure 2–. Most classification errors have a short duration and tend to be located: *a)* where the ground truth reference PAI levels oscillate rapidly (for our example, around 1.5, 8.5 and 18.0 h, where the circuit bouts from *Exp. 2* include 'active rests' for 5 min); or *b)* around sudden transients (especially from 'REST' to 'VIGOR' or vice versa, e.g. approx. at 0.5 and 9.0 h). Hence, on a 24 h basis the overall impact of this type of errors should be very limited in practice, with warm-up and cool-down exercising, etc.

4 Discussion

The accuracy achieved by our approach is remarkable (86.97% for k-means) and outperforms other PAI classifiers using combined accelerometry and HR, like Munguia Tapia[7] (58.40% accuracy in subject-independent classification). However, it must be noted that our proposal is explicitly intensity-oriented; while theirs was activity type-oriented (with certain types allowing several intensities), so that their number of possible classes was considerably higher.

In concordance with the conclusions by different researchers from the sport sciences background[2, 4, 5], we encountered that heart rate –and the features deriving from it– played a prominent role in PCA and classification, as they contain valuable information regarding physiological responses to exercise. In our view, this notable potential of HR has not yet been sufficiently exploited by methods from the ML background, since authors tended to focus mainly on accelerometry as their signal source.

Besides, the HMM introduced additional robustness into the algorithms by capturing temporal relationships among PAI labels for neighbor instants.

We observed that the recognition behaved worst for moderate intensities, with most miss-classifications occurring between 'LIGHT' and 'VIGOR' labels. A possible explanation is that, in free-living conditions, ground truth had to be based on volunteers' self-reports, as it was the case for *Exp. 1*[2]. Despite periods with ambiguous annotations were removed from the dataset, this dependence on subjective PAI grading poses the problem of introducing certain degree of uncertainty which cannot be eliminated from the ground truth. Nevertheless, for our research we considered essential not to restrict the analysis to laboratory situations, but to include an important amount of time in free-living conditions, to obtain datasets which assemble more realistic scenarios.

The significant class imbalance may also be a major responsible for the classifiers suffering lower performance at those underrepresented PAI levels. However, we obtained remarkable F-measures for these classes, what leads us to think that the algorithms are capable of compensating for most of the imbalance.

In current clinical and research practise (e.g. in epidemiological studies, to determine individuals' adherence to exercise programs and their effects on health), physical activity monitoring in 24 h-based ambulatory scenarios utilizes often merely a single device: either a pedometer, accelerometer or HR monitor; thus dismissing the potential of combining information sources. In addition, manufacturers' software for data analysis (as in the case of ActiTrainer) relies generally on simple thresholding to differentiate active periods from rest, and in linear regression for the EE computation. In contrast, our method may provide a more robust assessment of time exercised and PAI performed.

Furthermore, Crouter et al. proved in [1] that the accuracy obtained by these commercial EE estimation formulae may decrease substantially if the activity under monitoring is not comparable with the particular exercise for which the

[2] Such limitation was not present in *Exp. 2*, where volunteers exercised under direct supervision by the researchers.

equation was derived and validated. To solve this issue, several authors developed activity-specific EE estimation schemes[6–8]. Conversely, we intend to explore PAI-specific estimators based on the algorithms presented here.

5 Conclusions

This work presents an automatic algorithm based on statistical machine learning techniques for explicit assessment of physical activity intensity by means of simultaneous multi-axial accelerometry and heart rate signals. Our algorithms yielded up to 86.97% accuracy in PAI classification and up to 77.88% F-measure for non-sedentary situations. In addition, errors appeared mostly as brief transients. We therefore believe that our approach can be used for 24 h-based monitoring of physical activity in ambulatory scenarios and we suggest it as a first step towards the development of intensity-specific energy expenditure estimators.

Acknowledgments. The authors thank the members of the PRONAF Study Group for their assistance with data collection. This work was partially funded by a research grant of the Universidad Politécnica de Madrid and by the Spanish grants of the Ministry of Science and Innovation 'APRIORI' (FIS PS09/01318) and 'PRONAF' (DEP2008-06354-C04-01).

References

1. Crouter, S.E., Churilla, J.R., Bassett, D.R.: Estimating energy expenditure using accelerometers. Eur. J. Appl. Physiol. 98(6), 601–612 (2006)
2. Freedson, P.S., Miller, K.: Objective monitoring of physical activity using motion sensors and heart rate. Res. Q Exercise Sport 71(2 Suppl), S21 (2000)
3. Gotshalk, L.A., Berger, R.A., Kraemer, W.J.: Cardiovascular responses to a high-volume continuous circuit resistance training protocol. J. Strength Cond. Res. 18(4), 760 (2004)
4. Strath, S.J., Brage, S., Ekelund, U.: Integration of physiological and accelerometer data to improve physical activity assessment. Med. Sci. Sport Exer. 37(11), S563 (2005)
5. Plasqui, G., Westerterp, K.R.: Accelerometry and heart rate as a measure of physical fitness: Cross-validation. Med. Sci. Sport Exer. 38(8), 1510 (2006)
6. Bonomi, A.G., Plasqui, G., Goris, A.H.C., Westerterp, K.R.: Improving assessment of daily energy expenditure by identifying types of physical activity with a single accelerometer. J. Appl. Physiol. 107(3), 655 (2009)
7. Munguia Tapia, E., Intille, S.S., Haskell, W., Larson, K., Wright, J., King, A., Friedman, R.: Real-time recognition of physical activities and their intensities using wireless accelerometers and a heart rate monitor. In: 2007 11th IEEE International Symposium on Wearable Computers, pp. 37–40. IEEE, Los Alamitos (2007)
8. Albinali, F., Intille, S.S., Haskell, W., Rosenberger, M.: Using wearable activity type detection to improve physical activity energy expenditure estimation. In: Proceedings of the 12th ACM International Conference on Ubiquitous Computing, pp. 311–320. ACM, New York (2010)

9. Bao, L., Intille, S.S.: Activity recognition from user-annotated acceleration data. In: Ferscha, A., Mattern, F. (eds.) PERVASIVE 2004. LNCS, vol. 3001, pp. 1–17. Springer, Heidelberg (2004)
10. Allen, F.R., Ambikairajah, E., Lovell, N.H., Celler, B.G.: An adapted Gaussian Mixture Model approach to accelerometry-based movement classification using time-domain features. In: 28th Annual International Conference Engineering in Medicine and Biology Society, EMBS 2006, pp. 3600–3603. IEEE, Los Alamitos (2008)
11. Ermes, M., Parkka, J., Mantyjarvi, J., Korhonen, I.: Detection of daily activities and sports with wearable sensors in controlled and uncontrolled conditions. IEEE T. Inf. Technol. B 12(1), 20–26 (2008)
12. Krause, A., Siewiorek, D.P., Smailagic, A., Farringdon, J.: Unsupervised, dynamic identification of physiological and activity context in wearable computing. In: Proceedings of the 7th IEEE International Symposium on Wearable Computers (ISWC 2003). IEEE Computer Society, Los Alamitos (2003)
13. Lester, J., Choudhury, T., Borriello, G.: A practical approach to recognizing physical activities. In: Fishkin, K.P., Schiele, B., Nixon, P., Quigley, A. (eds.) PERVASIVE 2006. LNCS, vol. 3968, pp. 1–16. Springer, Heidelberg (2006)
14. Duchêne, F., Garbay, C., Rialle, V.: Learning recurrent behaviors from heterogeneous multivariate time-series. Artif. Intell. Med. 39(1), 25–47 (2007)
15. Freedson, P.S., Melanson, E., Sirard, J.: Calibration of the Computer Science and Applications, Inc. accelerometer. Med. Sci. Sport Exer. 30(5), 777 (1998)
16. Brage, S., Brage, N., Franks, P.W., Ekelund, U., Wong, M.Y., Andersen, L.B., Froberg, K., Wareham, N.J.: Branched equation modeling of simultaneous accelerometry and heart rate monitoring improves estimate of directly measured physical activity energy expenditure. J. Appl. Physiol. 96(1), 343 (2004)
17. Ainsworth, B.E., Haskell, W.L., Whitt, M.C., Irwin, M., Swartz, A.M., Strath, S.J., O'Brien, W.L., Bassett Jr., D.R., Schmitz, K.H., Emplaincourt, P.O., et al.: Compendium of physical activities: An update of activity codes and MET intensities. Med. Sci. Sport Exer. 32(9 Suppl), S498 (2000)
18. Benito Peinado, P.J., Álvarez Sánchez, M., Díaz Molina, V., Peinado Lozano, A.B., Calderón Montero, F.J.: Aerobic Energy Expenditure and Intensity Prediction during a Specific Circuit Weight Training: A Pilot Study. J. Hum. Sport Exerc. 5(2), 134–145 (2010)
19. Lester, J., Choudhury, T., Kern, N., Borriello, G., Hannaford, B.: A hybrid discriminative/generative approach for modeling human activities. In: Proc. of the International Joint Conference on Artificial Intelligence (IJCAI), Citeseer (2005)
20. He, J., Li, H., Tan, J.: Real-time daily activity classification with wireless sensor networks using Hidden Markov Model. In: 29th Annual International Conference Engineering in Medicine and Biology Society, EMBS 2007, pp. 3192–3195. IEEE, Los Alamitos (2007)
21. García-García, F., Martínez-Sarriegui, I., Gómez, E.J., Rigla, M., Hernando, M.E.: Automatic assessment of physical activity using multi-axial accelerometry and heart rate. J. Diab. Tech. Therap. 13(2), 182 (2011)

A Data Mining Library for miRNA Annotation and Analysis

Angelo Nuzzo[1], Riccardo Beretta[2], Francesca Mulas[1], Valerie Roobrouck[3], Catherine Verfaillie[3], Blaz Zupan[4,5], and Riccardo Bellazzi[1,2]

[1] Centre for Tissue Engineering, University of Pavia, Pavia, Italy
[2] Department of Computer Engineering and Systems Science, University of Pavia, Pavia, Italy
[3] Stamcelinstituut, K.U.Leuven, Leuven, Belgium
[4] Faculty of Computer and Information Science, University of Ljubljana, Ljubljana, Slovenia
[5] Department of Molecular and Human Genetics, Baylor College of Medicine, Houston, TX, USA

{angelo.nuzzo,francesca.mulas,riccardo.bellazzi}@unipv.it,
blaz.zupan@fri.uni-lj.si,
{Catherine.Verfaillie,Valerie.Roobrouck}@med.kuleuven.be

Abstract. Understanding the key role that miRNAs play in the regulation of gene expression is one of the most important challenges in modern molecular biology. Standard gene set enrichment analysis (GSEA) is not appropriate in this context, due to the low specificity of the relation between miRNAs and their target genes. We developed alternative strategies to gain better insights in the differences in biological processes involved in different experimental conditions. We here describe a novel method to analyze and interpret miRNA expression data correctly, and demonstrate that annotating miRNA directly to biological processes through their target genes (which is nevertheless the only way possible) is a non-trivial task. We are currently employing the same strategy to relate miRNA expression patterns directly to pathway information, to generate new hypotheses, which may be relevant for the interpretation of their role in the gene expression regulatory processes.

Keywords: miRNA analysis, Data Mining, annotation tools.

1 Introduction

Recent studies revealed the importance of understanding the role that miRNAs play in the regulation of gene expression. [1].

Since our knowledge of this domain is still limited but at the same time constantly increasing, it is critical to develop new methods to efficiently retrieve, represent and manipulate the available information about known miRNAs. We developed an annotation tool to facilitate the retrieval of miRNA information, and to represent it in an effective way. The tool also allows applying novel analysis methods to miRNA data, which are needed to address the peculiarities of the biological processess in which miRNAs are involved.

M. Peleg, N. Lavrač, and C. Combi (Eds.): AIME 2011, LNAI 6747, pp. 80–84, 2011.

2 Methods

We developed a library, called *obiMirna*, for miRNA annotation and analysis, to be included as an analysis tool in the Bioinformatics module (called *obi*, i.e. "Orange BioInformatics) of the Orange Data Mining package [2].

The Bioinformatics modules rely on a central server, which is incrementally updated with data downloaded from miRBase [3][4] and Target Scan databases [5]. The update on the client installation of Orange is made at first use of the Bioinformatics module.

The obiMirna module provides tools to display the miRNA database information. It allows the user to easily retrieve the pre-miRNA and mature miRNA sequences, and to computationally identify target genes.

Moreover, the obiMirna module processes the data so that it can be directly connected to other Orange Bioinformatics tools for further analysis. In particular, dictionaries matching miRNA annotations with other entities of interest (GeneOntology terms, Kegg pathways, etc) have been implemented, so that Gene Set Enrichment Analysis (GSEA) can be performed using the GSEA tool already available in Orange [6].

However, due to the biological nature of the problem, i.e. the low specificity of the miRNA - target genes relation, the standard GSEA approach is not appropriate for miRNA data. Thus, we developed alternative strategies to better catch the differences in biological processes involved in different experimental conditions. We created an empirical null enrichment distribution of GO terms for each miRNA present in miRBase, as follows:

1. The null distribution is created by a permutation strategy that randomly assigns target genes to each miRNA, keeping the same number of target genes as in the database (Fig. 1).
2. A distribution of GO terms is then derived from these genes.

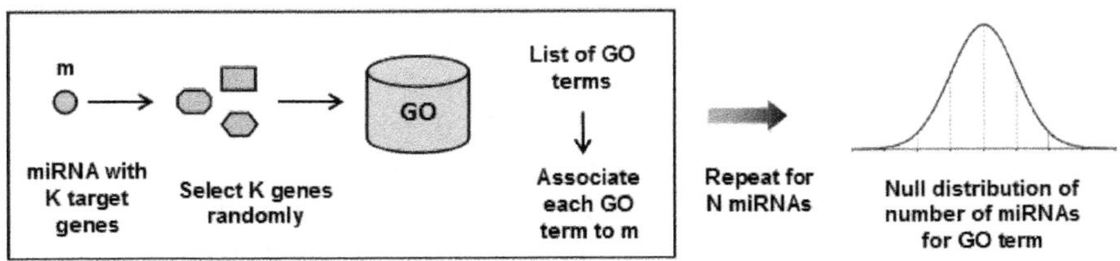

Fig. 1. The empirical null distribution construction for GO terms enrichment analysis

3. The experimental data are compared to this empirical null distribution computing a p-value as: i) the area under the curve (AUC) of the null distribution for the each miRNA and ii) a hypergeometric test on the differentially expressed miRNA with respect to all the miRNA annotated with the same GO terms (Fig. 2).

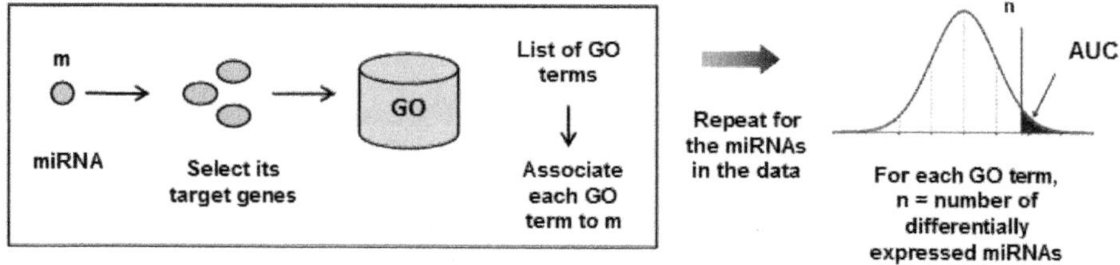

Fig. 2. Evaluation of experimental data with respect to the null distribution

4. Finally, we compute the rank correlation between the different experimental conditions for both strategies, in order to detect biological processes that are over-represented in the dataset.

3 Results and Discussion

We tested the functionality of obiMirna with a dataset containing 3 types of adult postnatal stem cells, namely Multipotent Adult Progenitor Cells (MAPC), Mesenchymal Stem Cells (MSC) and Mesoangioblasts (Mab), that was generated to identify which miRNAs regulate which biological processes in each cell population.

We performed first a standard GSEA with miRNAs that are differentially expressed between MAPC and MSC, and between MAPC and Mab, creating three different dictionaries: "GO terms – all miRNA", "GO terms – enriched miRNAs", and "GO terms – reduced miRNA set", where the reduced set was identified by a TF-IDF filtering method [7].

In all cases, we did not find significant p-values, suggesting that a standard enrichment analysis is not appropriate for this kind of data. This is mainly due to the fact that each miRNA targets a high number of genes, and once GO terms are derived from those genes none of them appears to be significantly over-represented with respect to the others.

On the contrary, with the alternative approaches described in the previous section, we identified 345 differentially expressed miRNAs in the MAPC vs. MSC comparison, with a 0.79 correlation rank, and 32 differentially expressed miRNA in the MAPC vs. Mab comparison, with a 0.82 correlation rank.

As the tool has been integrated in the Orange framework (Fig. 3), it is straightforward to use its network visualization module in order to easily investigate the annotation networks based on TF-IDF and highlight possible interesting relations (Fig. 4), both to confirm an original hypothesis and to suggest new possible relations to be investigated.

Finally, a validation of the proposed permutation-based analysis is ongoing on an independent published dataset, both to confirm the ability of this approach to overcome standard GSEA limitation in this context and to compare its performance to similar methods recently published [8].

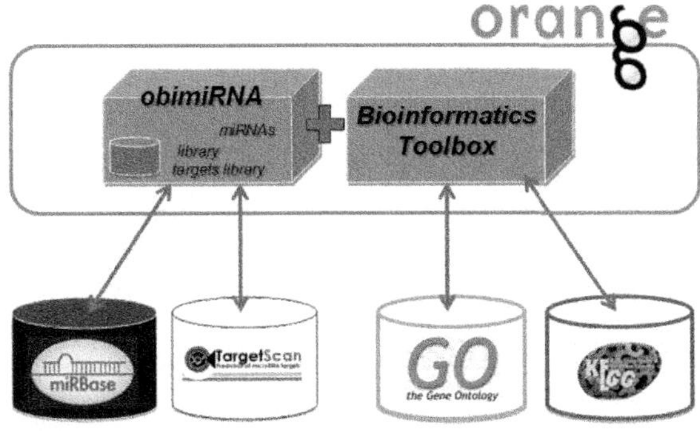

Fig. 3. Methods implementation and integration in Orange

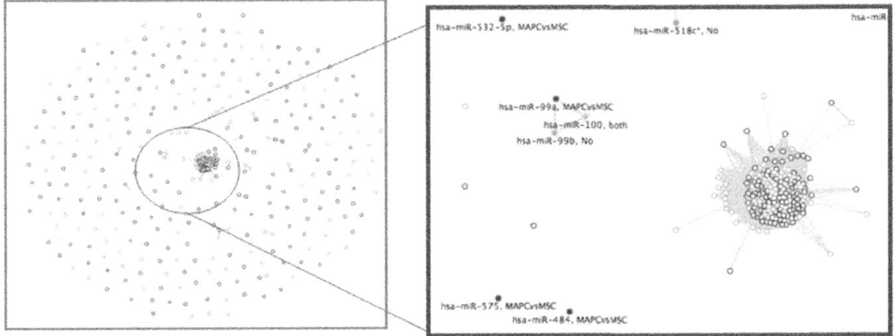

Fig. 4. Exploiting the Network Visualization tool for result exploration

4 Conclusion

Our results show how new methods have to be designed to analyse and interpret miRNA expression data correctly, and that annotating miRNA directly to biological processes through their target genes (which is nevertheless the only way possible) is a non trivial task. Traditional gene expression analysis indeed are affected by intrinsic biological features of miRNAs relationship with target genes. We showed how the research of statistical association can be improved both by a non-parametric approach (like the permutation-base that we proposed) and an appropriate annotation filtering step, which is crucial to exploit available knowledge to suggest new discovery.

We are currently employing the same strategy to try to relate miRNA expression directly to pathway information (retrieved from KEGG database), in order to generate new hypotheses which may be relevant for the interpretation of their role in the regulation of gene expression.

Acknowledgments. This work is a part of the project "Bioinformatics for Tissue Engineering: Creation of an International Research Group", funded by the "Fondazione Cariplo".

References

1. Mattick, J.S., Makunin, I.V.: Non-coding RNA. Human Molecular Genetics 15(1), R17–R29 (2006)
2. Curk, T., Demsar, J., Xu, Q., Leban, G., Petrovic, U., Bratko, I., Shaulsky, G., Zupan, B.: Microarray data mining with visual programming. Bioinformatics 21(3), 396–398 (2005)
3. Griffiths-Jones, S., Kaur Saini, H., van Dongen, S., Enright, A.J.: miRBase: tools for microRNA genomics. Nucleic Acid Research 36(Database Issue), D154–D158 (2008)
4. Griffiths-Jones, S., Grocock, R.J., van Dongen, S., Bateman, A., Enright, A.J.: miRBase: microRNA sequences, targets and gene nomenclature. Nucleic Acids Research 34, D140–D144 (2006)
5. Lewis, B.P., Burge, C.B., Bartel, D.P.: Conserved seed pairing, often flanked by adenosines, indicates that thousands of human genes are microRNA targets. Cell 120, 15–20 (2005)
6. GSEA in orange
7. Mulas, F., Curk, T., Bellazzi, R., Zupan, B.: On quality of different annotation sources for gene expression analysis. In: Combi, C., Shahar, Y., Abu-Hanna, A. (eds.) AIME 2009. LNCS, vol. 5651, pp. 421–425. Springer, Heidelberg (2009)
8. Gusev, Y.: Computational methods for analysis of cellular functions and pathways collectively targeted by differentially expressed microRNA. Methods 44(1), 61–72 (2008)

Ranking and 1-Dimensional Projection of Cell Development Transcription Profiles

Lan Zagar[1], Francesca Mulas[2], Riccardo Bellazzi[2], and Blaz Zupan[1]

[1] University of Ljubljana, Ljubljana, Slovenia
{lan.zagar,blaz.zupan}@fri.uni-lj.si
[2] University of Pavia, Pavia, Italy
{francesca.mulas,riccardo.bellazzi}@unipv.it

Abstract. Genome-scale transcription profile is known to be a good reporter of the state of the cell. Much of the early predictive modelling and cell-type clustering relied on this relation and has experimentally confirmed it. We have examined if this also holds for prediction of cell's staging, and focused on the inference of stage prediction models for stem cell development. We show that the problem relates to rank learning and, from the user's point of view, to projection of transcription profile data to a single dimension. Our comparison of several state-of-the-art algorithms on 10 data sets from Gene Expression Omnibus shows that rank-learning can be successfully applied to developmental cell staging, and that relatively simple techniques can perform surprisingly well.

Keywords: cell development, staging, temporal ordering, ranking, projection, regression.

1 Introduction

Rank learning has recently attracted much attention in both theoretical and practical branches of machine learning. Unlike standard prediction approaches, the problem of ranking is not concerned with the prediction of data's class values. Instead, its goal is to infer a predictive model from ranked data or from data with a list of ranked instance pairs, and apply the model to a set of new data instances. Rank learning is sometimes regarded as a part of the broader topic of preference learning [3].

First applications of this technology were in information retrieval [6,5], where the quality of search engines depended on appropriate ordering of search results. Today, however, other fields of research are recognizing the utility of the rank learning approach, and different tasks are emerging where the problems can be formulated as a ranking problem. Biomedicine is of course no exception. In this paper we show that the development of cells — a time-related process during which cells go through different development stages — can be considered by rank learning with the aim to develop stage-prediction models. We propose to consider cells from different stages through their characterization with whole-genome transcription profiles, and infer a function that can reconstruct the development stage based on microarray data and information on stage ordering.

M. Peleg, N. Lavrač, and C. Combi (Eds.): AIME 2011, LNAI 6747, pp. 85–89, 2011.

We show how this can be done with rank learning, and compare state-of-the-art techniques with more traditional approaches of regression and projection into one (temporal) dimension.

2 Methods

The goal of ordering samples with respect to their developmental stage can be approached from several different viewpoints. Standard projection methods project high-dimensional data into a lower dimensional subspace. We are interested in a specific case, where the projection maps the data into a one-dimensional space (*i.e.* a line). Regression algorithms can, in this particular case, be used for the same purpose since they also map high-dimensional data to a single number. Notice that while projection methods can be either supervised or unsupervised, regression always requires a numerical class in addition to the feature–description of samples. Ranking algorithms take ranked data as input and produce a function for ranking future sets of examples. Often the ranking function assigns a numerical utility score to samples and when it does not we can consider the rank itself as a predicted numerical label.

We have compared different types of inference methods to evaluate them on our ranking problem setting. The methods we have considered include:

PCA (Principal component analysis) is a very well known linear method for dimension reduction. It projects the data to a subspace where the maximum amount of variance is retained. Due to our interest in ranking, only the first principal component was considered, thus obtaining a linear transformation of the original data to a set of points on a line.

PLS (Partial least squares) also constructs a linear transformation, but additionally uses the numerical class vector, which makes it a supervised method. The directions it seeks have high variance and a high correlation with the class. We implemented the algorithm as described in [4].

LASSO and Ridge regression are extensions to the ordinary least squares regression. To avoid problems caused by too many or correlated features they impose additional constraints on the size of the coefficients. LASSO uses the L_1 norm: $\sum_i |\beta_i| < s$, while ridge regression uses L_2 norm: $\sum_i \beta_i^2 < s$. We used the implementation from scikits.learn[1].

SVMrank was proposed in [5] and is still considered a state-of-the-art approach for learning ranking functions. The algorithm aims at finding a ranking function that minimizes the number of discordant pairs. This task is approximated by considering the ranking problem as a binary classification problem on pairs of samples. In this context each pair is represented as a difference vector and plays the role of a single example in the standard classification SVM. We used the freely available implementation SVM^{rank}[2].

[1] `http://scikit-learn.sourceforge.net`

[2] `http://www.cs.cornell.edu/People/tj/svm_light/svm_rank.html`

3 Experiments and Results

3.1 Data

The methods were evaluated on multiple publicly available data sets from the Gene Expression Omnibus (GEO) repository. These were selected among microarray data sets measuring gene expressions for samples from different time points (stages) in stem cell development with at least three replicates per stage and a minimum of six stages. The following data sets met the criteria and were used for the experiments: GDS2431, GDS2666, GDS2667, GDS2668, GDS2669, GDS2671, GDS2672, GDS2688, GDS586, GDS587. Preprocessing consisted of normalizing the expression values in each data set using quantile normalization [1]. For regression methods which need numerical class values the ranks $(1, 2, 3, \ldots)$ of the stages were used as labels for samples.

3.2 Evaluation Procedure

The inference methods were evaluated on each of the GEO data sets. For all possible pairs of stages, samples from the selected stage pair were taken as the test set, while all remaining samples were used for training. This is a slightly more stringent version than the more common leave-two-out approach where all possible pairs of samples would be withdrawn. For model scoring we have computed a variant of the area under the ROC curve (AUC). AUC is equal to the probability that the predicted ranking of a pair of samples corresponds to the true ranking. This interpretation combined with our particular testing procedure provides us with an efficient way of computing the AUC. For two samples in the test set we check if the prediction model ranks them correctly. The proportion of correctly ranked pairs gives us the AUC score. Formally, the computation of AUC is given by the following equation:

$$AUC = \frac{\sum\limits_{x \in T_i, y \in T_j, i<j} \delta(p(x) < p(y))}{\sum\limits_{i<j} |T_i| \times |T_j|}, \tag{1}$$

where $p(x)$ is the projection of x, T_i the set of samples from time point i, $|T_i|$ the size of T_i and $\delta(cond)$ equal to 0 or 1 if *cond* is $False$ or $True$, respectively.

3.3 Results

Evaluation results are presented in Table 1. The AUC scores are very high (60% of the scores are > 0.9) implying excellent prediction power. Apart from GDS2688, where all methods achieved their lowest scores, all other data sets enable very precise ranking (temporal ordering) of samples based only on their gene expression profiles.

To compare the methods, mean AUC scores over all data sets are reported. Additionally, for each data set, the methods were ranked from best to worst.

Table 1. AUC scores of internal validation on ten data sets from GEO. Results are summarized as mean AUC score across all the data sets. For each data set the methods were ranked and mean rank along with mean AUC is given for each method.

	GDS2431	GDS2666	GDS2667	GDS2668	GDS2669	GDS2671
Ridge	0.867	0.960	0.929	0.925	0.927	0.903
PCA	0.867	0.962	0.952	0.899	0.907	0.913
PLS	0.859	0.952	0.923	0.931	0.933	0.909
SVMrank	0.844	0.931	0.917	0.903	0.927	0.881
LASSO	0.956	0.949	0.863	0.901	0.921	0.812

	GDS2672	GDS2688	GDS586	GDS587	$\overline{AUC}$	$\overline{rank}$
Ridge	0.923	0.624	0.984	0.889	0.893	2.200
PCA	0.822	0.709	0.952	0.958	0.894	2.550
PLS	0.915	0.610	0.948	0.889	0.887	2.800
SVMrank	0.885	0.613	0.984	0.878	0.876	3.600
LASSO	0.865	0.657	0.948	0.778	0.865	3.850

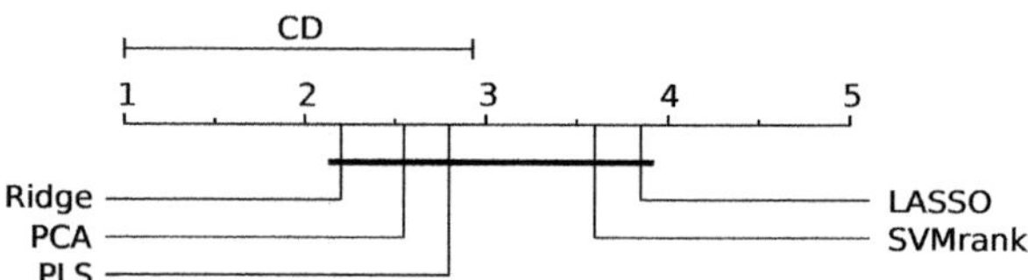

Fig. 1. Critical difference graph showing the mean ranks of the methods and the critical difference (CD). Pairwise differences between methods closer than CD (connected with a bar) are not statistically significant ($p = 0.05$).

The mean rank is given in the last column and is used in a statistical analysis [2] assessing the significance of pairwise differences between the methods. The result of the analysis is shown with a critical difference graph (Fig. 1), which tells us that the differences are not statistically significant (at $p = 0.05$).

4 Discussion

The results are somewhat surprising as one would expect the supervised regression algorithms or the specialized ranking approach of SVMrank to outperform an unsupervised method like PCA. Yet, apparently, this type of problem and the structure of the data sets enable PCA to be competitive in terms of the measured AUC. Because PCA's projection is unsupervised it has the additional benefit that it is not (over)fitted to the labels. The distances between the training samples on the projected line are therefore much more informative and representative of the inherent structure compared to projections of other methods that succeed "too well" in separating the labeled stages and result in their almost equidistant projections.

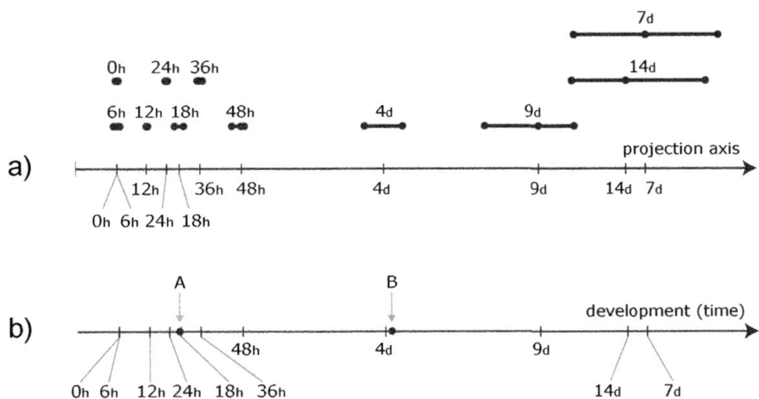

Fig. 2. a) One-dimensional projection of mouse embryonic stem cell data. Samples observed at the same development stage are connected with a line. Ticks mark the position of the median projection of a stage. b) Prediction of developmental stages of two new samples – A and B.

Besides simplicity, PCA also has an advantage of "discovery" of relation between development stages. Like in an example shown in Fig. 2, some stages are clustered together, and between other ones there is a substantial gap indicating a potentially large difference in stages and development of the cell. A visualization like this enables interpretation, and enhances understanding of the underlying phenomenon.

References

1. Bolstad, B.M., Irizarry, R.A., Åstrand, M., Speed, T.P.: A comparison of normalization methods for high density oligonucleotide array data based on variance and bias. Bioinformatics 19(2), 185–193 (2003)
2. Demšar, J.: Statistical comparisons of classifiers over multiple data sets. The Journal of Machine Learning Research 7, 1–30 (2006)
3. Fürnkranz, J., Hüllermeier, E. (eds.): Preference Learning. Springer, Heidelberg (2010)
4. Gutkin, M., Shamir, R., Dror, G.: SlimPLS: a method for feature selection in gene expression-based disease classification. PLoS One 4(7), e6416 (2009)
5. Joachims, T.: Optimizing search engines using clickthrough data. In: Proceedings of the Eighth ACM SIGKDD International Conference on Knowledge Discovery and Data Mining, KDD 2002, pp. 133–142 (2002)
6. Liu, T.Y.: Learning to Rank for Information Retrieval. Now Publishers (2009)

Comparing Machine-Learning Classifiers in Keratoconus Diagnosis from ORA Examinations

Aydano P. Machado[1,3], João Marcelo Lyra[2,3], Renato Ambrósio Jr.[3], Guilherme Ribeiro[2,3], Luana P.N. Araújo[1,3], Camilla Xavier[3], and Evandro Costa[1,3]

[1] IC - Universidade Federal de Alagoas, Campus A. C. Simões - Av. Lourival Melo Mota, s/n, 57072-970 Maceió-AL Brazil
aydano.machado@ic.ufal.br
[2] UNCISAL - Universidade de Ciências da Saúde de Alagoas
[3] BrAIn - Brazilian Study Group of Artificial Intelligence and Corneal Analysis

Abstract. Keratoconus identification has become a step of primary importance in the preoperative evaluation for the refractive surgery. With the ophthalmology knowledge improvement, corneal physical parameters were considered important to its evaluation. The Ocular Response Analyzer (ORA) provides some physical parameters using an applanation process to measure cornea biomechanical properties. This paper presents a study of machine learning classifiers in keratoconus diagnosis from ORA examinations. As a first use of machine learning approach with ORA parameters, this research work presents a performance comparison of the main machine learning algorithms. This approach improves ORA parameters' analysis helping ophthalmologist's efficiency in clinical diagnosis.

Keywords: machine learning, keratoconus, and biomechanics.

1 Introduction

Keratoconus is a bilateral and non-inflammatory condition characterized by progressive thinning, protrusion and scarring of the cornea [1]. It can be located in the anterior and/or posterior cornea side, associated to a stromal thinning. The estimated prevalence in the general population is 1 per 1800 [2], but the increased number of eyes undergoing screening for laser refractive surgery suggests the prevalence may be higher.

With ophthalmology knowledge improvement, corneal physical parameters were considered important to its evaluation. Thus, it was arose the necessity of a dynamic analysis through the biomechanical corneal properties.

The Ocular Response Analyzer (ORA) measurement of these physical parameters has previously been reported to demonstrate good reproducibility and clinical reliability. Besides, the significance of these ORA parameters is not fully understood, and some studies have shown intersection in normal and keratoconus values of these parameters. Thus, yet, it is not possible to set a cutoff between the groups [3].

M. Peleg, N. Lavrač, and C. Combi (Eds.): AIME 2011, LNAI 6747, pp. 90–95, 2011.

There are other parameters that are not yet well studied, so an improvement in ORA parameters' analysis can make ORA more effective in clinical diagnosis. Due to the fact that, this paper brings a fresh approach to ORA parameters' analysis we put the choice on a firmer basis, based on an incremental methodology study:

- We explain how ORA works and what is currently used in clinical diagnoses (Section 2.1).
- Biomechanical corneal analysis affects the process as a whole and can open new possibilities and improves results. With this in mind, we propose a new approach in ORA parameters' analysis based on Machine Learning (ML) (Section 2.2). To the best of our knowledge, this has not been done before.
- In order to better understand how each ML algorithm contributes to problem solution and how each category of ORA parameters affects the classification process, we proposed an incremental methodology (Section 3).
- The results obtained have showed that our approach is sound (Section 4), and that we can improve ORA parameters' analysis helping ophthalmologist's efficiency in clinical diagnosis.

In terms of its impact on ORA parameters' analysis, machine learning classifiers seem superior, mainly because these algorithms can handle a substantial amount of parameters at same time, as one can see in the following sections.

2 Keratoconus Diagnosis from ORA Examinations

To set the scene for this paper, we begin with a brief overview showing of how ORA works and which parameters are really used by ophthalmologists, followed by a discussion about current difficulties and how we can help to solve them.

2.1 The Ocular Response Analyzer (ORA)

The ORA uses a dynamic bi-directional applanation process to measure the biomechanical properties of the cornea and the intraocular pressure. The ORA measurement produces a morphological signal in complex waveforms. Although they are not yet completely understood, it is clear that there is clinically valuable information contained in them [4].

The ORA uses a precisely metered collimated-air-pulse, which applies force to the cornea making it moves inwards, past applanation, and into a slight concavity. The air pump shuts off milliseconds after applanation and the pressure declines. The cornea begins to return to its normal configuration as long as the pressure decreases. An advanced electro-optical system is responsible to monitor deformations of the cornea. [4,5]

Two independent pressure values are derived from inward and outward applanation events. Due to the dynamic nature of the air pulse, the viscous damping in the cornea causes delays in these events, resulting in two different pressure values [4,5]. The difference between these two pressures is the CH, that is an indication of cornea's viscosity. The mean of these two pressures is the IOPg. IOPcc is an intraocular pressure measurement. CRF is an empirically determined parameter that is thought to represent the overall resistance of the cornea [4,5].

Only these four basic outputs (CH, IOPg, IOPcc, and CRF) of the measurement process are commonly used in clinical diagnosis. Besides, some studies have shown intersection in normal and keratoconus values of these parameters. Thus, yet, it is not possible to set a cutoff between the groups [3].

However, the ORA measurement process produces 41 outputs calculated from waveforms. So, there are 37 parameters that are not yet used in clinical diagnosis. It seems clear to us that these parameters should be thoroughly studied. Due to the number of parameters to be considered and the characterization problem, we have chosen a machine learning approach to create a classifier. This classifier can be seen as the 5th basic output of the measurement process and makes ORA more effective in clinical diagnosis.

2.2 Machine-Learning Classifiers in Keratoconus Diagnosis from ORA Examinations

The task of classification occurs in a wide range of human activity, and it represents an important process in medical care. To help with this task, predictive models are used in a variety of medical domains, including diagnostic. Machine learning algorithms can build these models based on knowledge acquired from actual cases stored in databases.

Machine learning algorithms have already been used to keratoconus detection. However they were based on image keratoconus diagnosis [6,7,8,9], which means information from imaging devices without biomechanical corneal properties. Most of them just has been used multi-layer perceptron (MLP) and anterior topographic data, only [6] added other common supervised learning methods such as support vector machine (SVM) and radial basis function neural network (RBFNN).

In this work we also included other methods like decision tree (DT), linear regression (LR) and naive Bayes (NB) in order to evaluate the performance of some of the most widely used learning algorithms in keratoconus diagnosis from ORA examinations.

The purpose of evaluate these different types of classifiers is that they have different features that will be roughly adequate to solve the current problem.

3 Experimentation Methodology

In order to better evaluate the performance of different learning algorithms, we have chosen an incremental approach to perform the first experiments. Thus, the parameters were divided into four different groups, then these groups were analyzed one by one and also combined. The groups created follow ORA logic:

- The Group P contains two pressure values. The first one (P1) is measured in the inward and the second one (P2) in the outward applanation event.

- The Group O consists of original ORA parameters, i.e. the parameters that are currently used in clinical diagnostic (IOPg, CH, CRF, and IOPcc).
- The Group C1 have information obtained from the upper 75% of the applanation peak, this groups is composed by the parameters: aindex, bindex, p1area, p2area, aspect1, aspect2, uslope1, uslope2, dslope1, dslope2, w1, w2, h1, h2, dive1, dive2, path1, path2, mslew1, mslew2, slew1, slew2, and aplhf.
- The Group C2 is derived from the upper 50% of the applanation peak and has the parameters: p1area1, p2area1, aspect11, aspect21, uslope11, uslope21 dslope11, dslope21, w11, w21, h11, h21, path11, and path21.

In a effort to understand the influence of each group in the learning process and results, these groups were analyzed separately and combined. This group combination has generated 15 different situations to be analyzed, as showed in first column of Table 1.

4 Results

The experiments have been performed on a dataset composed of 314 eyes (226 normal eyes and 88 eyes with keratoconus) examined making use of ORA. The machine learning algorithms were implemented using WEKA and RapidMiner.

The classifier's evaluation is most often based on prediction accuracy (the percentage of correct prediction divided by the total number of predictions). All experiments presented in this work were evaluated using cross-validation technique with 10 equal-sized subsets.

In order to have an idea about performance of selected learning algorithms, we have done, as a first step, a simple experiment with each one. So, we tested the algorithms mentioned in Section 2.2 on each group of Section 3.

The results of this first experiment point to C1 as the most significant group for keratoconus detection, unlike what happens in ORA examinations (where group O parameters are highlighted). Besides that, combination of group parameters improves the performance. We can say that because the best results, in these first experiments, were obtained with all groups together.

Another conclusion that can be extracted from these first results is that the neural networks algorithms (MLP and RBF) have reached the best results on average. Thus these algorithms were applied in all group combinations presented in Section 3 and the results are presented in Table 1. Aiming to provide a model with an easy interpretation by humans, we also added a decision tree algorithm. Therefore ophthalmologists may also analyze, interpret and validate the knowledge automatically learned.

Unfortunately due to space limitations, we will not be able to provide all details of our experiments like all confusion matrixes. The best results are achieved when group C1 is combined with a group that contains pressure parameters like group P and/or group O, and the best one was MLP on P + O + C1.

Table 1. Performance of DT, MLP and RBFNN algorithm on all group combinations

	DT	MLP	RBFNN
P	85.3% ±5.6%	87.2% ±6.2%	86.0% ±7.5%
O	85.0% ±6.6%	86.6% ±5.2%	87.3% ±5.8%
P + O	85.7% ±6.6%	86.0% ±4.6%	86.6% ±7.2%
C1	88.2% ±4.6%	89.8% ±6.0%	89.5% ±3.5%
C2	85.0% ±5.2%	88.2% ±4.8%	89.8% ±3.2%
C1 + C2	85.0% ±3.3%	91.7% ±3.3%	88.9% ±3.0%
O + C1	89.5% ±4.8%	93.6% ±3.2%	90.8% ±4.0%
O + C2	87.6% ±6.4%	87.3% ±5.1%	89.2% ±5.2%
O + C1 + C2	89.1% ±4.6%	92.0% ±2.9%	89.8% ±3.1%
P + C1	88.9% ±4.3%	91.4% ±3.5%	91.4% ±3.5%
P + C2	87.6% ±6.4%	91.4% ±3.5%	88.9% ±3.3%
P + C1 + C2	88.6% ±4.3%	93.3% ±3.0%	82.1% ±10.%
P + O + C1	88.8% ±5.9%	93.6% ±2.9%	90.8% ±3.3%
P + O + C2	90.8% ±6.7%	87.9% ±4.0%	90.8% ±3.3%
All	90.8% ±3.3%	92.7% ±3.2%	90.1% ±3.0%

5 Conclusion and Further Work

This paper described a first study of machine learning classifiers in keratoconus diagnosis from ORA examinations. This study compared the performance of the main machine learning algorithms using an incremental methodology. As a result, we built classifiers with 93.6% of accuracy. Other parameters that are not highlighted by ORA device analysis were considered, and they were pertinent to build the classifier. This approach proved that can benefits ophthalmologist's efficiency in clinical diagnosis.

There are three main directions for future work. First, to apply a attribute selection algorithm in order to remove as many irrelevant and redundant features as possible, removing irrelevant or redundant ORA parameter. Another important issue is to analyze the waveforms themselves, there are a lot of information that is ignored by the pre-calculated parameters. Also, this work results can be merged with a image keratoconus diagnosis method in order to build more accurate classifiers.

References

1. Belin, M.W., Krachmer, J.H., Feder, R.S.: Keratoconus and related noninflammatory corneal thinning disorders. Survey of Ophthalmology 28, 293–322 (1984)
2. Santodomingo-Rubido, J., Romero-Jimenez, M.: J.S. Wolffsohn. Keratoconus: A review. Contact Lens & Anterior Eye 23, 157–166 (2010)
3. Jardim, D., Fontes, B.M., Ambrosio Jr., R., et al.: Corneal biomechanical metrics and anterior segment parameters in mild keratoconus. Ophthalmology, 673–679 (2010)

4. Luce, D.A.: Determining in vivo biomechanical properties of the cornea with an ocular response analyzer. Journal of Cataract and Refractive Surgery 31, 156–162 (2006)
5. Choi, J.S., Oh, J.Y., Kim, M.K., Lee, J.H., Shin, J.Y., Wee, W.R.: Evaluation of corneal biomechanical properties following penetrating keratoplasty using the ocular response analyzer. Korean Journal of Ophthalmology 24, 139–142 (2010)
6. Souza, M.B., Medeiros, F.W., Souza, D.B., Garcia, R., Alves, M.R.: Evaluation of machine learning classifiers in keratoconus detection from orbscan ii examinations. Clinics 65, 1223–1228 (2010)
7. Smolek, M.K., Thompson, H., Maeda, N., Klyce, S.: Automated keratoconus screening with corneal topography analysis. Invest. Ophthalmol. Vis. Sci. 35(6), 2749–2757 (1994)
8. Pensiero, S., Accardo, P.: Neural network-based system for early keratoconus detection from corneal topography. J. Biomed. Inform. 35(3), 151–159 (2002)
9. Smolek, M.K., Klyce, S.D., Karon, M.D.: Screening patients with the corneal navigator. Journal Refractive Surgery 21(5 Suppl), 617–622 (2005)

HRVFrame: Java-Based Framework for Feature Extraction from Cardiac Rhythm

Alan Jovic and Nikola Bogunovic

Department of Electronics, Microelectronics, Computer and Intelligent Systems, Faculty of Electrical Engineering and Computing, University of Zagreb, Unska 3, 10000 Zagreb, Croatia
{alan.jovic,nikola.bogunovic}@fer.hr

Abstract. Heart rate variability (HRV) analysis can be successfully applied to automatic classification of cardiac rhythm abnormalities. This paper presents a novel Java-based computer framework for feature extraction from cardiac rhythms. The framework called HRVFrame implements more than 30 HRV linear time domain, frequency domain, time-frequency domain, and nonlinear features. Output of the framework in the form of .arff files enables easier medical knowledge discovery via platforms such as RapidMiner or Weka. The scope of the framework facilitates comparison of models for different cardiac disorders. Some of the features implemented in the framework can also be applied to other biomedical time-series. The thorough approach to feature extraction pursued in this work is also encouraged for other types of biomedical time-series.

Keywords: heart rate variability; computer framework; nonlinear features.

1 Introduction

Analysis of cardiac abnormalities usually starts with routine diagnostic procedure called electrocardiogram (ECG). Detection of anomalies in an ECG can indicate the existence of cardiovascular and other diseases [1]. Heart rate variability (HRV) analysis examines fluctuations in the sequence of cardiac interbeat (RR) intervals. In cardiac rhythm research there is a problem with the selection of features for optimal arrhythmia description, because of the infinite dimensionality of the feature space. Therefore, researchers base their work either on physiological explicability of the features or on proven mathematical properties of the time-series. Both of these approaches do not guarantee that the entire feature space had been searched.

HRV features can be grouped in several categories depending on the type of the time-series' analysis needed to be performed for their extraction. These include: linear, time-frequency, nonlinear features, and rhythm pattern analysis [2,3,4].

Linear time and frequency domain features include statistical properties of the heart rhythm and power spectral density estimates in clinically relevant frequency bands [2]. Time-frequency features are useful for finding nonstationarities in cardiac rhythm. The time-frequency methods mostly employed for arrhythmia detection from ECG and HRV time-series include discrete and continuous wavelet transforms [5].

M. Peleg, N. Lavrač, and C. Combi (Eds.): AIME 2011, LNAI 6747, pp. 96–100, 2011.

Numerous nonlinear features can be grouped into three categories: chaos and phase space quantification features, entropy-based features and other nonlinear features.

There are several programs known to us that implement some of the features used in the HRV analysis: ECGLab [6], KARDIA [7], and HRV Analysis Software [8]. In this work, we develop a novel framework for HRV analysis called HRVFrame that implements most of the previously mentioned features for HRV analysis. The framework is intended to act as a bridge between cardiac rhythm data records and medical knowledge discovery. The strong point of the framework is the number of implemented features, which allows researchers to easily compare the results with other authors. Our framework is still a work in progress, albeit at an advanced stage. From scientific perspective, the framework has been evaluated in a number of successful cardiac disorder classification tasks [9,10].

2 Framework Overview

HRVFrame is an extensive Java-based framework containing many features covered in the HRV analysis literature. Its main purpose is data preparation – it is used to extract features from cardiac rhythm records and store them as feature vectors prepared for further knowledge discovery. At present, the process of feature extraction is performed offline and the framework has not been integrated in any particular knowledge-based platform. The whole process of cardiac rhythm records analysis using HRVFrame is shown in Fig. 1. HRVFrame is organized into three major logical parts: input, feature calculation, and output.

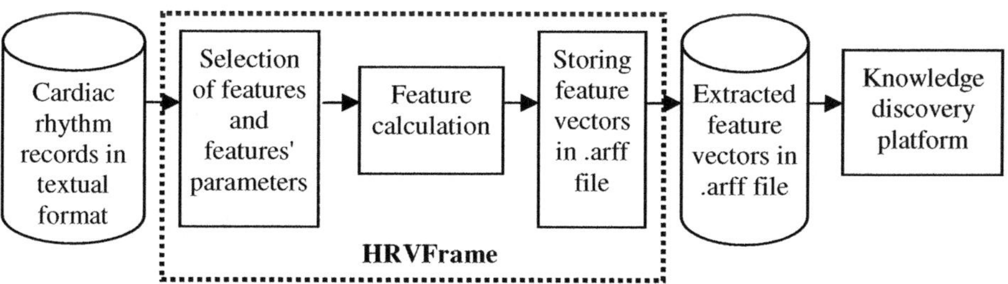

Fig. 1. Cardiac rhythm analysis using the HRVFrame computer framework

2.1 Data Input

The input part of the framework is designed to take cardiac rhythm records, to allow the selection of features and specification of features' parameters. Cardiac rhythm records in the form of textual ASCII files are acceptable as input files. The input file structure is the same as the one provided by the PhysioNet tool *rdann* [11]. The files should contain the information on the times of R peaks, types of beats, and optional rhythm annotations. All beat and rhythm annotations used in PhysioBank databases are supported by the framework. Also acceptable is the input format where only R peak times are known. Some features have parameters that determine the calculation procedure. Currently, the framework accepts a list of desired features and their parameters as arguments through a command line interface. Visual interface for feature and parameter selection is planned in the future. HRVFrame also accepts the list of cardiac rhythm files intended for analysis. Other system specifications include: start time or starting interval, end time or ending interval, RR interval series output, RR interval differences output, learning segment types from beats, etc. Features intended for extraction have to be specified by the researcher, currently there is no intelligent selection of appropriate features with respect to analyzed disorders or segment lengths, mainly because this area is still under research.

2.2 Feature Calculation and Output

HRVFrame is used to calculate values for the specified HRV features. The list of currently supported features is given in Table 1. A thorough search of the available literature was performed that resulted in implementation of most of the features applied in HRV research. Features are calculated for one record segment at a time.

The framework allows users to first create an .arff file that only contains the declaration of features. After the feature calculation process is complete, the framework creates output feature vectors and stores them in the .arff file. Data are appended to the end of the file as long as the new segments and records are continued to be analyzed. The .arff file can then be used by several data mining and knowledge discovery platforms like Weka [16] and RapidMiner [17] for disorder classification.

Table 1. Features implemented in the HRVFrame framework

Feature(s)	Category	Parameters
Mean; SDNN; RMSSD; SDANN; SDSD; pNN*X*; Fano factor; Allan factor; HRV triangular index; TINN; Total PSD; ULF; VLF; LF; HF; LF/HF [2,5]	Linear, time and frequency	SDANN: number of segments; pNN*X*: miliseconds *X*; Fano and Allan factor: counting time; Fast Fourier Transform; window (Hanning, Hamming, none); Burg AR model; model order
Discrete Haar wavelet standard deviation [5]	Time-frequency	Scale
Largest Lyapunov exponent; correlation dimension; spatial filling index; central tendency measure; SD1/SD2; CSI, CVI; sequential trend analysis [4,5,6,12]	Nonlinear - phase space	Embedding dimension, trajectory length, lag
Detrended fluctuation analysis (DFA) α_1, α_2; Hurst exponent; Higuchi's fractal dimension [5,13]	Nonlinear - fractal estimates	Higuchi's kmax
Entropies: approximate (ApEn), sample (SampEn), multiscale sample (MSampEn), Rényi, spectral [4,14]	Nonlinear - entropy	ApEn, (M)SampEn: embedding dimension, radius, maximum (Y/N); Rényi: order; spectral: frequency band
Multiscale asymmetry index [15]	Other	Scale

3 Related Work and Framework Applications

ECGLab [6] and KARDIA [7] are Matlab-based tools for ECG and HRV analysis. Both tools extract some of the simple linear time and frequency domain features. In addition, current version of ECGLab implements time-frequency features, and KARDIA implements DFA scaling analysis. Both tools lack direct implementation of more recent nonlinear HRV features and depend on Matlab for execution. HRV Analysis Software [8] is freely-available Windows software with support for basic HRV analysis (linear and SD1/SD2 features) and is not intended for scientific data exploration, but rather as a decision support system for medical professionals.

The main application of HRVFrame is in cardiac data preparation for automated classification tasks. HRVFrame is oriented toward scientific exploration of different feature combinations for optimal models of cardiac abnormalities. It can be used for result comparison from different authors and for investigation of the research results reported by the authors. It should be however noted that this type of analysis requires that the protocol was clearly stated by the authors and that the used data is publicly available, which is often not a case. The framework can be used both for the analysis of cardiac disorders and for cardiac rhythm description in each record segment with arrhythmia detection in mind [10]. The framework always designates one rhythm type per segment based on rhythm priority, which can be specified by the user.

HRVFrame contains many features used by researchers in HRV analysis. It is interesting that the majority of the features are not specific for cardiac rhythm analysis and can be used in the analysis of other biomedical series (ECG, EEG, EMG, gait, skin resistance...). Application of our framework in non-cardiac domain is possible, e.g. if one investigates couplings between several different biomedical time-series.

Biomedical data analysis presents significant scientific challenges. Finding the appropriate feature combination for cardiac disorder detection and description is difficult. It includes both obtaining a significant number of feature vectors for valid conclusions as well as finding the optimal feature selection method and classifier models for each diagnosis. Any efficient and accurate methodology that would perform such a task would have to rely on a carefully selected subset of appropriate domain features. It would also need to integrate a number of features from diverse biomedical time series. Constructing thorough frameworks such as HRVFrame for each biomedical domain might be a favorable way for accomplishing such a task.

The current version of the framework is available free-of-charge, and only for non-commercial, scientific purposes. The framework is not open source at the moment. Please contact the author by e-mail: alan.jovic@fer.hr for further instructions.

4 Conclusion

A novel framework for HRV analysis is presented in this work. The framework allows researchers to thoroughly analyze cardiac rhythm records with different linear and nonlinear features and their combinations. It can be used in the analysis of cardiac disorders, arrhythmias, and in other biomedical domains. The main advantage of the framework compared to the existing solutions lies in the larger number of implemented HRV features and features' parameters. Future work will be focused on improving the interface of the framework and on implementation of other existing nonlinear methods for cardiac rhythm analysis.

References

1. Garcia, T.B., Holtz, N.E.: 12-Lead ECG: The Art of Interpretation. Jones and Bartlett Publishers, Sudbury (2001)
2. Malik, M., Bigger, J.T., Camm, A.J., Kleiger, R.E., Malliani, A., Moss, A.J., Schwartz, P.J.: Heart rate variability guidelines: Standards of measurement, physiological interpretation, and clinical use. Eur. Heart J. 17(3), 354–381 (1996)
3. Yang, A.C.-C., Hseu, S.-S., Yien, H.-W., Goldberger, A.L., Peng, C.-K.: Linguistic Analysis of the Human Heartbeat Using Frequency and Rank Order Statistics. Phys. Rev. Lett. 90(10), 108103 (2003)
4. Acharya, R.U., Joseph, K.P., Kannathal, N., Lim, C.M., Suri, J.S.: Heart rate variability: a review. Med. Bio. Eng. Comput. 44, 1031–1051 (2006)
5. Teich, M.C., Lowen, S.B., Jost, B.M., Vibe-Rheymer, K., Heneghan, C.: Heart-Rate Variability: Measures and Models. In: Akay, M. (ed.) Nonlinear Biomedical Signal Processing. Dynamic Analysis and Modeling, vol. II, ch. 6, pp. 159–213. IEEE Press, New York (2001)
6. de Carvalho, J.L.A., da Rocha, A.F., Nascimento, F.A.O., Neto, J.S., Junqueira, L.F.: Development of Matlab Software for Analysis of Heart Rate Variability. In: Proc. 6th Int. Conf. Sig. Proc. ICSP 2002, pp. 1488–1491. IEEE Press, Beijing (2002)
7. Perakakis, P., Joffily, M., Taylor, M., Guerra, P., Vila, J.: KARDIA: A Matlab software for the analysis of cardiac interbeat intervals. Comp. Meth. Prog. Biomed. 98, 83–89 (2010)
8. Niskanen, J.-P., Tarvainen, M.P., Ranta-aho, P.O., Karjalainen, P.A.: Software for advanced HRV analysis. Comp. Meth. Prog. Biomed. 76, 73–81 (2004)
9. Jovic, A., Bogunovic, N.: Random Forest-Based Classification of Heart Rate Variability Signals by Using Combinations of Linear and Nonlinear Features. In: Bamidis, P.D., Pallikarakis, N. (eds.) Proc. XII Mediterranean Conf. Medical and Biological Engineering and Computing MEDICON 2010, pp. 29–32. Springer, Berlin (2010)
10. Jovic, A., Bogunovic, N.: Electrocardiogram analysis using a combination of statistical, geometric, and nonlinear heart rate variability features. Artif. Intell. Med. (in press), doi:10.1016/j.artmed.2010.09.005
11. PhysioNet tool rdann, `http://www.physionet.org/tutorials/physiobank-text.shtml#ann`
12. Faust, O., Acharya, R.U., Krishnan, S.M., Min, L.C.: Analysis of cardiac signals using spatial filling index and time-frequency domain. BioMedical Engineering OnLine 3, 30 (2004)
13. Peng, C.-K., Havlin, S., Stanley, H.E., Goldberger, A.L.: Quantification of scaling exponents and crossover phenomena in nonstationary heartbeat time series. Chaos 5(1), 82–87 (1995)
14. Costa, M., Goldberger, A.L., Peng, C.-K.: Multiscale entropy analysis of biological signals. Phys. Rev. E 71, 021906 (2005)
15. Costa, M., Goldberger, A.L., Peng, C.-K.: Broken asymmetry of the human heartbeat: Loss of time irreversibility in aging and disease. Phys. Rev. Lett. 95, 198102 (2005)
16. Witten, I.H., Frank, E.: Data mining: Practical machine learning tools and techniques. Morgan Kaufmann, San Francisco (2011)
17. RapidMiner, `http://rapid-i.com/content/view/181/190/`

Lessons Learned from Implementing and Evaluating Computerized Decision Support Systems

Saeid Eslami[1], Nicolette F de Keizer[1], Evert de Jonge[2], Dave Dongelmans[3], Marcus J. Schultz[3,4], and Ameen Abu–Hanna[1]

Academic Medical Center, University of Amsterdam,
P.O. Box 22660, 1100 DD, Amsterdam, The Netherlands:
[1] Department of Medical Informatics
[3] Department of Intensive Care
[4] Laboratory of Experimental Intensive Care and Anesthesiology
Leiden University Medical Center, P.O. Box 9600 RC, Leiden, The Netherlands:
[2] Department of Intensive Care
n.f.keizer@amc.uva.n, e.de_jonge@lumc.nl,
{s.eslami,d.a.dongelmans,m.j.schultz,a.abu-hanna}@amc.uva.nl

Abstract. A potentially effective IT intervention to implement guidelines and evidence based practice consists of the use of computerized decision support systems (CDSS). CDSSs aim at providing meaningful feedback to professionals in order to positively influence their behavior. Intensive care medicine, with its heavy reliance on information and the advanced information infrastructure in intensive care units (ICUs), is an attractive specialty and environment for applying and investigating CDSSs. In particular, antibiotic prescription, control of the tidal volumes in the lungs, and control of glucose levels in the blood form hot topics in intensive care medicine and provide opportunities for decision support applications. However, issues pertaining to the design, implementation, critical success factors, as well as the evaluation of CDSSs are largely still open, especially in these domains. This work describes important issues learned from designing and implementing CDSSs in these domains based on our literature reviews and lessons learned from conducting various trials in our ICU.

Keywords: Computerized Decision Support Systems, Intensive Care Units, lesson learned.

1 Introduction

Information technology (IT) is increasingly used to address information problems in medicine. A particularly interesting IT intervention to implement guidelines and evidence based practice is the use of computerized decision support systems (CDSS) that provide meaningful feedback to professionals in order to influence their behavior. CDSSs are computer programs that are intended to support healthcare workers in making their decisions [1].

Intensive care units provide life-sustaining therapies, but are also a place where harm lurks [2]. ICUs are highly complex environments in which clinicians make

M. Peleg, N. Lavrač, and C. Combi (Eds.): AIME 2011, LNAI 6747, pp. 101–108, 2011.

time-pressured decisions for patients with limited physiological reserve. This combination of conditions makes intensive care at times risky for critically ill patients.

Therefore ICU forms an important area for CDSS implementation. However, issues pertaining to their design, implementation, critical success factors, as well as their evaluation are largely still open. This work describes six important issues for designing and implementing computerized decision support systems for the ICU tasks of blood glucose control, tidal volume control, and antibiotic prescription. We draw on our literature reviews and lessons learned during conducting trials that we designed and implemented in these domains.

In the rest of this paper, we describe the ICU setting and the three CDSS studies along with the specific issues pertaining to these studies. Next we provide a discussion of lessons learned and conclude the paper.

2 Study Description

2.1 Setting

In our "closed–format" ICU, all types of critically ill patients are under the direct care of the ICU–team. The ICU–team comprises 10 full–time intensivists, 8 subspecialty fellows, 20 residents and occasionally 1 intern. On average, more than 1500 patients are admitted per year and more than 60,000 orders are prescribed each month. Since 2002, the ward started using a commercial Patient Data Management System (PDMS). The PDMS is a point-of-care Clinical Information System, which runs on a Microsoft Windows platform and includes computerized order entry, automatic data collection, clinical documentation, electronic medication administration record, some clinical decision support and a data storage repository. The ICU–teams use the PDMS to complete all patient charting and documentation such that no information has paper as its primary storage mechanism. This commercial system is used in more than 100 large hospitals around the world.

2.2 Study One: Default Dose for Aminoglycosides [3]

In our system, like many other computerized physician order entry (CPOE) systems, when a drug is selected and a dosage is to be entered, the system displays an initial patient-nonspecific default dose value that can be selected or otherwise overridden. Regardless of the choice of this default, it will always stay a constant that is not related to the patient's specific situation. In this sub-study we focused on the narrow-therapeutic range and hence potentially dangerous, antibacterial medications Gentamycin and Tobramycin. For almost all drugs, and especially for dangerous and narrow-therapeutic range ones, there are special prescribing guidelines that have to be followed. One important section of these guidelines is dose adjustment, which contains the recommended dose mainly based on the patient's ideal body weight and renal function. In our ICU a dose adjustment guideline based on ideal body weight and renal function is available on paper and on the hospital Intranet, but not yet formalized in a CDSS. To understand ordering behavior we investigated the effects of a CPOE system that displayed an initial default dose for Gentamycin and Tobramycin administration, which can be regarded as a simple form of CDSS, on the frequency of medication errors and potential adverse drug events (ADEs) in patients with renal insufficiency. Three hundred and ninety two prescriptions, relating to 253 patients (of whom 184 had renal insufficiency), were analyzed. A markedly high frequency of prescriptions with the default dose value (which would prove too high for renal insufficiency patients) was observed resulting in a high frequency of doses exceeding the guideline recommendation for patients with renal insufficiency. Hence initial CPOE dose values for prescribing Gentamycin and Tobramycin, which are based on a fixed (high) default value, form a source of potential ADEs. It seems that the physicians are overly trustful of the system's suggestions perhaps because of the widely reported advantages of decision support for dose adjustment. In addition, when the default dose was actually overridden it still resulted in many errors and potential ADEs. We hence learn that physicians, when unsupported, make many prescribing mistakes when overriding the default dose and do not seem to consult the paper-based guidelines.

In general, we learned that there is a need for patient-specific computerized suggestions and that there is indication that physicians would probably follow these suggestions. Software developers and patient safety investigators should be aware of the possibility of introducing new kinds of errors and eventually leading to more complex problems by introducing a computerized system. Therefore evaluation of DSS implementations is an imperative task to uncover unintended effects.

2.3 Study Two: Adherence to Tidal Volume Recommendations [4]

Mechanical ventilation with high tidal volumes may induce or aggravate lung injury in critical ill patients. A guideline on tidal volume, for lung protection is available in paper form and on intranet in our ICU. It simply specifies that the tidal volume (VT) should not exceed 6 ml/kg of the predicted body weight (PBW). PBW is calculated as 50in men or 45.5in women + 0.91* (centimeters of height – 152.4). One regards PBW because it is better correlated with the volume of the lungs than the actual body weight is. We implemented the guideline into a CDSS and conducted two studies to investigate the effect of this CDSS on adherence to a tidal volume guideline that was in place.

The first study4, a prospective before–after evaluation, implied that once a day the CDSS showed the recommended tidal volume in a pop–up window irrespective of the actually applied tidal volume. This was done for each patient connected to a ventilator at the bedside or on the computer screen of the physicians' working room. This patient–specific recommendation appeared only the first time on each day that an ICU–physician or ICU–nurse selects the "respiratory page" in the PDMS which shows all respiratory–related settings and results. Clinicians cannot change the mechanical ventilation setting through the PDMS but they usually first check the respiratory–related settings and results on the respiratory page in the PDMS and then, if necessary, change the setting on the machine. Therefore clicking on the respiratory page seems to be the best point for supporting the clinician or nurse. The pop-up window could be closed by a button, otherwise it would disappear within 15 seconds. In order to not disturb the stabilization process, the abovementioned messages were not shown in the first 2 hours after admission. A total of 3,663,674 VT records of 696 patients were analyzed. We showed that the use of a computerized decision support system, integrated in a patient data management system, does improve implementation of a lower tidal volume mechanical ventilation strategy for patients ventilated >24 hours.

The second study had a prospective off–on–off–on design. The study evaluated the effect of an active consulting vs. critiquing computerized decision support system on adherence to VT recommendations. Implemented active consulting CDSS in this study was a slightly modified version of the above described system in the first phase of this study. In the critiquing phase, when an ICU–physician or ICU–nurse selects the "respiratory page" in the PDMS, the recorded VT during the previous 60 minutes were queried. The system calculated the percentage of time that VT was above the guideline recommended VT. Only when VT was above the guideline recommended VT for more than 25% (15 minutes) of the previous 60 minutes, a pop–up window was shown displaying the guideline, patient's height, gender, PBW, as well as the percentage of time in which VT was above 6 ml/kg PBW.

In conducting these tidal volume studies one better appreciates the importance of addressing the questions below pertaining to the when, where and how clinicians should be supported.

2.3.1 When and Where

In a medication oriented process the time of ordering forms an appropriate trigger point for decision support. However, there is no such clear trigger point for the tidal volume adjustment CDSS for tidal volume. VT adjustment is a continuous process and repeatedly performed during the period that the patient is mechanically ventilated. In ICUs like ours, which do not have central monitoring rooms, a fixed triggering time is not appropriate because one cannot assure that a clinician is at the bedside and that he/she is logged in the system at a predefined time. In this way many alerts will be missed and, worse yet, one might not know if this was the case. The event of logging in and clicking the ventilation tab in the PDMS provide another triggering moment. Logging in was not selected as a triggering point because perhaps the clinicians log in to check other clinical parameters than ventilation, in which case showing VT related messages would be annoying. The respiratory page in the PDMS showed all respiratory–related settings and results. Clinicians usually click on the respiratory page to check the currently applied VT and therefore adjust the VT if necessary. Our message appeared at this moment. However one cannot be sure that the clinicians actually check the respiratory tab at all or only when they feel it is necessary to do so.

2.3.2 How: Critiquing vs. Consulting CDSS

Developing, integrating and maintaining a critiquing CDSS, which provides feedback based on a comparison between a physician's behavior with a guideline, is more complicated and technically demanding than a consulting CDSS. Therefore, when equally effective, the consulting mode seems to be more practical and generalizable. A potential advantage of active critiquing systems, in contrast, may be that they do not provide unnecessary "support". This might increase the acceptance of healthcare workers and thereby increase the effect of the CDSS. On the other hand, in the critiquing style, launching an alert is based on an assessment whether the physicians are adhering to the guideline or not but it is unclear how to verify the adherence status. If we used different definitions of adequate adherence to the guideline (for example when VT was above the guideline recommended VT for more than 35% instead of 25% of the previous 60 minutes) our results would have differed. This underlies the importance of performing a sensitivity analysis to scrutinize the effects of adherence thresholds (used to trigger the feedback) on the resulting adherence. In addition, we note that in our patients the mean of excess VT was already relatively low before using the CDSS. Therefore there was a limited room for improvement. Hence it is fair to hypothesize that the effect of a CDSS in situations where larger VT is being applied could be much higher than in our patients.

2.4 Study Three: Glucose Regulation

Glucose regulation is a hot item in intensive care. A majority of glucose regulation guidelines, like the one in our ICU, recommend insulin dosage and time of next blood glucose measurement according to patient previous blood glucose levels and response to treatment. In two systematic reviews, we showed that there is no uniform indicator set (e.g. mean blood glucose, percentage of hypoglycemia etc.) of glucose regulation used in the reviewed studies [5], [6], [7]. Most indicators, in addition, differed in their definitions among the studies, although they are all meant to measure the same underlying concept. Thus reproducibility and comparability of research results are hampered by this lack of unambiguous definitions. The choice of quality indicators used was not explicitly motivated in any of the studies and this raises the possibility that reporting bias was at play: researchers could have reported only the indicators which significantly changed from the baseline. We also showed that while most studies evaluating the effect of CDSS on the quality of the tight glycemic control (TGC) process did find improvement when evaluated on the basis of the quality indicators used, it is impossible to define the exact success factors, because nearly all studies simultaneously implemented the CDSS with a new or modified glucose control guideline [5]. In addition there were hybrid solutions used to integrate the CDSS into the clinical workflow.

3 Discussion and Lessons Learned

The projects performed during the last years taught us how complex CDSS implementation can be and the absence of an agreed upon methodology or best practices for designing these systems. It is imperative that one had to carefully decide which specific care process needs, and perceived as needing, improvement and is suitable for CDSS application. One has also to take many measures to guarantee the safety of the ICT intervention: not every intervention (like the default dose in our antibiotics study) is beneficial. To optimize the success chances of the implementation, one has to integrate the CDSS with the current workflow and the existing technical infrastructure not only to facilitate the implementation of the system but also to facilitate the analysis of the data. For example, the respiratory machine is not integrated in the PDMS, making it hard to define the best triggering point or to verify that the operator had the exposure to the CDSS's feedback. We address these issues below.

3.1 Lesson One: Applicability

The selection of a clinical practice for CDSS development should be based on a perceived necessity as well as applicability. The existence of a guideline which describes how the clinical practice should be organized is a first prerequisite. The selected clinical guideline should be widely accepted by users and the level of adherence to them should show room for improvement. With this condition one could hypothesize that the CDSS could improve adherence to the guideline and therefore improve the safety and quality of care. But this is not the whole story. Formalization of the selected guideline into a formal, specifically a computer language, should be possible and the necessary data used in the guideline should be available in a structured and standardized (coded) way. For example, in our academic medical center antibiogram results were only available in free text and extracting the preferred and most effective antibiotic to support the physician's antibiotic therapy would be difficult and hazardous (guaranteeing safety becomes a major issue). As another example, the tidal volume strategy is especially recommended for patients with an acute lung injury (ALI) or acute respiratory distress syndrome (ARDS) diagnosis. But diagnosing ALI/ARDS is often challenging and difficult. As ALI/ARDS diagnoses were not available in the PDMS, we could not show the message explicitly for these patients. The selection of the CDSS mode, supporting level and communication style also depend on technical issues and data availability. If VT for example was not sufficiently repeatedly recorded, a critiquing CDSS implementation would not be possible as it would be practically impossible to tell whether there is adherence to the guideline at the time of CDSS triggering.

3.2 Lesson Two: Safety of Safety Approach

One should avoid the introduction of new kinds of errors by implementing CDSSs. A wrong suggestion, e.g. the default dose for aminoglycosides or low tidal volumes while the patients are severely suffering from low arterial O2 and high CO2, could introduce new kinds of errors and hence result in potential ADEs. It is important to ensure that the specification of a system accurately reflects the real needs of the users of that system [8]. Even when the specifications of a CDSS are accurate, still the system could be unsafe. Therefore it is important to understand the risks faced by the system and generate dependability requirements to cope with these risks. A recommended way to cope with the safety of the software, which we followed, is to draw a fault tree, clearly define all possible risks in these fault categories, explain the effects and find the best way to manage them. After implementation, the system should also carefully be monitored. An error logging system should be implemented by the developers and regularly controlled. As an example, in our tidal volume adjustment critiquing CDSS, possible communication problems between the CDSS and the mechanical ventilation database (where VT measurements reside) at the time of triggering form a risk. If communication problems happen, the adherence level to the guideline cannot be assessed because the latest tidal volumes are not accessible. For these situations we decided to inform the users about the communication problem and just showed, in a consulting mode, the guideline recommended VT.

3.3 Lesson Three: Technical Aspects

There are several technical issues which should be systematically considered when a CDSS is developed. When a CDSS is integrated with other systems, determining which system has priority is an important issue. In case of any unexpected problem in the CDSS, developers should define which system has higher priority, and hence should take over. The system should be designed in a way that the most important system always continues to work. Connections to the databases also should be defined in the most secure way and should not slow down and reduce the performance of the host system. Especially when running a query to extract data from a database is time consuming, the best approach is recording the data in a second database and just adding the new data to it to be ready for each new request. In the testing phase, the CDSS usually is tested on one workstation. But when employed in practice, it usually works on a network; therefore the data are possibly queried from more than one station at the same time. This should be considered in the development phase. Any problem in the CDSS and the host system may influence the net effect and acceptance of and trust in the system.

3.4 Lesson Four: Integration

To reach an optimal effect, the CDSS should be integrated into the existing clinical workflows9. It should exploit the knowledge for clinical decision making at the point of care. The question is however what is the best place and time for presenting the information to the user. More research is needed to investigate the most appropriate implementation location (bedside, nursing station etc.), target user and time of advice. However, based on local circumstances such as technical infrastructure, developers should select the most efficient place and time for supporting the user. For example, we analyzed the VT adjustment workflow in our ICU and decided to show a message when an ICU–physician or ICU–nurse clicks on the "respiratory page" in the PDMS. In other ICUs with different circumstances, possibly other triggering points should be selected.

3.5 Lesson Five: Evaluation Issues

In performing an evaluation study one should attempt to isolate the effect of the CDSS and be aware of transition periods before the behavior of care professionals arrives at a steady state. Simultaneous implementation of the CDSS with a new or modified guideline blurs the effect of the system. One should hence isolate the effect of the CDSS from the underlying guideline. One should also be aware that introducing the CDSS may imply a transition phase in which users go through a learning curve and/or some structural changes in the long term. This highlights the importance of monitoring the effect of the system over time. We endorse the use of time series analysis, such as statistical process control, to scrutinize effects over time. These approaches may reveal transition periods in adherence to guidelines.

3.6 Lesson Six: Quality Indicators

Uniform, unambiguous and well-motivated quality indicators should be used for evaluating the effect of the CDSS. The choice of quality indicators used should be explicitly motivated. Whenever possible, surrogate indicators should be replaced by true outcomes, such as mortality or morbidity. For example, in antibiotic therapy the true outcome indicators may be mortality and bed-days, with appropriate antibiotic as a surrogate outcome with a strong proven relation to mortality. The level of adherence to guideline is a weaker choice unless the relation between adherence to guideline and outcome was previously proven.

Our review on blood glucose control indicators we showed that this was not the case, raising concerns for reporting bias (that is, reporting the indicators which were associated with significant changes).

4 Conclusion

In conclusion, our experience shows that decision support systems can indeed have an important role in increasing adhering to guidelines but that their employment in practice is far from trivial. We have gained a lot of insight into their design and effects and learned various lessons that we share in this paper with other interested parties.

References

1. Shortliffe, E.H.: Computer programs to support clinical decision making. JAMA 258, 61–66 (1987)
2. Marcucci, L., Martinez, E.A., Haut, E.R., Slonim, A.D., Suarez, J.I.: Avoiding common ICU errors. Wolters Kluwer/Lippincott Williams & Williams, Philadelphia (2007)
3. Eslami, S., Abu-Hanna, A., de Keizer, N.F., de Jonge, E.: Errors associated with applying decision support by suggesting default doses for aminoglycosides. Drug Saf. 29, 803–809 (2006)
4. Eslami, S., de Keizer, N.F., Abu-Hanna, A., de Jonge, E., Schultz, M.J.: Effect of a clinical decision support system on adherence to a lower tidal volume mechanical ventilation strategy. J. Crit. Care 24, 523–529 (2009)
5. Eslami, S., Abu-Hanna, A., de Jonge, E., de Keizer, N.F.: Tight glycemic control and computerized decision-support systems: a systematic review. Intensive Care Med. 35, 1505–1517 (2009)
6. Eslami, S., de Keizer, N.F., de Jonge, E., Schultz, M.J., Abu-Hanna, A.: A systematic review on quality indicators for tight glycaemic control in critically ill patients: need for an unambiguous indicator reference subset. Crit. Care 12, R139 (2008)
7. Eslami, S., Taherzadeh, Z., Schultz, M.J., Abu-Hanna, A.: Glucose variability measures and their effect on mortality: a systematic review. Intensive Care Med. 37, 583–593 (2011)
8. Sommerville, I.: Software engineering, 8th edn. Addison Wesley, Reading (2006)
9. Kawamoto, K., Houlihan, C.A., Balas, E.A., Lobach, D.F.: Improving clinical practice using clinical decision support systems: a systematic review of trials to identify features critical to success. BMJ 330, 765 (2005)

CARDSS: Development and Evaluation of a Guideline Based Decision Support System for Cardiac Rehabilitation

Niels Peek[1], Rick Goud[2], Nicolette de Keizer[1], Mariëtte van Engen-Verheul[1], Hareld Kemps[1,3], and Arie Hasman[1]

[1] Dept. of Medical Informatics, Academic Medical Center, University of Amsterdam, The Netherlands
[2] Gupta Strategists, Ophemert, The Netherlands
[3] Maxima Medisch Centrum, Veldhoven, The Netherlands
n.b.peek@amc.uva.nl

Abstract. Cardiac rehabilitation is a multidisciplinary therapy aimed at recovery and secondary prevention after hospitalization for cardiac incidents (such as myocardial infarctions) and cardiac interventions (such as heart surgery). To stimulate implementation of the national guidelines, an electronic patient record system with computerised decision support functionalities called CARDSS (cardiac rehabilitation decision support system) was developed, and made available to Dutch rehabilitation clinics. The system was quantitatively evaluated in a cluster randomised trial at 31 clinics, and qualitatively by interviewing 29 users of the system. Computerised decision support was found to improve guideline concordance by increasing professional knowledge of preferred practice, by reducing inertia to previous practice, and by reducing guideline complexity. It was not effective when organizational or procedural changes were required that users considered to be beyond their responsibilities.

Keywords: clinical decision support systems, guideline implementation, cardiac rehabilitation.

1 Introduction

One of the main challenges in contemporary health care is to increase the application of sound clinical evidence to routine care [1]. The development and implementation of clinical practice guidelines is considered essential for this purpose. But although clinical practice guidelines are designed to promote effectiveness and discourage the use of ineffective treatments, adherence to guidelines in practice is often poor [1,2]. Dissemination of practice guidelines on paper alone has generally proved to be insufficient. Instead, carefully designed methods for change are usually required for effective implementation of guidelines [3,4].

Computerised decision support (CDS) to individual professionals at the point of care is one of the most effective methods of improving clinical decision making [1,3,4,5]. It has been shown to improve the decisions of individual professionals in

M. Peleg, N. Lavrač, and C. Combi (Eds.): AIME 2011, LNAI 6747, pp. 109–118, 2011.

screening for cancer, in vaccination, in management of diabetes, for ordering (laboratory) tests, and in other settings [6]. However, CDS has also failed to improve practitioners' performance [5,6]. There still remain many questions about the circumstances and settings in which it is optimally effective [6].

This paper describes the development and evaluation of CARDSS, an electronic patient record system with guideline based CDS functionalities. CARDSS was developed to stimulate implementation of the Dutch national guidelines for cardiac rehabilitation, by encouraging professional teams to harmonize their treatment decisions with these guidelines. The system was used in approx. 40 Dutch rehabilitation clinics, and it was evaluated in a cluster randomised trial at 31 clinics and by interviewing 29 end-users. Sec. 2 gives a brief overview of cardiac rehabilitation and the Dutch guidelines in this field; Sec. 3 describes guideline modeling, development, and pilot testing of the CARDSS system. Sec. 4 describes the results of the two evaluation studies. Sec. 5, finally, discusses and integrates the various findings and presents an outlook to future developments.

2 The Dutch Guidelines on Cardiac Rehabilitation

Cardiac rehabilitation (CR) is a multidisciplinary therapy for outpatient recovery after hospitalization for cardiac incidents (such as myocardial infarctions) and cardiac interventions (such as heart surgery) [7]. A typical CR programme lasts for 6-12 weeks, and may consist of exercise training, relaxation and stress management training, education about the disease and its consequences, lifestyle change interventions, and psychosocial counseling, mostly provided in group therapy. The aim of CR is to ensure that patients are in the best possible physical and psychosocial condition to return to and maintain their normal place in society and to reduce their future cardiovascular risk [8]. To this end, CR teams usually include physical therapists, nurses, psychologists, dietitians, social workers, rehabilitation physicians, and cardiologists. CR has been shown to be cost effective by reducing future medical consumption [7]. However, in many Western countries CR practice is poorly standardised and does not follow the available scientific evidence [9].

To stimulate evidence based CR services, the Netherlands Heart Foundation (a patients' interest organisation) and the Netherlands Society for Cardiology (a professional organisation) published national guidelines for CR in 2004 [10]. These guidelines state that patients should be offered an individualised rehabilitation programme, built up from four possible group-based therapies (exercise training, relaxation and stress management training, education therapy, and lifestyle change therapy) and if needed, different forms of individual counseling (e.g. by physical therapists, psychotherapists, or dietitians). Patients should only receive therapies and forms of counseling that they really need, and not others. For instance, to decide whether a patient should receive exercise training, the patient's desired level of exercise capacity should be compared with the results of a maximal exercise capacity test. Compared to earlier guidelines from the mid 1990s, relaxation and stress management training and lifestyle change interventions were additions to the CR therapy bundle, and many clinics did not yet have the facilities, experience and personnel to provide these therapies when the new guidelines appeared in 2004.

To assist CR professionals in developing an individualised rehabilitation programme for each patient, the guidelines were accompanied by a clinical algorithm for the needs assessment and therapy selection procedure. This procedure requires 15 to 40 data items concerning the patient's physical, emotional, and social condition and lifestyle to be gathered. It generally takes place two weeks after discharge from the hospital, after which, during weekly meetings, the multidisciplinary CR team formally decides on the content of the patient's rehabilitation programme. The algorithm is described by nine decision trees, with each of the branches leading to one or more therapeutic indications.

3 The CARDSS System

To stimulate implementaton of the CR guidelines in the Netherlands, it was decided to develop a decision support system called CARDSS (cardiac rehabilitation decision support system). The system was to actively provide its users with patient-specific, guideline-based therapy recommendations at the onset of a patient's rehabilitation trajectory. As no electronic patient record (EPR) system was yet in use in Dutch CR clinics, the system had to provide EPR functionalities as well. To maximize the chances of acceptance, CARDSS also needed to provide explanations of therapy recommendations and give insight into relevant guideline information and scientific evidence. Furthermore, the system was required to take the working procedures specific to multidisciplinary outpatient care into account [11].

3.1 Guideline Modeling

Clinical practice guidelines often contain ambiguities, inconsistencies, and logical errors that hamper their translation to formal guideline models that can be used in CDS systems. To avoid this problem, a concurrent guideline development and modeling strategy was applied in the CARDSS project. Existing methodologies for guideline development [12] and formal guideline modeling [13,14] were analyzed and used as a basis to develop this strategy, which is described in more detail elsewhere [15]. In brief, a guideline development team (consisting of 23 clinical experts from the field of CR) and a guideline modeling team (consisting of a medical informatician, two computer scientists, and the coordinator from the guideline development team) worked in parallel on separate but related tasks such summarization of scientific evidence, guideline text authoring, development of a formal domain ontology, and formal guideline modeling. A crucial and joint effort was the development of the clinical algorithm, which formed the basis for the formal guideline model. The involvement of the guideline modeling team ensured that several vague and inconsistent recommendations and impracticabilities were identified in the initial draft of the algorithm. These were subsequently removed or reformulated in collaboration with the guideline development team.

To develop the CDS functionalities of the CARDSS system, the GASTON framework and toolset [16] were used. GASTON is consists of (i) an ontology-based guideline representation language, (ii) a graphical guideline-modeling tool that enables CDS developers to formally describe and modify guideline models, and (iii) a guideline execution engine. The developers of GASTON were willing to provide personal assistance in the development of CARDSS.

3.2 System Development

To provide all the required functionalities, CARDSS consists of an EPR for outpatient CR, a structured dialogue module for gathering the information that is required to assess patient needs, a decision support module that generates guideline-based therapy recommendations, and several information management services. The EPR and information management functionalities were developed in Microsoft's .NET framework with an SQL server database that is accessible to multiple CARDSS clients within the same clinic. The structured dialogue and decision support modules were developed in GASTON. The system facilitates a genuine multidisciplinary needs assessment, where different clinical users can start, interrupt, and continue the structured dialogue at any time. Fig. 1 displays a sample CARDSS screen with therapy recommendations.

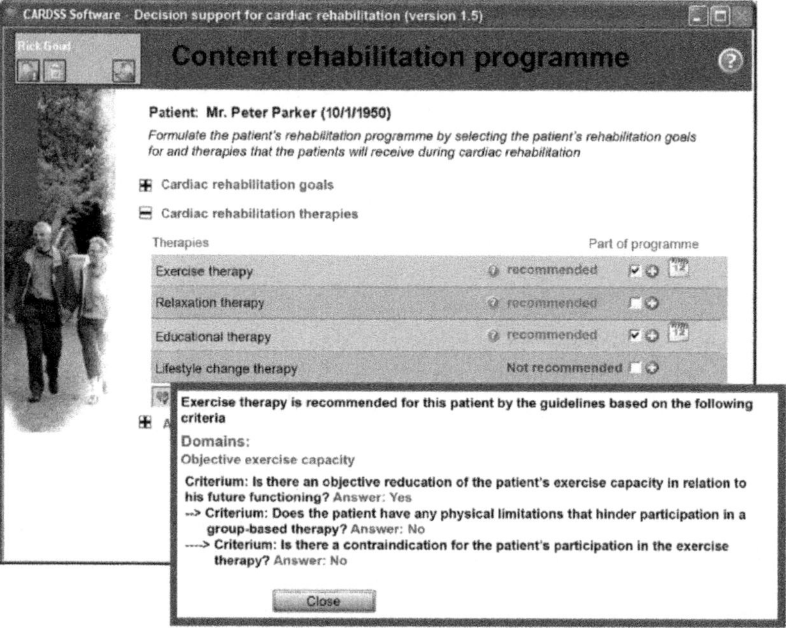

Fig. 1. Screen from the CARDSS system in which the rehabilitation programme is formulated based on therapy recommendations by the guidelines. The pop-up window displays the explanation why the system recommends giving exercise training for this particular patient.

3.3 Pilot Testing

A prototype version of CARDSS was tested during a two-month pilot study in four CR clinics. The number of patients enrolled in the pilot study was 134, and there were eleven different users of the system. After the pilot study, all users were requested to fill in a questionnaire. In addition, all data stored in CARDSS, including log files, anonymized patient data, guideline recommendations, and therapy decisions were analyzed. Five system bugs were identified which all could be resolved in one day.

Concordance to therapy recommendations by the system was 68%. The users were generally positive about system usability and usefulness, and found that CARDSS increased their understanding of the CR needs assessment procedure. In addition, all users indicated they wanted to continue using CARDSS, provided that several additional functionalities were implemented. Based on their recommendations CARDSS was extended with a module for generating summary statistics on patients enrolled in the system, and a message board to facilitate communication between users.

4 System Evaluation

CARDSS was made available at low cost to all 101 Dutch CR clinics. The system was used in approx. 40 clinics.

4.1 Quantitative Evaluation: Cluster Randomised Trial

The ultimate test for any guideline-implementation method is an evaluation of its causal effect on decision making in clinical practice. Causal effects can only be assessed in randomised studies. It was therefore decided to evaluate the effect of CARDSS on concordance to the Dutch CR guidelines in a randomised trial [18]. Thirty-one Dutch CR clinics agreed to participate.

There exist several potential sources of bias when empirical studies are carried out with information systems [17]:

- "Hawthorne effect": human performance may improve as a result of attention from investigators, a psychological phenomenon;
- "carry-over effect": clinical decisions may be influenced by earlier system advice given to the same professional or to a colleague from the same clinic;
- "checklist effect": the structuring of information (e.g. dialogue structure) by an information system may improve the quality of decision making of its users;
- registration bias: information entered into the system may reflect socially desirable behaviour and not actual clinical practice; and
- "clustering effect": observations on decision making that were made within the same clinic may be correlated.

In randomised studies the "Hawthorne effect" will cancel out when the study groups are contrasted. To avoid "carry-over effects" resulting from professionals or teams learning from the CARDSS system, we chose a cluster randomised design [19]. Participating clinics worked with either of two versions of CARDSS: an intervention version (having full functionality) or a control version which comprised the EPR, needs assessment dialogue, and information management services but did not provide therapeutic recommendations. We thereby controlled for the "checklist effect", because the structuring of information was equal for both groups. During the trial, one or more members of the multidisciplinary CR team, usually a specialised nurse or therapist, recorded needs assessment data into CARDSS during a 30-60 minute meeting with the patient. The data were subsequently used as input for the weekly multidisciplinary team meeting, where all decisions about the patient's rehabilitation programme were made. In intervention clinics also the guideline-based therapy recommendations from CARDSS were available during such meetings. Teams recorded their final therapeutic decisions in CARDSS at the end of the meetings. Each participating clinic worked for at least six months with CARDSS in this manner.

From fifteen clinics allocated to work with the control version of CARDSS, four discontinued participation due to a lack of motivation (n=3) or a lack of personnel (n=1). After the trial, data audits were conducted in all participating clinics to assess the quality and completeness of record keeping in CARDSS. The results of these audits were used to correct for registration bias. During the data audits we randomly selected 10 patients receiving cardiac rehabilitation during the trial period, and compared their CARDSS records to data from an independent source. If we found discrepancies in the recorded information for more than two patients, we considered all the data of the clinic in question to be unreliable and excluded them from the analysis. This occurred with four intervention clinics. In addition, three intervention clinics had not recorded all their clinical decisions properly into CARDSS, and one clinic had too much missing data. These clinics were also excluded from the analysis. One control clinic, finally, accidentally erased its database and was also excluded.

The resulting data set from 21 centres (12 intervention, 9 control) comprised 2787 CR patients (1655 intervention, 1132 control). The numbers of patients enrolled per clinic ranged from 78 to 171; the median number of patient per month per clinic was 14. The mean (SD) age of patients was 60.8 (11.4), and the number of male patients was 2060 (73.9%). The main reasons for referral to CR were heart surgery (n=1104, 39.6%), acute coronary syndrome (n=1086, 39.0%), and hospitalisation and treatment for stable angina pectoris, including percutaneous coronary intervention (n=454, 16.3%). Table 1 lists the results of the trial in terms of concordance to the guideline recommendations.

Table 1. Results of trial: differences in concordance with guideline recommendations between intervention and control clinics. Values are percentages.

Therapy	Concordance (intervention)	Concordance (control)	Crude difference	Adjusted difference [95% CI]
Exercise training	92.6	84.7	7.9	3.5 [0.1 to 5.2]
Education	87.6	63.9	23.7	23.7 [15.5 to 29.4]
Relaxation	59.6	34.1	25.5	41.6 [25.2 to 51.3]
Lifestyle change	57.4	54.1	3.3	7.1 [-2.9 to 18.3]

Concordance was generally high for exercise training and education therapy, and low for relaxation therapy and lifestyle change interventions. To control for "clustering effects", the differences between intervention and control groups were statistically analysed with generalised estimation equations [20] using three patient level variables (age, sex, and indication for cardiac rehabilitation) and two clinic level variables (weekly volume of new patients, and type of clinic) as covariates to adjust for differences in case mix between the intervention and control groups. CDS increased guideline concordance for exercise training, education therapy, and relaxation therapy, but not for lifestyle change interventions. Both cases of over- and undertreatment were reduced by CDS, but reduction in undertreatment (i.e., not receiving guideline-recommended therapy) occurred more often. Concordance with recommendations for lifestyle change interventions was poor across both study arms: only 26% of the patients for which it was recommended actually received it. Similarly, despite the positive effect of the CDS, there remained still considerable undertreatment for relaxation therapy. In addition, there was a large variation between clinics in their levels of guideline concordance for all four therapies, in both intervention and control groups.

4.2 Qualitative Evaluation: Semi-structured Interviews with End-Users

While randomised clinical trials can be used to study the magnitude of change in decision making behaviour, they do not provide insight into the reasons why professional behaviour changes. For this reason, it was decided to also study the effect of CARDSSs on factors that hamper guideline implementation with qualitative research methods [21]. This study consisted of in-depth, semi-structured interviews with end-users of the system, focusing on reasons for improved concordance or persistent non-concordance to the guidelines after successful adoption of CARDSS. Interviews were transcribed verbatim, and all remarks regarding guideline implementation were extracted, and classified using the conceptual framework from Cabana et al. [2]. This framework distinguishes between external barriers (patient factors, guideline factors, and environmental factors) and internal barriers (lack of awareness, familiarity, agreement, outcome expectancy, self-efficacy, or motivation, and inertia to previous practice) to guideline implementation.

Twenty-nine rehabilitation nurses and physiotherapists from 21 Dutch clinics were interviewed, resulting in the identification of 18 barriers. Seven barriers had vanished since the introduction of CARDSS. Table 2 lists five examples, including the barrier type, whether or not the barrier was removed by CARDSS, and a sample comment.

Table 2. Examples of reported barriers to following the CR guidelines, with barrier type, effect of CARDSS (r = reduced, p = persistent), and sample comment from interviews

Barrier	Type	Effect	Sample comment
Guideline complexity	External	r	"We now use the quality-of-life questionnaire with every patient."
Lack of familiarity	Internal	r	"Since CARDSS we focus more on [lifestyle related] questions."
Inertia to previous practice	Internal	p	"We don't offer lifestyle change interventions in this clinic. We haven't thought about it yet. I think that is just because of a lack of time."
Lack of resources	External	p	"[Exercise training] is currently full due to a lack of accommodation. The physiotherapist says he just wants five patients in his group, because otherwise the hall is too small for sports activities."
Lack of reimbursement	External	p	"The insurance companies do not reimburse relaxation therapy."

Interviewees reported that CARDSS increased their familiarity with the guidelines' recommendations and decision logic, stimlated them to abandon their conventional way of reasoning, and helped them to apply the guideline in practice, for example by calculating and interpreting of quality-of-life scores. If the system's recommendations were shared with patients, these were more often willing to participate in psychosocial therapies. Interestingly, none of the participants reported that their decision making for exercise training and education therapy had changed because of the introduction of CARDSS. However, these were two of the three therapies for which the trial had shown that the CDS increased concordance to guideline recommendations. Many clinics lacked the facilities and resources to offer all patients all recommended therapies. This fact explained the considerable undertreatment of patients with lifestyle change interventions and relaxation therapy. Similar problems existed with lacking reimbursements and difficult collaboration with other departments. CARDSS was not effective in solving these organizational barriers.

5 Discussion

In this paper we have described the development and evaluation of CARDSS, a guideline based decision support system for therapy recommendation in cardiac aftercare. Although CARDSS's reasoning module is built on relatively simple branching logic, a cluster randomized trial showed that it was an effective instrument to improve guideline concordance of multidisciplinary CR teams. Guideline concordance increased for three out of the four CR therapies, but CDS was not evenly effective in all participating clinics and not for all therapies. A subsequent qualitative study indicated that CDS improved guideline implementation by increasing the knowledge of guideline recommendations, by reducing inertia to previous practice, and by reducing guideline complexity. However, CDS was not effective when organizational or procedural changes were required that users considered to be beyond their tasks and responsibilities. In that case additional guideline implementation methods should be used to empower CDS users to invoke such changes, or to involve the actual decision makers. Users seemed not fully aware of the effect of the system on their decision making behaviour.

Many projects have aimed to implement clinical practice guidelines using CDS technology, with varying results [3,5,6]. We believe that the CARDSS project was successful for a number reasons. A parallel guideline/CDS development strategy was followed, ensuring perfect consistency between the paper guidelines and the CDS guideline model. The system was supported by two major stakeholders in the Dutch CR field, the Netherlands Heart Foundation and the Netherlands Society of Cardiology. Furthermore, thorough pilot testing with professional end-users preceded the system's widespread introduction to clinical practice. Whereas most researchers confine themselves to a quantitative evaluation of system effectiveness, we have applied both quantitative and qualitative research methodologies. Triangulation of the resulting data has allowed us to gain a firm understanding of the effect of CARDSS on professional behaviour. Finally, we believe that our quantitative evaluation study stands out in methodological rigour.

A limitation of the CARDSS project was the absence of an existing information infrastructure in most Dutch CR clinics. For this reason a complete system with EPR functionalities had to be built from scratch. But consequently the clinics that already did have an EPR system were not interested in using CARDSS. Others were disappointed because there was no possibility to make local adaptations to the guideline model in CARDSS. Other limitations are the fact that development and evaluation of CARDSS were carried out by the same team, which is a potential bias in outcome assessment [5], and the fact that a considerable number of clinics dropped out from our trial. Dropouts from the control group due to a lack of motivation could probably have been avoided by applying a balanced incomplete block design [22]. Finally, we only measured the impact of CDS on concordance with guideline recommendations, and not on patient outcomes. When evaluating the effect of quality improvement interventions, such process measures are commonly used, and they are even preferable over patient outcomes if they are based on evidence or on accepted standards of care, as is the case in our work.

The CARDSS system was made permanently available to all Dutch CR clinics after our study was completed. Currently, there are still 10-15 clinics that use the system on a routine basis. However, it was not possible to obtain funding for ongoing support and maintenance of the system. In addition, the Dutch guidelines for CR were recently revised using new scientific evidence and findings from the CARDSS project. For these reasons, it was decided to collaborate with a Dutch IT company to develop a new version of CARDSS based on the revised guidelines. In future research we will evaluate a multifaceted strategy to implement the revised guidelines. This strategy encompasses both CDS and a benchmark-feedback loop which is targeted at organizational barriers [23].

Acknowledgment. This project was funded by ZonMW, the Netherlands Organisation for Health Research and Development, Health Care Efficiency Research Program 2004, subprogram Implementation, under project no. 945-14-205.

References

1. Institute of Medicine: Crossing the quality chasm: a new health system for the twenty-first century. National Academy Press, Washington, DC (2001)
2. Cabana, M.D., Rand, C.S., Powe, N.R., et al.: Why don't physicians follow clinical practice guidelines? A framework for improvement. JAMA 282, 1458–1465 (1999)
3. Grimshaw, J.M., Thomas, R.E., MacLennan, G., et al.: Effectiveness and efficiency of guideline dissemination and implementation strategies. Health Technol. Assess 8(6), 1–72 (2004)
4. Grol, R., Grimshaw, J.: From best evidence to best practice: effective implementation of change in patients' care. Lancet 362, 1225–1230 (2003)
5. Garg, A.X., Adhikari, N.K., McDonald, H., et al.: Effects of computerized clinical decision support systems on practitioner performance and patient outcomes: a systematic review. JAMA 293, 1223–1238 (2005)
6. Shiffman, R.N., Liaw, Y., Brandt, C.A., Corb, G.J.: Computer-based guideline implementation systems: a systematic review of functionality and effectiveness. J. Am. Med. Inform. Assoc. 6, 104–114 (1999)

7. Ades, P.: Cardiac rehabilitation and secondary prevention of coronary heart disease. N. Engl. J. Med. 345, 892–902 (2001)
8. World Health Organization: Needs and Action Priorities in Cardiac Rehabilitation and Secondary Prevention in Patients with CHD. WHO, Copenhagen (1993)
9. Short, R.: Access to cardiac rehabilitation varies widely across Europe. BMJ 336, 1095 (2008)
10. Rehabilitation Committee Netherlands Society of Cardiology and Netherlands Heart Foundation. In: Guidelines for Cardiac Rehabilitation 2004, Netherlands Heart Foundation, The Hague (2004)
11. Goud, R., Hasman, A., Peek, N.: Development of a guideline-based decision support system with explanation facilities for outpatient therapy. Comput Methods Programs Biomed. 91(2), 145–153 (2008)
12. Shekelle, P.G., Woolf, S.H., Eccles, M., Grimshaw, J.: Clinical guidelines: developing guidelines. BMJ 318(7183), 593–596 (1999)
13. De Clercq, P.A., Blom, J.A., Korsten, H.H., Hasman, A.: Approaches for creating computer-interpretable guidelines that facilitate decision support. Artif. Intell. Med. 31(1), 1–27 (2004)
14. Peleg, M., Tu, S., Bury, J., Ciccarese, P., Fox, J., Greenes, R.A., et al.: Comparing computer-interpretable guideline models: a case-study approach. J. Am. Med. Inform. Assoc. 10(1), 52–68 (2003)
15. Goud, R., Hasman, A., Strijbis, A.M., Peek, N.: A parallel guideline development and formalization strategy to improve the quality of clinical practice guidelines. Int. J. Med. Inform. 78(8), 513–520 (2009)
16. De Clercq, P.A., Hasman, A., Blom, J.A., et al.: Design and implementation of a framework to support the development of clinical guidelines. Int. J. Med. Inform. 64, 285–318 (2001)
17. Friedman, C.P., Wyatt, J.C.: Evaluation Methods in Medical Informatics, 2nd edn. Springer, New York (2006)
18. Goud, R., de Keizer, N.F., ter Riet, G., Wyatt, J.C., Hasman, A., Hellemans, I.M., Peek, N.: Effect of guideline based computerised decision support on decision making of multidisciplinary teams: cluster randomised trial in cardiac rehabilitation. BMJ 338, b1440 (2009)
19. Donner, A., Klar, N.: Design and Analysis of Cluster Randomization Trials in Health Research. Arnold, London (2000)
20. Zeger, S.L., Liang, K.: Longitudinal data analysis for discrete and continuous outcomes. Biometrics 42, 121–130 (1986)
21. Goud, R., van Engen-Verheul, M.M., de Keizer, N.F., Bal, R., Hasman, A., Hellemans, I.M., Peek, N.: The effect of computerized decision support on barriers to guideline implementation: a qualitative study in outpatient cardiac rehabilitation. Int. J. Med. Inform. 79(6), 430–437 (2010)
22. Verstappen, W.H., van der Weijden, T., ter Riet, G., Grimshaw, J., Winkens, R., Grol, R.: Block design allowed for control of the Hawthorne effect in a randomized controlled trial of test ordering. J. Clin. Epidemiol. 57(11), 1119–1123 (2004)
23. Van Engen-Verheul, M.M., de Keizer, N.F., Hellemans, I., Kraaijenhagen, R.A., Hasman, A., Peek, N.: Design of a continuous multifaceted guideline-implementation strategy based on computerized decision support. Stud. Health Technol. Inform. 160(Pt 2), 836–840 (2010)

Using Formal Concept Analysis to Discover Patterns of Non-compliance with Clinical Practice Guidelines: A Case Study in the Management of Breast Cancer

Nizar Messai[1], Jacques Bouaud[2], Marie-Aude Aufaure[1], Laurent Zelek[3], and Brigitte Séroussi[4]

[1] École Centrale Paris, MAS, Châtenay-Malabry, France
[2] AP-HP, STIM, Paris, France; INSERM UMR_S 872 éq. 20, CRC, Paris, France
[3] Université Paris 13, UFR SMBH, Bobigny, France; AP-HP, Hôpital Avicenne, Service d'Oncologie Médicale, Bobigny, France
[4] UPMC, UFR de Médecine, Paris, France; AP-HP, Hôpital Tenon, Département de Santé Publique, Paris, France; Université Paris 13, UFR SMBH, LIM&BIO, Bobigny, France; APREC, Paris, France

Abstract. Clinical decision support systems (CDSSs) may be appropriate tools to promote the use of clinical practice guidelines (CPGs). However, compliance with CPGs is a multifactorial process that relies on the CPGs to be implemented, the physician(s) in charge of the decision, and the patient to manage. Formal concept analysis (FCA) allows to derive implicit relationships from a set of objects described by their attributes, based on the principle of attribute sharing between objects. We used FCA to elicit patient-based formal concepts related to the non-conformity of multidisciplinary staff meetings (MSMs) decisions with CPGs in the domain of breast cancer management. We developed a strategy for selecting attributes and make lattices manageable. We found that when not using the guideline-based CDSS OncoDoc2, patients with bad prognostic factors were associated with non-compliant decisions. This was corrected when the system was used during MSMs.

Keywords: Formal Concept Analysis, Clinical Practice Guideline Adherence, Breast Cancer Management, Routine Decision Data.

1 Introduction

Developed by health professional societies and national health agencies, clinical practice guidelines (CPGs) are intended to improve the quality of clinical care by reducing inappropriate variations, producing optimal patient outcomes, and promoting cost-effective practices. Usually elaborated in a narrative format, they may be disseminated either as paper-based or electronic documents. However, despite their wide dissemination, CPGs have had limited effect in changing physician behavior. There is indeed a variety of barriers to physician compliance with CPGs [1]. Some barriers such as lack of awareness, lack of familiarity,

M. Peleg, N. Lavrač, and C. Combi (Eds.): AIME 2011, LNAI 6747, pp. 119–128, 2011.

lack of agreement, lack of self-efficacy, lack of outcome expectancy, the inertia of previous practice are physician-related. Others are "external barriers" and may be either guideline-related, patient-related, or environmental. Tu and Musen [2] have previously analysed the guideline effect when making the difference between "consultation guidelines", *i.e.* one-shot simple guidelines such as large vaccination campaigns or management of acute diseases guidelines, and "management guidelines" used for the more complex management of patients with, for instance, chronic diseases. Some authors of this article already studied the patient effect in primary care with the ASTI system [3].

Several reviews [4] suggest that because clinical decision support systems (CDSSs) provide patient-specific guideline-based recommendations, they may be appropriate tools to impact physician-related barriers to CPGs implementation such as lack of familiarity and lack of agreement, and thus promote CPG use. Nevertheless, reviews of computer-based guideline intervention strategies report mixed conclusions about the actual effectiveness of CDSSs to improve physician compliance with CPGs. Many studies showed positive effects, but others found only a limited impact of these systems upon physician practices. Very few have studied the impact of CDSSs over the time [5]. Delivering patient-specific recommendations at the point of care appears to be "neither necessary nor sufficient" to ensure compliance [6]. A great amount of research is thus currently carried out to better understand the factors responsible for the success or the failure of CDSSs. Beyond variations in clinical setting, culture, training, and organisation, research is mainly being conducted to explore the CDSS effect and elicit technical features, *e.g.* design, implementation, and level of description, that would predict their effectiveness to increase clinician compliance with CPGs.

Since several years, a long term political action, known as "Cancer Plan", has been initiated in France. In order to guarantee best patient-specific care, therapeutic decisions should now be taken by multidisciplinary staff meetings (MSMs) according to CPGs. MSMs are thus the place where therapeutic decisions are collectively taken by physicians that represent all medical specialties involved in the management of breast cancer. CPGs would preferably be evidence-based and nationwide, but when evidence and national consensus are lacking, then "local reference guidelines" can be applied. OncoDoc2 [7] is a guideline-based CDSS providing patient-specific recommendations in the management of non-metastatic breast cancer according to CancerEst local reference guidelines. A randomised clinical trial (RCT) including 6 hospitals in Paris (France) and suburb is currently carried on to evaluate the impact of using OncoDoc2 upon the compliance of decisions with the system recommendations.[1] OncoDoc2 has been used during MSMs where and when medical decisions are made.

Formal Concept Analysis (FCA) [8] is a data analysis method allowing to derive and graphically represent implicit relationships from a set of objects described by their attributes. Based on attribute sharing between objects, the data are structured into units called formal concepts. These concepts are partially

[1] The study has been funded by the Assistance Publique - Hôpitaux de Paris, France.

ordered and form a special hierarchy of concepts, or "concept lattice", which emphasizes the relationships between objects, attributes, and formal concepts.

Apart from the RCT, we have analysed the decisions of one of the 3 centres of the intervention arm, in the preliminary observational phase where decisions were made without using OncoDoc2, and in the intervention phase using OncoDoc2. This work aims at evaluating the application of FCA to elicit formal concepts related to the non-compliance of MSM decisions with CancerEst CPGs without and with OncoDoc2, and to estimate how using a guideline-based CDSS could impact the compliance rate and improve the quality of MSM decisions.

2 Material and Methods

2.1 Material

OncoDoc2 [7] has been developed according to the documentary paradigm of decision support. This approach allows physicians to contextualize both guideline medical knowledge and patient information thus improving a flexible use of guidelines for any given patient and optimizing the patient-specificity of the recommended therapeutic propositions. OncoDoc2 relies on a formalised knowledge base (KB) structured as a decision tree designed to be browsed where nodes represent patient-centred decision criteria, or attributes. From the root of the decision tree, the physician is asked to characterize her patient clinical profile by clicking at each tree level of the KB to select the appropriate value of attributes (medical history, clinical examination, pathology results, etc.). While navigating through the KB, all instantiated patient characteristics are collected to incrementally build a summary which corresponds to the best equivalent "formal patient" derived from the actual patient. When this hypertextual navigation is completed, *i.e.* a leaf is reached, the therapeutic advices associated with this patient profile are displayed. A path of the decision tree is a conjunction of statements such as attribute = value. All paths are numbered (*node*). Figure 1 displays the path corresponding to node 70650, as a set of patient attributes leading to the CPGs recommendations. When the MSM decision is chosen among the system propositions, it complies by construction with CPGs and the field "MSM Decision" is automatically colored in green.

2.2 Data Set of Breast Cancer Management Decisions

In the studied hospital, breast cancer MSMs occur every Monday afternoon. This is the place where physicians conjointly determine patient-specific care plans for all presented clinical cases. The design of the RCT currently carried on involved a first observational period where MSM decisions were made without using OncoDoc2, denoted the "without" period, and a second period where MSMs of the intervention arm used OncoDoc2, denoted the "with" period. In the without period, OncoDoc2 has been used retrospectively to formalise the profiles of patients for which therapeutic decisions had been made by MSMs and to assess the compliance of recorded MSM decisions with CPGs. In the with period, the

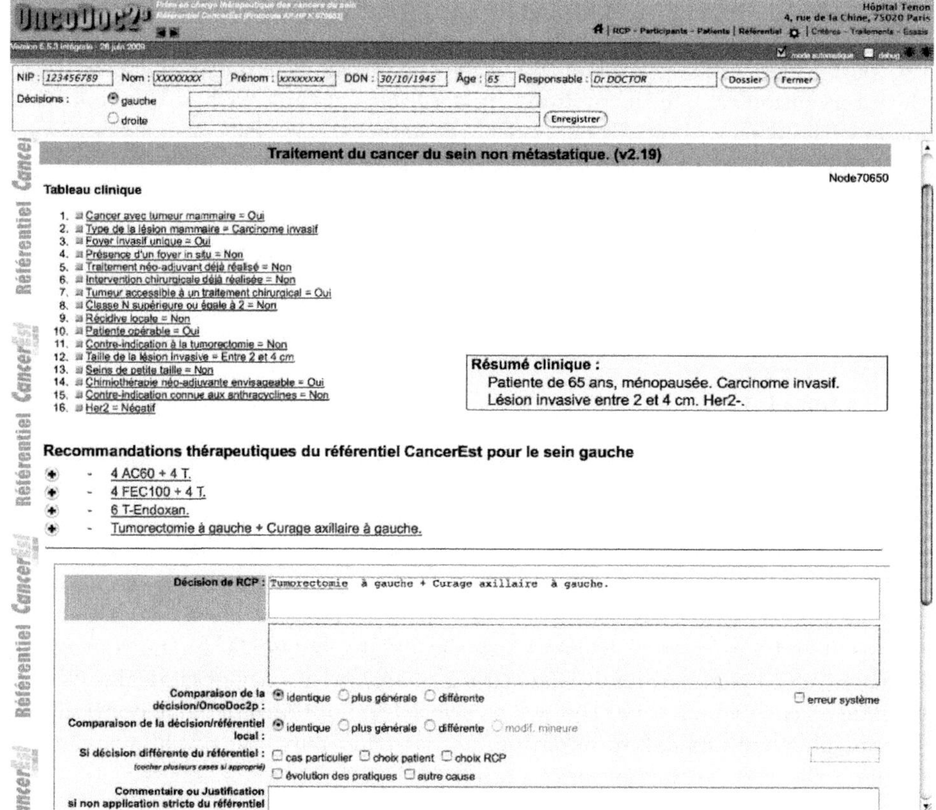

Fig. 1. Formalised patient profile displayed when completing the navigation with the node identifying the path of the decision tree

same data are directly recorded by the MSM secretary at the time the patient case is discussed and the decision made. The data set to be analysed consists in two subsets collected during the without and with periods composed of (*i*) a decison identifier, (*ii*) the MSM decision itself, (*iii*) its compliance with CPGs, and (*iv*) the patient profile number in OncoDoc2's KB.

3 Method

3.1 Basic Notions of Formal Concept Analysis

Used as an unsupervised clustering technique, FCA has been successfully applied to many fields, in particular to medicine and psychology [9,10]. FCA (see [8] for more details) takes as input a data set represented as a formal context and produces the set of all the formal concepts which form a concept lattice. A formal context is denoted by $\mathbb{K} = (G, M, I)$ where G is a set of objects, M is a set of attributes, and I is a binary relation between G and M ($I \subseteq G \times M$). $(g, m) \in I$ denotes the fact that the object $g \in G$ is in relation through I with the attribute $m \in M$ (also read as g *has* m). A formal context can be encoded as a table where rows correspond to objects and columns to attributes. When an object g has an attribute m, the corresponding table entry contains a cross ($\times$). Table 1 shows an example of a formal context. The objects correspond to the patient cases for which decisions were made. The attributes are of two types, either clinical to describe patient profiles or related to the conformity of the decision with respect to CPGs.

Table 1. An example of formal context

Objects \ Attributes	INDEX_MITO:1	HER2:1	SBR:1	SBR:2	SG_INFLAM:0	T4_INIT:0	TYPE_LESION_MAM:3	CONFORMITE:YES	CONFORMITE:NO
4	×		×				×		×
8		×					×		×
9	×	×	×				×		×
19				×			×	×	
20					×	×	×	×	

Formal concepts are computed based on the relation I as maximal sets of objects having in common maximal sets of attributes. These maximal sets are obtained by the means of two dual derivation operators, $' : \mathfrak{P}(G) \rightarrow \mathfrak{P}(M)$ and $' : \mathfrak{P}(M) \rightarrow \mathfrak{P}(G)$, defined as follows for any $A \subseteq G$ and $B \subseteq M$:

$$A' = \{m \in M \mid (g, m) \in I \; \forall g \in A\}$$

$$B' = \{g \in G \mid (g, m) \in I \; \forall m \in B\}$$

$\mathfrak{P}(G)$ and $\mathfrak{P}(M)$ denote the powersets of G and M, respectively. A' is the set of all objects which have all attributes in B and B' is the set of all attributes common to all objects in A. For example, $\{8, 9\}' = \{$HER2:1, TYPE_LESION_MAM:3, CONFORMITE:NO$\}$ and $\{$HER2:1, TYPE_LESION_MAM:3, CONFORMITE:NO$\}' = \{8, 9\}$.

Formal concepts are then defined as pairs (A, B) such that $A \subseteq G$, $B \subseteq M$, $A' = B$, and $B' = A$. A and B are respectively called the *extent* and B the *intent* of the concept (A, B). For example, ($\{$8,9$\}$,$\{$HER2:1, TYPE_LESION_MAM:3, CONFORMITE:NO$\}$) is a formal concept.

A concept $(A1, B1)$ is called a subconcept of $(A2, B2)$ when $A1 \subseteq A2$ (or equivalently $B2 \subseteq B1$). In this case, $(A2, B2)$ is called a superconcept of $(A1, B1)$ and we write $(A1, B1) \leq (A2, B2)$. For example, ({8,9},{HER2:1, TYPE_LESION_MAM:3, CONFORMITE:NO}) $\leq$ ({4,8,9}, {TYPE_LESION_MAM:3, CONFORMITE:NO}). The set of all concepts in a context (G, M, I) ordered using the partial order "$\leq$" forms a concept lattice denoted by $\underline{\mathfrak{B}}(G, M, I)$. The concept lattice of the context given in Table 1 is represented by the so-called line diagram (or Hasse diagram) shown in Figure 2 and computed using Conexp (http://conexp.sourceforge.net/). This representation follows *reduced labelling* where objects and attributes are mentioned only once.

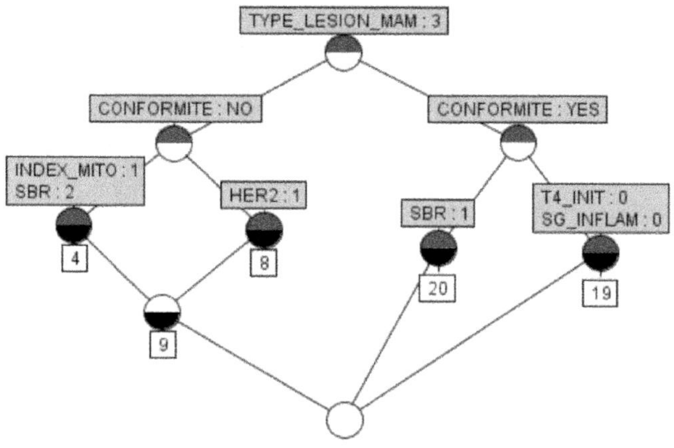

Fig. 2. The concept lattice corresponding to the formal context given in Table 1

3.2 Protocol of the Study

Data Preparation. With respect to FCA, objects are patient profiles for which decisions have been taken, and attributes are made of the decision conformity and of the clinical criteria used in OncoDoc2 that correspond to patient profiles. Criteria have been first extracted from the system KB from the profile number (node). Because of the tree structure of the KB, each profile does not contain the same criteria, so that each object is not characterised by the same set of attributes. Thus, since criteria are often bi- or tri-valued, some attributes may contain such values or not. The tabular representation of such data set does not produce a formal context and requires a transformation process called conceptual scaling in the FCA jargon. Conceptual scaling consists in replacing each multi-valued attribute by a set of binary attributes. In our case, as the attribute values represent independant modalities, we adapt a classical conceptual scaling, called plain scaling, which consists in considering each value as a binary attribute. For example, the criterion SBR which has three possible modalities (1,2,3) is transformed into three binary attributes SBR:1, SBR:2 and SBR:3. This yields two different formal contexts for both with and without periods.

Attribute Selection with Respect to Conformity. When we first ran the FCA algorithm on both formal contexts, the number of formal concepts that were obtained was too high, and the size of the lattice was not manageable. No relationship between the attribute CONFORMITE:NO, respectively CONFORMITE:YES, was easily found. Thus, we decided to simplify the contexts. Since the aim is to identify patient-based concepts (made of attributes) that are related either to non-conformity or to conformity with CPGs, we partionned attributes to keep only those with a value only for objects with CONFORMITE:NO or with CONFORMITE:YES which are exclusive. Every attribute used in either conformant or non-conformant decisions was removed. This yields two simplified formal contexts for both with and without periods.

4 Results

We collected two MSM decision sets: 22 from the 3-month without period, and 69 the 10-month with period. The compliance rate significantly increased from 41% in the without period to reach 83% in the with period (Chi^2, $p < 10^{-3}$).

4.1 Full Contexts

When applied to full contexts, *i.e.* without selecting attributes, results of FCA were hardly interpretable. On the 22 decisions of the without period, we got 61 active attributes, 212 concepts, 566 edges in the lattice and 130 implication sets were generated. On the 69 decisions of the with period, we got 81 attributes, 2,199 concepts, 8,551 edges and a total of 344 implication sets. Figure 3 displays the formal concept lattice obtained for the 69 decisions of the with period.

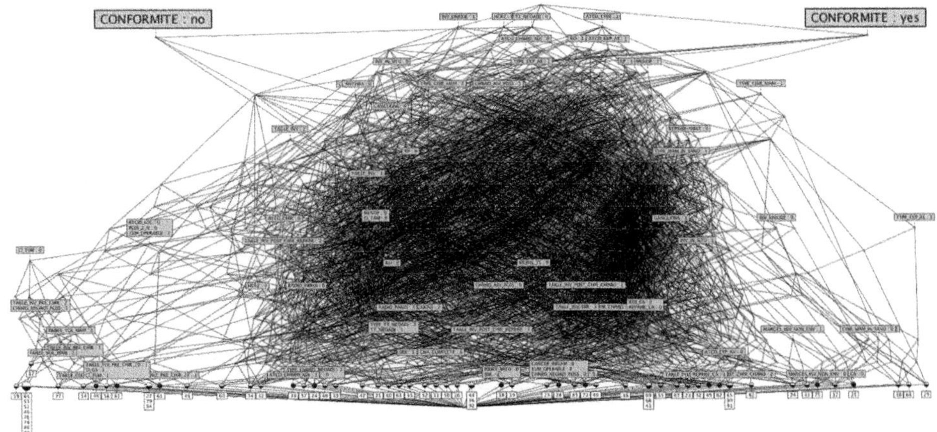

Fig. 3. Original formal concept lattice obtained for the with period on 69 decisions

4.2 Partitioned Context in the Without Period

When selecting attributes, 24 attributes remained. This simplified context was ran with Conexp and yielded the concept lattice shown in figure 4 made of 17 concepts and 25 edges. Twenty-three implication sets were generated, among them, 12 (52%) implies COMFORMITE:NO, for instance: HER2:1$\Longrightarrow$COMFORMITE:NO.

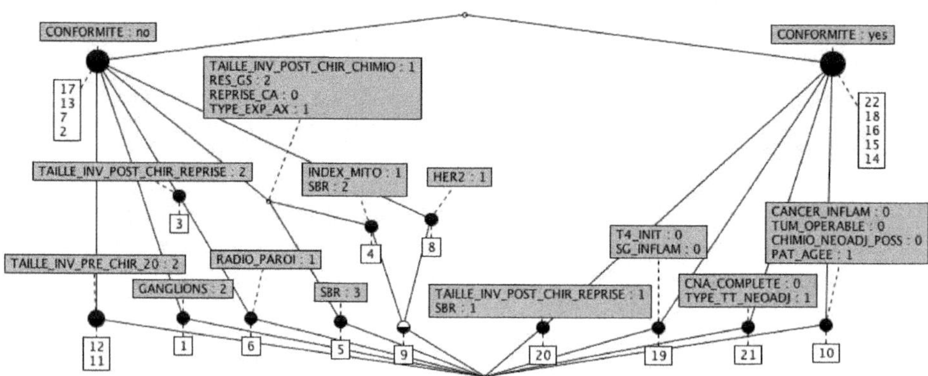

Fig. 4. Simplified formal concept lattice obtained after selecting attributes on the 22 decisions of the without period

4.3 Partitioned Context in the with Period

After selecting attributes, 39 remained. The resulting concept lattice (Figure 5) contains 56 concepts and 108 edges. It must be noticed that implications sets (n=62) contains nearly no implication leading to COMFORMITE:NO, except: MARGE_INV_NON_ENV:1 $\Longrightarrow$COMFORMITE:NO.

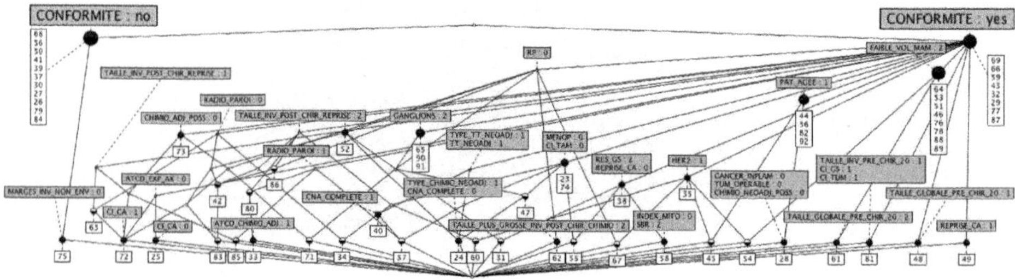

Fig. 5. Simplified formal concept lattice obtained after selecting attributes on the 69 decisions of the with period

5 Discussion and Conclusion

Our hypothesis is that the different explaining factors for physicians' non-compliant decisions when they use a CDSS are related to the physicians, the patient, the CPGs to be implemented, and the CDSS itself. To evaluate the patient effect, we applied FCA to two sets of breast cancer management decisions issued by a French MSM on actual patients. Since analysed decisions came within the same CPGs (CancerEst local reference guidelines), we concentrated our analysis on the patient, MSM participants, and OncoDoc2, without taking into account second-order interactions (MSM-patient, MSM-OncoDoc2 and patient-OncoDoc2).

We applied FCA on two sets of breast cancer management decisions issued by a French MSM for actual patients. In the first set of 22 decisions, MSM participants did not use any decision support, whereas they used OncoDoc2 in the second set of 69 decisions.

Without OncoDoc2, formal concepts leading to compliance were *SBR = 1, T4 = NO and Inflammatory = NO*, *Neoadjuvant chemotherapy = Yes but incomplete and with anthracyclines as first-line therapy*, and *elderly with no possibility of surgery or neoadjuvant chemotherapy*. All these scenarios concern common and "easy" patient cases. For these patients, chemotherapy is either not recommended, or recommended but obviously contraindicated (patients of more than 80 years old), or recommended but already partly given so that the choice of the protocol has already been resolved. On the contrary, formal concepts leading to non-compliance cover more serious patient situations, with either a highly proliferative tumor (*SBR = 3* or *SBR = 2 with a high mitotic index*) or with overexpression of HER2/neu (*HER2 = 1*), or with axillary lymph nodes invasion (*GANGLIONS = 2*) or when radiotherapy of chest wall is recommended although there was a surgery by mastectomy (*RADIO-PAROI = 1*). For these patients, the difficulty is twofold, first to realise that chemotherapy is recommended, then to determine the appropriate protocol. In such cases, non-compliance is essentially explained by physicians' lack of familiarity with CPGs.

With OncoDoc2, profiles that lead to compliant decisions without OncoDoc2 were still associated with compliant decisions and those that lead to non-compliant decisions without OncoDoc2 resulted then in compliant decisions: (*HER2 = 1*, *GANGLIONS = 2* and *RADIO-PAROI = 1*) are formal concepts of compliance. The use of OncoDoc2 that provides physicians with patient-specific guideline-based recommendations improved the implementation of CPGs. However, even with OncoDoc2, the compliance rate of physicians decisions is not 100%. In particular although surgical margins were invaded with breast cancer, a criteria that recommends re-excision as proposed by OncoDoc2, MSMS physicians decided not to renew surgery. In these cases, non-compliance of physicians is related to lack of self-efficacy and lack of outcome expectancy.

Apart from quantitative methods, FCA can be considered as a qualitative investigation method to build concepts from data. With large contexts, as it was the case with breast cancer management, the method leads to some complexity and may lack of clarity. However, we implemented a strategy to make the structure manageable, *i.e.* selection of attributes. When applying FCA to detect formal concepts responsible of non-compliance in the management of breast cancer patients we noted that indications of chemotherapy were not properly identified by MSM physicians. This was *de facto* corrected when using OncoDoc2.

References

1. Cabana, M.D., Rand, C.S., Powe, N.R., Wu, A.W., Wilson, M.H., Abboud, P.A.C., et al.: Why Don't Physicians Follow Clinical Practice Guidelines? A Framework for Improvement. 282(15), 1458–1465 (2009)
2. Tu, S.W., Musen, M.A.: A flexible approach to guideline modeling. J. Am. Med. Inform. Assoc. 6(suppl), 420–424 (1999)
3. Séroussi, B., Bouaud, J.: Reminder-based or on-demand guideline-based decision support systems: a preliminary study in primary care with the management of hypertension. In: Kaiser, K., Miksch, S., Tu, S. (eds.) Computer-based Support for Clinical Guidelines and Protocols. Actes Symposium on Computerized Guidelines and Protocols (CGP 2004). Studies in Health Technology and Informatics, vol. 101, pp. 142–146. IOS Press, Amsterdam (2004)
4. Garg, A., Adhikari, N., McDonald, H., Rosas-Arellano, M., Devereaux, P., Beyenne, J., et al.: Effects of computerized clinical decision support systems on practitioner performance and patient outcomes: a systematic review. JAMA 293(10), 1223–1238 (2005)
5. Abu-Hanna, A., Eslami, S., Schultz, M.J., de Jonge, E., de Keizer, N.F.: Analyzing effects of providing performance feedback at ward rounds on guideline adherence - the importance of feedback usage analysis and statistical control charts. Stud. Health Technol. Inform. 160(Pt 2), 826–830 (2010)
6. Shiffman, R.N., Liaw, Y., Brandt, C.A., Corb, G.J.: Computer-based guideline imple- mentation systems: a systematic review of functionality and effectiveness. J. Am. Med. Inform. Assoc. 6(2), 104–114 (1999)
7. Séroussi, B., Bouaud, J., Antoine, E.-C.: OncoDoc, a successful experiment of computer- supported guideline development and implementation in the treatment of breast cancer. Artif. Intell. Med. 22(1), 43–64 (2001)
8. Ganter, B., Stumme, G., Wille, R. (eds.): Formal Concept Analysis. LNCS, vol. 3626. Springer, Heidelberg (2005)
9. Schnabel, M.: Representing and Processing Medical Knowledge Using Formal Concept Analysis. Methods of Information in Medicine 41(2), 160–167 (2002)
10. Jay, N., Napoli, A., Kohler, F.: Cancer Patient Flows Discovery in DRG Databases. In: Proceedings of MIE 2006, The XXst International Congress of the European Federation for Medical Informatics, Maastricht, The Netherlands, August 27-30, vol. 124, pp. 725–730. IOS Press, Amsterdam (2006)

Integrating Clinical Decision Support System Development into a Development Process of Clinical Practice – Experiences from Dementia Care

Helena Lindgren

Department of Computing Science, Umeå University,
SE-90187 Umeå, Sweden
helena@cs.umu.se

Abstract. This paper describes the process of developing the decision-support system DMSS (Dementia Management and Support System) and some lessons learned. An action research and participatory design approach has been adopted during development, with a strong research focus on optimizing support to physicians in dementia diagnosis assessment, involving a number of physicians and clinics in the process. A stand-alone version is currently used in 11 clinics distributed over four countries. Results from evaluation studies show that the system and the physician comply in 84,6% of the patient cases and that reasons for non-compliance lie primarily in physician's insufficient knowledge. The impact the system has had on the individual physician's diagnostic procedure in observation studies, factors identified enabling the integration and obstacles to use are presented and discussed. The system's support for assessing basic cognitive functions is being improved, primarily as a feature for personalization of a future web-based version of DMSS.

Keywords: Clinical decision-support system, dementia, evaluation, knowledge management.

1 Introduction

Developing clinical decision support (CDS) for health and medical care is essentially a process of developing the clinical practice in which the system will be used [1]. This means that there is several stakeholders that need to become involved who have influence on the results. Furthermore, the organization of clinical practice differs between clinics and countries. Local routines, work division, amount and characteristics of teamwork, etc., affect who may benefit from the support provided by a CDS. Such factors need also to be taken into account when the use environment is assessed and requirements for a CDS are formulated.

In a larger perspective of developing sustainable knowledge-based system in the health domain, results from iterative user evaluations are ideally fed into new versions of the system [2]. Due to the safety-critical nature of health and medical decision-support systems, the integration of prototypes of such systems in their earlier stages are commonly troublesome (e.g., [3]). As a consequence, the ecological validity of the

M. Peleg, N. Lavrač, and C. Combi (Eds.): AIME 2011, LNAI 6747, pp. 129–138, 2011.

support provided can not be properly assessed, which is particularly important when developing systems for supporting a continuing medical education in individuals. In order to overcome this constraint on the development, efforts have been done to develop methods to integrate early prototypes in clinical practice using an action research and participatory design approach, e.g., [4]. Another example is DMSS-R (Dementia Management and Support System - Revised version) in focus for our work [5]. DMSS is a system currently in use in controlled evaluation settings in Asia and Scandinavia. The main purpose of the system is to provide aid to less experienced physicians in the process of diagnosing a suspected dementia disease, for the patient to receive a correct diagnosis (to the extent the domain knowledge supports this), leading to appropriate interventions. Another aim is to design this aid in such a way so that the physician develops his or her knowledge and skills in the process of use (ideally, after a period of use, the system would become superfluous) [6].

This paper is organized as follows. In the next section the dementia domain with the motivations for developing the system, and the process of developing the system with domain professionals involved at different stages is described. The system and the knowledge engineering process are presented and discussed in Section 3 leading to a presentation of the effectuation of four lessons learned in Section 4. Finally, Section 5 concludes the paper.

2 Integrating CDS Development into Dementia Care

Dementia care is characterized by the involvement of a wide range of professionals distributed over municipality, primary care and hospital organizations. In addition, relatives and next-of-kin are to a high degree involved in the care of a person with dementia [7]. From a societal perspective, dementia diseases are costly, in such proportion that if dementia care would have been a country, it would been the world's 18th largest economy [7]. By increasing the proportion of early, correctly assessed diagnoses, interventions can be provided, which is a way to increase capacity in the patient, which in turn increases the quality of life and reduces the need (and cost) for care during the years when the disease is progressing. The symptoms to investigate range over psychological, neurological, behavioral, physical and cognitive symptoms. The diseases causing dementia are many and they may co-exist in an individual, which adds complexity when differentiating between dementia types. Studies have shown that only 25% of persons with suspected dementia receives a specific dementia diagnosis when they meet the physician [8]. The domain knowledge is evolving and sometimes ambiguous, with different views on diagnoses, such as whether or not view mild cognitive impairment as a pre-stage of dementia. Consequently, this incomplete knowledge causes difficulties in the formalization of the knowledge.

The organization of care is also different in different parts of the world. A few of the clinics that we have collaborated with have had fully developed ICT-infrastructure for administration of patients and care, while others have been small private clinics, which have invested in their first computer for the purpose of using DMSS. The system is currently in use for evaluation purposes in 11 clinics distributed over three Asian countries and one Scandinavian country.

An action research and participatory design methodology was applied in the project, typical for the Scandinavian tradition. In an initial phase, early prototypes were developed and evaluated as part of an activity analysis of clinical practice. A so-called socio-technical perspective was adopted (e.g., [3], [9]). Organizational as well as personal factors were investigated. By introducing prototypes, which the physicians used in patient cases, while the researchers investigated contextual factors influential on the success of a CDS, a common perception of the system's purpose and content was created and re-created during the development process [10]. Similar factors as those identified in [11] concerning barriers for guideline adherence were observed, relating to knowledge, attitude and behavior change.

A product development process was not the primary goal when the project started in 2001, initiated by physicians who were experts in the dementia domain and active researchers. The goal was to develop a proof-of-concept system, which would function as a demonstrator showing in what way a CDS could contribute to a continuing medical education and improving the assessment of diagnoses in individual users at the point of care, partly to reduce the number of patients being referred to expert teams at long distances from home. However, when physicians in primary care became involved, their desire and need of using the system inspired and paved way to the current goal to develop the system into a product integrated in or with existing ICT-systems. From this perspective, the development process was analyzed in retrospect and the results will be summarized in the following sub-sections. The most important lessons learned will be described and discussed.

2.1 A participatory Action Research Project

The development of DMSS has been conducted in iterations, with cycles of design, knowledge acquisition and formalization, developing prototypes, testing, evaluation and re-design. Formative evaluation studies have been conducted for different purposes at different stages, with the results fed into re-design and adjustments of the system. In all studies physicians have been using the system while considering actual patients currently in focus for their work, in order to increase the ecological validity of the studies. An overview of nine evaluation studies is provided in [12].

Lesson Learned 1: An individual's motive for start using a CDS is primarily generated in a local collaborative development of clinical practice. What has been characterizing the fruitful periods of development is that it has then primarily been integrated into health-care providing organizations' roadmap for improving dementia care in a local perspective. This has proven to be successful, since then implications for physicians to change their routines have existed and sometimes been imposed by the organization. This was not the case during the first years of development. In this phase the participating primary care physicians saw obstacles to the integration of the system in economic structures, limitations in resources, organizational structures, etc. The implications for changing routines have been increased resources for improvements (such as for using DMSS-R and for participating in studies), possible acknowledgement and attention in research communities, or simply a demand from their organization to alter their routines [5].

Lesson Learned 2: Availability of a CDS alone does not imply its use or that it may improve care. The conducted evaluation studies have been mainly qualitative and formative, in order to assess phenomenon observed and reasons for why the system is used in a certain way. To summarize the results, it has been observed that when the system is integrated into clinical use, it has the potential to change the routine by which the physician do the dementia workup [6]. Nurses, care personnel and relatives became more involved in the assessments, and the physicians asked the patient about difficulties to a higher extent. There was also seen an increase in the use of standardized and validated assessment instruments. The physician used the system as a checklist of phenomenon to assess, as a verification of own assessments, and as a base for discussing symptoms with other professionals involved. For these purposes they found the system highly valuable. In some work places they use the system as a base for education of team members in order to distribute the assessment work to offload the responsible physician. The nurses were very pleased with their increased involvement, and the physicians were satisfied with the feedback provided by the system. The main complaint expressed, by primarily physicians in the position to govern the production of care, was that there are too many things to investigate and enter into the system when there may be only three minutes available for a physician for assessing a patient. The time recorded for physicians using the system is the following. In the first patient case they spend 15-20 minutes to go through the different parts of the system, reading the definitions and interpret the findings in the patient case into data to be entered. After the first case or two, it took between 5-35 minutes for a physician to assess a patient case while using the system depending on the circumstances in the patient case (e.g., to what extent cognitive screening instruments were used).

Since the past year a quantitative study is ongoing, with the system in use in clinical practice in four countries. The purpose is to collect data in a multicentre study and we present preliminary results from this study to frame the qualitative results.

The quantitative study was initiated by a qualitative study in all countries except one. The system was introduced "hands-on" to physicians while they were considering actual patient cases. They were observed and interviewed in order to create a baseline for the quantitative study. In one country this introductory study was not conducted, which affected the initial set of data that was collected from this hospital. A comparison was made of the data (comprising of 67 patient cases) with data collected from the other study environments (218 patient cases). The results showed that the procedure by which the system was introduced made a significant difference in the quality. Of the 67 patient cases 42 were shown to have no cognitive disorder, 12 had a cognitive disease but all were incomplete so that the type could not be assessed. The remaining 13 cases were too incomplete to tell whether or not they were affected by a cognitive disease. This makes 37,3% of these cases incomplete. The physicians who had at least seen the system in use in a patient case, provided more complete information about each patient case. Of 218 cases only 8,1% were incomplete [13] and in these cases it was clear at least whether there were a cognitive disorder present or not. Before more data was collected from this use environment, an introduction was given to the involved physicians similar to the one provided in the other use environments. The quality was increased in the following 61 cases where there was enough data to generate at least weak support for a diagnosis in all cases.

Several factors could have explained the difference, however, it is clear that learning takes place in the introductory sessions where the physicians gain an affirmation of what they know and may have a chance to express what they do not know or do not understand. The emphasis that is put on the dementia workup during the introductory sessions with visiting researchers, who are experts in the domain and who were putting interest in the individual physician's work, probably made the physicians aware of the importance of the assessments, leading to a change in priorities among daily tasks. In the action research perspective, the physicians became more personally involved in the collaborative work of collecting data for improving both their clinical routines and the system. The conclusion was made that it is not obvious that simply providing access to this particular CDS improve dementia assessments, even if the aim has been to make the system as easy to use as possible through a purposefully designed interaction. The learning aspects and organizational (cultural) issues will be further discussed in the next section.

3 DMSS and Integrating Expert Clinicians into CDS Development

DMSS-R is based on clinical practice guidelines (CPGs) for dementia diagnosis and care with a primary focus on differential diagnosis, which represents the physician's perspective, e.g. [6]. Additional support is integrated for assessing severity levels and for selecting interventions suitable for the individual patient. International terminologies and classifications are used for the concepts in the system, with associated terms and definitions to aid the user on what is being asked for. Inferences are implemented using production rules, with structures based on formal argumentation theory [14] and activity theoretical analyses of clinical practice [6, 15].

The support is divided into two supplementary lines of inferences. The first one is based on a set of core and necessary features that are analyzed in an abductive heuristic process. This set of features has been extracted from the different guidelines, and the process results in a Boolean assessment of one unambiguous cognitive disorder and a dementia disease as explanation if there is a dementia syndrome. If the assessment of core features does not result in one unambiguous suggestion of diagnosis, this inference points to the fact that the information is insufficient for assessing a typical case of dementia and refers to the second inference mechanism, developed to handle atypical and ambiguous cases. This line of inference also generates information in a heuristic manner, but uses modal values as expressed in clinical guidelines for assessing different levels of support to hypothetical diagnoses.

DMSS-R works essentially as an interactive checklist of necessary and supplementary features to investigate, while providing analyses of the findings in a patient case. The user can choose to enter all the known information and use the system to verify assessments and diagnoses, or let the system guide the process following a set of steps visualized by three questions to be answered. In this case, the system shows what information needs to be assessed and suggests conclusions, such as diagnoses based on the information. One suggested diagnosis is provided in the typical patient cases while in the atypical cases, the system presents the features supporting different diagnoses possibly manifested in a patient case based on a set of certain CPGs, without suggesting one particular diagnosis in the way the system does in the typical, unambiguous cases (Figure 1). The purpose is to illuminate the limited domain knowledge, making the physician aware of the ambiguities in the assessment and different possible interpretations. Explanations are also provided when there is insufficient information to assess a diagnosis.

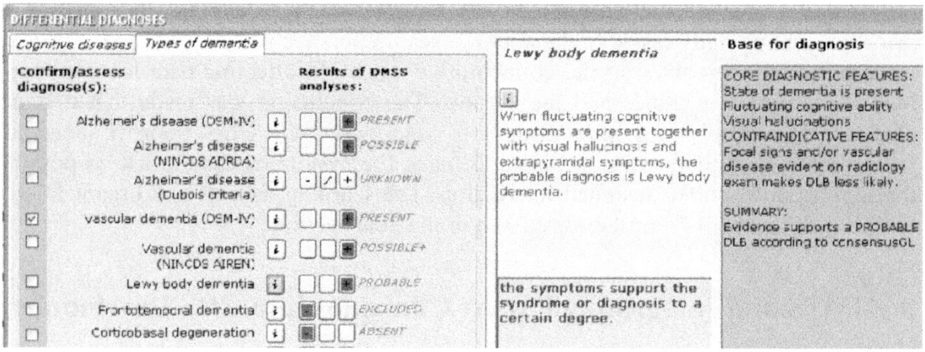

Fig. 1. Part of an overview of diagnoses and their strengths in an atypical patient case

The DMSS prototype was developed as a proof-of-concept demonstrator for clinicians and stakeholders in different use contexts. Therefore, focus was primarily on interaction design and formalizing the underlying knowledge and not on preparing the system to be integrated into a health information infrastructure. DMSS-R is developed using Visual Studio 2008 as a stand-alone application with a database, primarily designed for ongoing evaluation studies. As such it is limited in that requested data needs to be entered by the health care professional manually and the data is stored separately. The benefits have been that it is easily installed and can be quickly taken into use also in clinics without ICT-infrastructure.

Clinicians who are experts in the domain have been taking an active part in the modeling of knowledge to be integrated during different phases. However, a critical limitation in the system is the difficulty to manage the knowledge content and adjust the interaction design. The limiting factors will be discussed in the following sub-sections as lessons learned that motivate ongoing development of alternative methods.

Lesson Learned 3: Apply transparent methods for managing and communicating the formalized knowledge. In the DMSS project decision tables, decision trees and patient case scenarios were used in the modeling in different phases. What has been observed during the project is that the status of the knowledge was changing, both with respect to how the individual physicians interpret the knowledge and how the research community views the knowledge. Obviously, there is a need for an alternative knowledge acquisition method, which facilitates also the management of the knowledge. In addition, the evolving status of the domain knowledge creates an interest in some end user physicians to have the possibility to view the interpretation made by the expert physicians involved in the knowledge acquisition and modeling.

Lesson Learned 4: Remember that experts operate at a higher level of complexity in their reasoning. Provide support also for basic data collecting activities to support novices. Another observation made is the important difference in what we call culture between the domain experts and the potential end users. While the domain experts know well the complex aspects of the diagnostic process and aim at providing support for these, they are commonly overestimating the end users' ability to assess e.g., basic cognitive functions in patients. When integrating aid in the form of definitions of concepts, these were also shown to be too abstract to be of practical use for some not familiar with observable consequences of cognitive dysfunctions. The reasons for noncompliance between physicians' assessment and DMSS-R assessments were investigated [15, 12]. In a majority of cases this was due to a misconception in the physician about primarily memory and its relation to diagnosing Alzheimer's disease. A few physicians diagnosed Alzheimer's disease based on intact episodic memory function, which should be significantly affected as one of the main diagnostic criteria. Similar tendencies were seen in the assessments of other cognitive functions and their characteristics. In another qualitative evaluation study, it was observed that the physician neglected visible symptoms of parkinsonism, and did not enter information about ongoing Parkinson's disease [6]. The reason given by the physician was that he did not know about this type of disease. This lead to agreement between the system and the physician, based on the partly incorrect information entered into the system. Reasons why contradictory information was entered may be stressful work situations, or lack of knowledge about dementia diagnosis, or simply that the interaction design of the system does not provide enough support to complete the task in a satisfactory way. We take these possible reasons into account in further development of the system, mainly in providing aid for assessing these basic functionalities. Consequently, what the domain experts aimed for at the startup of the DMSS project (to computerize the different guidelines that need to be used when diagnosing a suspected case of dementia) is not sufficient as aid in the patient encounter. In order to make correct diagnostic assessments, the assessment of basic functionalities need to be done in a proper way, in order to have correct base for diagnosis. Consequently, these tasks need to be supported as well.

Lesson Learned 5: To make a CDS support simple patient cases it has to also be able to differentiate between simple and difficult patient cases, which means that it can never be "simple". In the startup of the DMSS project the expert physicians were aiming at providing a system for supporting the novice physicians in assessing the "easy" (typical) cases, while more difficult cases were to be referred to experts. However, this starting point turned out to have two major flaws. This view was sprung from the local organization where they operated, and did not necessarily comply with how dementia workup was performed in other organizations within the same country or compared to other countries [15]. Another obstacle with this view, turned out to be the feedback provided by the system to the physician in the atypical cases. In a study comprising of 21 patient cases with high proportion of atypical cases, the feedback was unsatisfactory in some of these cases, mainly due to the fact that the distribution of symptoms in the atypical cases overlaps with the typical cases [12]. Consequently, the system suggested common dementia diagnoses in some atypical cases and could not differentiate between common dementia diagnoses and the rare types, since the expert physicians had excluded these from being in the set supported by the system. As a consequence, support also for identifying rare types were integrated into the system.

4 Lessons Learned Crystallized in the Development Process

During the years when the DMSS project has been active, a shift has been taking place from viewing the CDS as a product that is one of several ways to improve dementia care, towards viewing the CDS as a service that comes with a set of services, differently composed and tailored to the local organization and its need for development. In practice, this is seen in that a close collaboration is taking place between developers and researchers involved in development, and medical associations at different levels, and with care providing organizations. DMSS-R is not presented as the CDS product, but as a continuing medical education service, which comes equipped with an initial lecture in dementia for not only the responsible physician, but also for the whole team. DMSS-R is introduced by discussing current patient cases using the CDS as a tool at this occasion, where the health professionals become familiar with the system. Thus, the first step towards use is taken as a teamwork exercise. This way the individual physician may gain confidence in the content of the system and become aware of personal as well as organizational motives for using the system.

Regarding the content of the system the investigation of alternative methods for knowledge acquisition and management is being explored. It is necessary to involve health professionals in the knowledge acquisition process in order to verify the accuracy of the transformation of informal knowledge expressed in CPGs into formal structures in a CDS. However, this has been proven to be difficult, therefore modeling languages have been developed especially for formalizing CPGs into CDSs [16]. The task-network modeling languages have been evaluated for this purpose, however, the choice was made to use ACKTUS, a service-oriented architecture using Semantic Web technology that is being developed for modeling knowledge and interaction with knowledge-based systems in the health domain [17]. The aim is to translate the knowledge content and functionality of the stand-alone application DMSS-R to a web-based application in order to extend the system and make it easy to tailor to local organizations and individuals' need for assessment support and education.

ACKTUS makes use of an ontology, which captures components used for tailoring interaction with the resulting knowledge applications, components of argument-based reasoning and components for modeling the user agents as actors in a reasoning process [17]. Ongoing work involves knowledge acquisition, formalization and validation of knowledge, which is done by domain professionals using the modeling application ACKTUS-dementia in a distributed, collaborative setting (a pilot-evaluation study is presented in [18]). Transparency is improved in that a semi-formal interpretation of the underlying knowledge source is created and included in the knowledge modeling, which is visible also to the end user. In addition, expert physicians' "rules-of-thumb" can be included (i.e., commonly used knowledge which cannot be verified by an internationally established and published guideline).

The same mechanism will be used to assess users' reasons for deviating from CPG-based suggestions of diagnoses provided by the system, which is information that may lead to improving the system and be used for medical research.

Besides knowledge modeling, ongoing work also includes interaction design of the end user application, which is done in a structured form also by domain professionals using ACKTUS-dementia. Support for different levels of reasoning is being included such as the assessment of basic cognitive functions, which supplements the higher-level diagnostic reasoning. Experiments for evaluation purposes have been made, such as composing a minimal assessment protocol for dementia based on the request for support for a 3-minute assessment (which is, however, in practice impossible) [19]. This was accomplished by one of the domain experts within 30 minutes by reusing components imported from DMSS-R and creating a few new rules. The new assessment protocols were displayed in a prototype end user interface, providing the physician the possibility to test and evaluate the outcome. This is a significant improvement from developing the stand-alone system, since at this point, local medical professionals appointed to develop the care produced by their organization, can easily compose a set of assessment instruments and protocols to be used by their health care professionals.

Based on our experiences, we aimed at adopting the most flexible solution, which may become easily adopted and adapted to each local organization and culture, while still being rooted in the internationally developed and developing domain knowledge. Therefore, the increasing possibilities to share and develop knowledge repositories, reuse assessment protocols and instruments between organizations will be explored in future work. One important part of the ongoing development of the ACKTUS architecture is the use of ontologies and standards for communicating data between the ACKTUS-applications and local ICT-infrastructures. This would solve the obvious limitation of current version of DMSS-R, in the lack of integration and communication with existing ICT-systems.

5 Conclusions

The development and integration of knowledge-based systems in health care poses demands on methods used during the development process as well as the system's content and interaction design. This has been illustrated in this paper by describing the development of DMSS-R, a clinical decision-support system for dementia diagnosis, and the lessons learned in the process. By integrating the CDS development into a general development of clinical practice, driven by local medical associations and health care organizations, individual end users' motivation for using the system is increased. Using a participatory action research methodology that involves health care professionals in the development allows for identifying the local cultures and need for support at different levels of care. Tools, technology and methods that facilitate this active participation are needed. Therefore, ongoing and future work focuses on developing DMSS-R into a collaborative management and use environment.

Acknowledgments. The author would like to thank the professionals participating in studies and development work. The project is partly funded by VINNOVA (Sweden's innovation agency), the Swedish Brain Power and Emil and Wera Cornell foundation.

References

1. Kaplan, B.: Evaluating informatics applications – clinical decision support systems literature review. Int. J. Med. Inf. 64, 15–37 (2001)
2. Kaplan, B.: Evaluating informatics applications – some alternative approaches: theory, social interactionism, and call for methodological pluralism. Int. J. Med. Inf. 64, 39–56 (2001)
3. Goorman, E., Berg, M.: The contextual nature of medical information. Int. J. med. Inf. 56, 51–60 (1999)
4. Hertzum, M., Simonsen, J.: Positive effects of electronic patient records on three clinical activities. Int. J. Med. Inf. 77(12), 809–817 (2008)
5. Lindgren, H., Eriksson, S.: Sociotechnical Integration of Decision Support in the Dementia Domain. Stud. Health Technol. Inform. 157, 79–84 (2010)
6. Lindgren, H.: Towards personalised decision support in the dementia domain based on clinical practice guidelines (2011), doi:10.1007/s11257-010-9090-4
7. Wimo, A., Prince, M.: World Alzheimer Report 2010. The Global Economic Impact of Dementia. Alzheimer's Disease International, ADI (2010)
8. Ólafsdóttir, M., Marcusson, J., Skoog, I.: Mental Disorders among Elderly People in Primary Care: The Linköping Study. Acta Psychiatrica Scandinavica 104, 12–18 (2001)
9. Engeström, Y.: Expansive visibilization of work: An activity-theoretical perspective. Computer Supported Cooperative Work 8, 63–93 (1999)
10. Singh, G., Hawkins, L., Whymark, G.: An Integrated Model of Collaborative Knowledge Building. Interdisciplinary Journal of Learning Objects 3, 85–105 (2007)
11. Cabana, M.D., Rand, C.S., Powe, N.R., Wu, A.W., Wilson, M.H., Abboud, P., Rubin, H.R.: Why Don't Physicians Follow Clinical Practice Guidelines? A Framework for Improvement. JAMA 282(15), 1458–1467 (1999)
12. Lindgren, H.: DMSS – a Dementia Management and Support System for providing Tailored Advice in the Dementia Workup. Technical report, UMINF 10.02, Umeå University, Sweden (2010)
13. Lindgren, H.: Limitations in physicians' knowledge when assessing dementia diseases – an evaluation study of a decision-support system. Tentatively (accepted for publication)
14. Lindgren, H., Eklund, P.: Differential diagnosis of dementia in an argumentation framework. Journal of Intelligent & Fuzzy Systems 17(4), 387–394 (2006)
15. Lindgren, H.: Decision Support System Supporting Clinical Reasoning Process – an Evaluation Study in Dementia Care. Stud. Health Technol. Inform. 136, 315–320 (2008)
16. Wang, D., Peleg, M., Tu, S., Boxwala, A., Greenes, R., Patel, V., Shortliffe, E.: Representation primitives, process models and patient data in computer-interpretable clinical practice guidelines: A literature review of guideline representation models. Int. J. Med. Inf. 68(1-3), 59–70 (2002)
17. Lindgren, H., Winnberg, P.: A Model for Interaction Design of Personalised Knowledge Systems in the Health Domain. In: Grasso, F., Paris, C. (eds.) Proc. 5th International Workshop on Personalisation for e-Health 2010, Casablanca, Morocco (2010)
18. Lindgren, H., Winnberg, P.: Evaluation of a Semantic Web Application for Collaborative Knowledge Building in the Dementia Domain. In: Proc. E-Health 2010, Casablanca, Morocco (2010)
19. Lindgren, H., Winnberg, J.P., Winnberg, P.: Domain Experts Tailoring Interaction to Users – an Evaluation Study. To appear in: proc. Interact 2011 (2011)

Personalized Techniques for Lifestyle Change

Jill Freyne, Shlomo Berkovsky, Nilufar Baghaei, Stephen Kimani, and Gregory Smith

Tasmanian ICT Centre, CSIRO
GPO Box 1538, Hobart, 7001, Australia
{jill.freyne,shlomo.berkovsky,gregory.smith}@csiro.au,
nbaghaei@unitec.ac.nz, stephenkimani@googlemail.com

Abstract. Online delivery of lifestyle intervention programs offers the potential to cost effectively reach large cohorts of users with various information and dietary needs. Unfortunately, online systems can fail to engage users in the long term, affecting their ability to sustain positive lifestyle change. In this work we present the initial analysis of a large scale application study of personalized technologies for lifestyle change. We evaluate the stickiness of an eHealth portal which provides individuals with three personalized tools – meal planner, social network feeds, and social comparison – to make change a reality in their lives. More than 5000 Australians took part in a 12 week study and provided solid empirical evidence for how the inclusion of personalized tools can assist and motivate users. Initial results show that the personalized tools boost user interaction with the portal, simplify information access, and assist in motivating users.

1 Introduction

The World Health Organisation is predicting that the number of obese adults worldwide will reach 2.3 billion by 2015 and the issue is attracting increased attention [13]. Much of this attention is being paid to online diet and lifestyle monitoring systems, which have been replacing traditional pen-and-paper programs. These systems include informative content and services, which persuade users to alter their lifestyle as well as tools and features which allow users to plan and record their progress. By the nature of these planning and recording tools, they gather a vast amount of information pertaining to dietary and exercise preferences of users. We propose harnessing this valuable user preference data to personalize the provided interactive features in order to reduce the work load of the individual and increase engagement with the system, and, in turn, the chances of sustained lifestyle change.

To investigate the role of personalized technologies in online lifestyle change systems, we designed and developed an experimental eHealth portal supported by an online social networking system and trialed it with a large cohort of users from across Australia. We implemented a number of intelligent personalized tools in the portal, some directly related to assisting users in their diet goals and some aimed at sustaining and increasing their interaction with the system. Specifically we added a *Personalized Meal Planner*, a *Personalized Network Activity Feed,* and a *Personalized Social Comparison* tool. The meal planner combines both explicit ratings on recipes

M. Peleg, N. Lavrač, and C. Combi (Eds.): AIME 2011, LNAI 6747, pp. 139–148, 2011.

and implicit feedback learned from a user's interaction with the planner to predict recipes liked by a user and produce meal plans relevant to a given day, based on food consumption patterns, frequency, and sequencing observed for that user. The network activity feeds highlight social network activities, which are highly relevant to a user, based on the observed relationship strength between the target user and the user who performed the activity and the user's interest in this type of activity. Finally, the social comparison tool also exploits user relationship strength and action relevance to select a set of highly relevant users and actions to ask social comparison questions about, in order to drive competition and positive feedback in the social network.

We conducted a large scale user evaluation of our lifestyle portal and the personalized tools. More than 5000 users participated in the study for a period of 12 weeks. We logged all interactions with the portal and analysed several parameters addressing the uptake of the personalized tools. Initial results show that the personalized tools boost user interaction with the portal, simplify information access, and assist in motivating users. Hence, the contributions of this paper are: 1) presentation of three personalized features for lifestyle change, 2) initial analysis of interaction with these features in a large scale live user study, and 3) report on learnings from the study on a range of topics from popularity of various features in the activity feeds to weight loss.

2 Related Work

Personalization and recommender technologies have been the proposed solution to the information overload for a number of years. It is well accepted that user modeling and the exploitation of user models to predict user needs and desires is an effective way of reducing the burden of users in domains such as information retrieval, e-commerce and entertainment. Here we touch on related work which employs personalization in the areas of meal planning, information access and social competition.

The use of implicit interaction and explicit rating data have both recently been explored in the area of food recommendations. Svensson *et al.* [10] report on their recommender system which judges the relevance of recipes based on the browsing patterns of users. Freyne *et al.* concentrate on explicit rating data on recipes and investigated three recommender strategies, which break down meals into ingredients to generating recommendations [2].

Social networking systems are continually changing and the challenge for individuals is keeping up with the actions and updates of their friends. Social Networking systems try to assist users by aggregating the actions of friends into Network Feeds which show in chronological order the activities of others. These feeds however do not consider the interests of the user or the relationship dynamics between friends on the system. Recently works have appeared which address the development of predictive models for computing the relevance of items within activity feeds. Gilbert and Karaholios developed a *tie strength* model [4], which classified the strength of the relationship between users as weak or strong based on 74 Facebook factors, divided into seven categories: intensity, intimacy, duration, reciprocal services, structure, emotion, and social distance. Paek *et al.* used SVM-based classifiers to elicit a set of most predictive features and then used these features to compute the importance of activities included in Facebook news feeds [5]. The predictive models were accurate in both cases, but the evaluations were conducted with small cohorts of users. In contrast, our work reports on a large-scale evaluation.

Wu *et al.* developed a model for computing professional, personal, and overall closeness of users of an enterprise SN [14]. 53 observable SN factors were derived and divided into five categories: user factors, subject user factors, direct interaction factors, mutual connection factors, and enterprise factors. Freyne *et al.* developed a system for recommending SN activities of an interest based on long- and short-term models of content viewed and activities performed by users [14]. These systems were both evaluated using offline logs, whereas our work aims at live user evaluation.

Social comparison works by comparing the contribution of users to contribution of other users. Vassileva *et al.* used social visualization to increase participation by displaying the contribution made by each user and facilitating social comparison [11]. Harper et al. discovered that emails informing users whether their contributions was above or below average prompted users to rated more movies [5]. Michinov et al. showed the prolific impact of social comparison feedback on productivity of group members in an online collaborative brainstorming system [7]. To the best of our knowledge, no research addressed personalization aspects in social comparison.

3 Personalized Tools for Lifestyle Change

In our earlier work we investigated the role of social technologies for families interested in lifestyle change [1]. The study highlighted that the attitude towards health was correlated with engagement with the system. This prompted further investigation into increasing the value of the portal to individuals through personalized features, in order to prolong their interaction with the portal and, in turn, sustain the lifestyle change.

3.1 Meal Planner

Changing lifestyle primarily requires changing the types and amounts of food consumed and physical exercises performed. This is often a daunting task, as dietary habits are built over time and are hard to break. To combat this, some programs explicitly tell people what to eat or even supply the foods required. While this might be a short term solution, specified plans are often restrictive and may deter users. More importantly however, users do not acquire the diet management skills which they need to achieve long term success. The current alternative is to ask users to plan from scratch, which can be a daunting task. Our meal planner aims to assist people in planning desirable meal plans by acquiring a small amount of explicit meal preferences and learning from interactions of the users.

The domain of food is varied and presents a challenge for recommender systems. We gather explicit and implicit user preferences for recipes. We gather initial explicit recipe ratings on a 5-Likert scale, deliberately spanning a number of recipe categories to maximize the information gain. Also, we learn an implicit user profile with each meal planned by the user. We determine the implicit relevance of each recipe to the target user by examining how often the recipe appears in the user's meal plans. Finally, we combine the explicit ratings and implicit data in a weighted manner.

Our user profile is structured as a ratings vector, where each rating represents a recipe on which we have either explicit or implicit knowledge. We use a traditional collaborative filtering algorithm [6] to compute predictions for unrated recipes based on the ratings of N most similar neighbours. Briefly, neighbours are identified using Pearson's correlation algorithm shown in Equation 1 and predictions for recipes not rated by the target user are computed using Equation 2.

$$sim(u_a, u_b) = \frac{\sum_{i=1}^{k} \left(u_{ai_i} - \overline{u_a}\right)\left(u_{bi_i} - \overline{u_b}\right)}{\sqrt{\sum_{i=1}^{k} \left(u_{ai_i} - \overline{u_a}\right)^2} \sqrt{\sum \left(u_{bi_i} - \overline{u_b}\right)^2}} \quad (1)$$

$$pred(u_a, r_t) = \frac{\sum_{n \in N} sim(u_a, u_n) rat(u_n, r_t)}{\sum_{n \in N} sim(u_a, u_n)} \quad (2)$$

We employ a decay strategy for each recipe which takes into consideration how often a recipe appears in the user's meal plan and when it last occurred. Equation 3 shows the exponential decay algorithm which determines the score for a target recipe r_t for user u_a on day D where $k<0$. The final processing of the recommendation list occurs as the user interacts with the planner, such that recommendations that would break the diet rules based on the current partial plan disappear from the recommendation list.

$$score(u_a, r_t, D) = pred(u_a, r_t) * e^{kD} \quad (3)$$

Figure 1 illustrates the interface of the meal planner. The daily plan is shown in the centre, a structured tree of recipes is on the left, and the recommended recipes are on the right. Users can drag their preferred recipes to/from the daily plan and the recommended list changes accordingly.

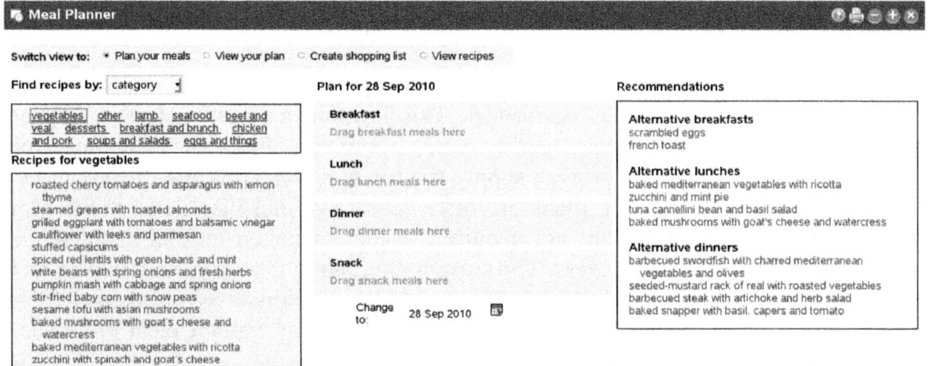

Fig. 1. Meal planner interface

3.2 Network Activity Feeds

One of the burdens on social networking systems (SNS) is their success. Typically SNS's are used for communication and sharing but billions of actions are carried out daily making keeping up to date extremely difficult. Although network feeds aggregate the activities of friends and deliver updates, they normally disregard the user's interests and the relevance of the feed content, leaving the viewer to search for interesting updates. Our personalized network feeds aim to reduce the burden of identifying interesting activities by computing the relevance of each activity and ordering the feed, such that the relevant activities are presented higher in the feed.

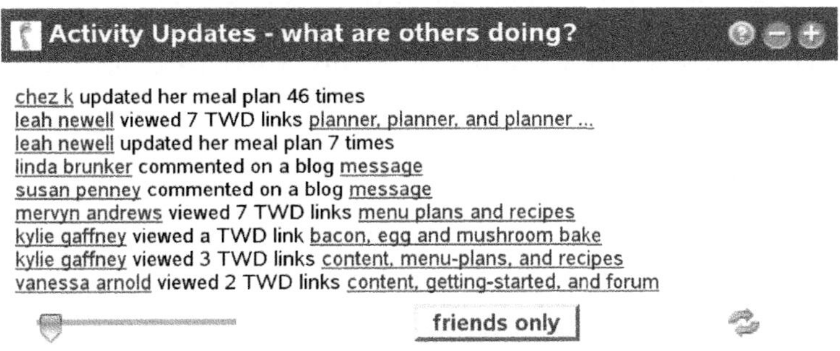

Fig. 2. Activity feed interface

We propose scoring feed activities based on previously observed interactions of the target user T with the social network. In short, the relevance score of a feed item (e.g., "*Bob added a photo*" in *Alice*'s feed), is computed as a weighted combination of the user-to-user score between *Alice* and *Bob* and user-to-action score between *Alice* and *adding photos*. Hence, the overall relevance score $S(T,I)$ is computed as a weighted combination of the user-to-user $S_U(T,u_x)$ and user-to-action relevance score $S_A(T,a_z)$:

$$S(T,I)=w_1 S_U(T,u_x)+w_2 S_A(T,a_z) \tag{4}$$

where w_1 and w_2 denote the relative weights of the components. In our case, we assign more weight to w_1, in order to emphasise activities performed by relevant users.

To compute the user-to-user relevance score $S_U(T,u_x)$, we adopt the model of [14] and use four categories of factors: (1) user factors (UF) – online behaviour and activity of the target user, (2) subject user factors (SUF) – online behaviour and activity of the subject user, (3) direct interaction factors (DIF) – direct communication between the two users, and (4) mutual connection factors (MCF) – communication between the users and their common network friends. Overall user-to-user relevance score $S_U(T,u_x)$ is computed as a weighted combination of the category scores:

$$S_U(T,u_x)=w_3 S_{UF}(T,u_x)+w_4 S_{SUF}(T,u_x)+w_5 S_{DIF}(T,u_x)+w_6 S_{MCF}(T,u_x) \tag{5}$$

In our case, we assign more weight to w_{DIF}, in order to emphasise the importance of direct communication between the users. In turn, category scores $S_{UF}(T,u_x)$, $S_{SUF}(T,u_x)$, $S_{DIF}(T,u_x)$, and $S_{MCF}(T,u_x)$ are computed as a weighted combination of the individual scores of observable network interaction factors in each category. Overall, we use 32 factors for the UF/SUF categories and 28 factors for the DIF/MCF categories.

The frequency of performing actions is the main indicator of user-to-action relevance scoring. We denote by $f(T,a_z)$ the frequency of user T performing action a_z, by $f(T)$ the average frequency of all actions performed by T, by $f(a_z)$ the average frequency of all users performing a_z, and by *f()* the average frequency of all actions performed by all users. The user-to-action relevance $S_A(T,a_z)$ is computed as the relative relevance of a_z for T and normalised by the relevance of a_z for all users:

$$S_A(T,a_z) = \frac{f(T,a_z)}{f(T)} / \frac{f(a_z)}{f()} \quad (6)$$

Figure 2 illustrates the interface of the activity feeds. Both the user and action are hyperlinked, facilitating access to the profile of the user who performed the activity and the content viewed/contributed by the activity. Users have the facility to adjust the number of items shown and seek for further items of interest.

3.3 Social Comparison

Social comparison, as a persuasive technique to affect user behavior and increase their engagement, has recently received much attention. Social comparison works by asking users to compare their friends in relation to a specific question, which can relate to either a user's online or offline activity. For example, "*Who spends more time on the site, Alice or Bob*?" or "*Who is more outgoing, Alice or Bob?*". The selected user (Alice or Bob) then receives feedback on this from the system. Although social comparison has been shown as an effective technique in changing online behavior and increasing user engagement, the reach and uptake of social comparison could be further improved through personalization. We implemented a personalized social comparison tool, which selects the topics and users which are best suited for the target user to compare, in order to maximize the chances of uptake and the generation of positive feedback from the system.

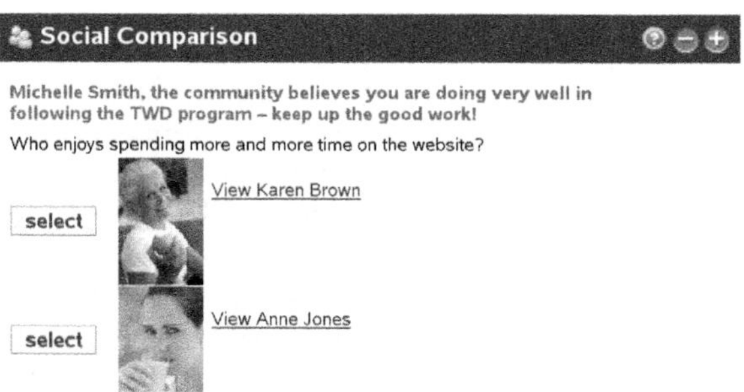

Fig. 3. Social comparison interface

We re-use the user-to-user $S_U(T,u_x)$ and user-to-action $S_A(T,a_z)$ relevance scores detailed above to personalize the questions and subjects that are presented to an individual. Our personalized social comparison tool aims to select candidates for comparison who meet the following criteria: (1) high user-to-user relevance $S_U(T,u_x)$, (2) high user-to-action relevance, and (3) low number of received feedback $fb(u_x)$ from system. The personalized social comparison initially selects M users ($u_1,\ldots,u_M$) with the highest user-to-user score $S_U(T,u_x)$. In order to prioritize users who received less feedback from the system, the relevance score of each of them is adjusted as in Equation 7 and two users with the highest prioritized score $S'_U(T,u_x)$ are selected as the candidate users CU_1, CU_2.

$$S'_U(T,u_x)=fb(u_x)(1-S_U(T,u_x)) \tag{7}$$

Then, we select candidate questions which meet the following criteria: (1) high user-to-action score $S_A(T,a_z)$, (2) high user-to-action scores $S_A(CU_1,a_z)$ or $S_A(CU_2,a_z)$ for either CU_1, or CU_2, and (3) not asked in previous K days, $lastask(T,q_x)$>K. We combine the user-to-action score of the target user and two candidate users as follows:

$$S_A(T,CU_1,CU_2,a_z)=S_A(T,a_z)S_A(CU_1,a_z)+ S_A(T,a_z)S_A(CU_2,a_z) \tag{8}$$

The action with the highest score is chosen as the candidate action to ask about. Each action is associated with a set of questions. If the question associated with the candidate action was not asked in previous K days, it is selected and asked. Figure 3 illustrates the interface of the social comparison.

4 Evaluation and Analyses

The eHealth portal we developed is a diet compliance system, providing users with skills, information, and tools designed to sustain and enhance their interaction with the portal in order to assist them with diet compliance and lifestyle chance. The core dietetic information was extracted from the CSIRO's Total Wellbeing Diet [8]. We evaluated the three personalized tools in a live study involving the users of the portal. More than 5000 users participated in the study for a period of 12 weeks, from September to November of 2010. Interaction with website features was optional, thus the number of users who interacted with each tool varied, we report here on the subsets of users who interacted with the features detailed above. The users were uniformly divided into several experimental groups, such that half of the groups were exposed to the personalized and half to non-personalized tools. As such, half of the users used the personalized and half the standard planner with no recommendations; half were exposed to personalize and half to non-personalized activity feeds; and lastly half were asked personalized and half randomized social comparison questions. No personalization was applied during the first week, due to the bootstrapping phase of the recipe preferences and relevance scores.

4.1 Meal Planner

Users in the personalized groups received recommendations on a daily basis through the meal planner. The recommendations were limited to three recommendations for *breakfast*, *lunch*, and *dinner* and were determined using the algorithms presented in Section 3.1. The recipes with the highest weighted relevance to the user were deemed recommendation candidates. Different users planned with different levels of granularity, i.e., for individual meals, a set of meals, or even for multiple days. For the sake of simplicity, we report on planning at the level of meals and days with plans.

Note that users who received personalized recommendations did not plan for a larger period of days than those who had no assistance. However, we do note that the plans created by those with assistance were more detailed with an average of 4.93

entries per day (including snacks) in comparison to 4.42 when no assistance was offered. Again, the total number of user interactions with the planner was comparable, as well as the number of required user interactions per meal planned.

Table 1. Uptake of the meal planner

	users	days planned	meals per day	interactions	interaction per meal planned
non-personalized	*512*	*9.17*	*4.42*	*100.69*	*2.11*
personalized	*515*	*9.11*	*4.99*	*102.48*	*2.13*

The meal planner system was designed to provide recommendations from a set of recipes associated with the diet program. We assumed that users would base their meal plans primarily around these recipes but in fact users primarily planned around recipes that they manually added to the planner. The first change requested by users was the facility to add their own recipes to the planner. Many users added their own recipes, others added combinations of foods (e.g., work lunch), and some simply worked with individual food groups (breads, proteins, etc). Overall, more than 12,000 extra meals were inserted to the plans. Thus, about 80% of all meals planned were from these additional items and our recommender could potentially only be effective in 20% of cases. Further to this, the interface did not allow users to easily browse recipes in the recommendation panel which was likely to have impacted the uptake.

4.2 Network Activity Feeds

Users in the personalized groups were exposed to feeds, in which the relevance scores were computed as presented in Section 3.2, and the activities with the highest score were presented high in the feed. Users in the non-personalized groups were exposed to non-personalized feeds, which presented the activities in reverse chronological order. The feeds were generated upon a user's login to the portal, such that the predicted scores of the activities were not re-computed until the next login. Table 2 summarises the number of users, sessions with feed clicks, clicks observed, and two click-through rates (CTR_u – number of clicks per user and CTR_s – number of clicks per session with clicks), computed for both groups from week 2 onwards. As can be seen, the uptake of the personalized feeds was higher than that of the non-personalized feeds.

Table 2. Uptake of the feeds

	users	sessions	clicks	CTR_u	CTR_s
personalized	*1397*	*390*	*901*	*0.6450*	*2.3103*
non-personalized	*1416*	*382*	*805*	*0.5685*	*2.1073*

Generally, the uptake of the activity feeds was not as high as we expected. There are several possible explanations to this. Firstly, unlike in other online social networks, users of our portal had no offline familiarity with each other. As a result, the friending level was low and the establishment of strong user-to-user relationships took longer. Secondly, many users requested to include a thumbnail image of users in the activity feeds. Supposedly, this could have increased the attractiveness of the feed items and boost the uptake of the feeds. Finally, about half of the feed clicks were observed for the first week of the study, for which we ignored the observed users' interaction due to the required bootstrapping of the user-to-user and user-to-action scores. This is in line with previous works on social network, which observe the highest drop-off rates at the initial stages of interaction [1].

4.3 Social Comparison

The personalized social comparison feature was the least useful feature of the portal, resulting in low response rates to the questions posed. Overall, we obtained only 315 questions received responses from a cohort of 44 users, who answered on average 7.15 questions each (stdev 19.7). The obtained feedback (i.e., users that were selected in the answers) addressed 254 users, averaging at 1.2 messages per user (stdev 1.09).

The social comparison feature was not well received by the users, with many of them feeling that the system was asking them to pass judgement on other users, which they were often uncomfortable with. The lower acceptance of social comparison tools in general was also observed in [12], which reports only a 5% update by users in traditional social networking systems. We observed a 7.2% initial uptake rate, but very few users re-used the feature afterwards. 1349 users were given the opportunity to engage with the social comparison tools, however only 44 took up the opportunity. Generally interaction with the feature was low but one user answered every question (over 100) which was generated for him. Due to the low uptake, it is difficult to asses the impact of the personalization, but there seem to be differences in uptake of questions: users shown non personalized questions responded to an average of 2.53 questions and users shown personalized questions responded to on average 2.89 questions. A further separate analysis of this tool in a different environment is required.

The social comparison feature did not have the desired impact on users and, in fact, it had quite an opposite impact. Some users were unsure as to how and why they should respond to the questions. Many of them were uncomfortable with comparing other users with respect to their performance on the portal. Again, several users complained that the social comparison interface was cumbersome and inconvenient. Since social comparison was not directly related to the tasks associated with the diet, users felt that it was unproductive for them.

5 Conclusions and Future Work

In this paper we report on a large scale live user study on the impact of personalization in an online portal for lifestyle change. We examine the update of three personalized tools with differing roles in the portal. Our meal planning tool was central to the portal and diet, the activity feeds were central to maintaining awareness and interaction with the portal, and the social comparison was an experimental tool aimed to motivate users. More than 5000 users from across Australia participated in the study for a period of 12 weeks. We have presented in the paper our initial findings, which suggest that personalized tools have the ability to boost user interaction, simplify information access, and motivate users. We also presented our observations and feedback obtained from users on the personalized tools and interaction with them.

Next steps for this work are obviously to carry out a more in-depth analysis of the overall impact of all of the features evaluated in this study. In this work, we have looked at each feature individually, whereas the larger picture can only be known by looking at the portal in its entirety. Thus, we will analyse how the combination of the provided tools impacted weight loss, attitude of users, duration and intensity of interaction, and engagement with the portal and lifestyle change program.

Acknowledgements

This research is funded by the Australian Government through the Intelligent Island Program and CSIRO Food and Nutritional Sciences. The Intelligent Island Program is administered by the Tasmanian Department of Economic Development, Tourism, and the Arts. The authors acknowledge Mealopedia.com and Penguin Group for permission to use their data.

References

1. Baghaei, N., Kimani, S., Freyne, J., Brindal, E., Smith, G., Berkovsky, S.: Engaging Families in Lifestyle Changes through Social Networking. International Journal of Human-Computer Interaction (2011) (in press)
2. Freyne, J., Berkovsky, S.: Recommending Food: Reasoning on Recipes and Ingredients. In: Proceedings of UMAP (2010)
3. Freyne, J., Berkovsky, S., Daly, E.M., Geyer, W.: Social Networking Feeds: Recommending Items of Interest. In: Proceedings of RecSys (2010)
4. Gilbert, E., Karahalios, K.: Predicting Tie Strength with Social Media. In: Proceedings of CHI (2009)
5. Harper, F.M., Li, S., Chen, Y., Konstan, J.: Social Comparisons to Motivate Contributions to an Online Community. In: de Kort, Y.A.W., IJsselsteijn, W.A., Midden, C., Eggen, B., Fogg, B.J. (eds.) PERSUASIVE 2007. LNCS, vol. 4744, pp. 148–159. Springer, Heidelberg (2007)
6. Konstan, J., Miller, B., Maltz, D., Herlocker, J., Gordon, L., Riedl, J.: GroupLens: applying collaborative filtering to Usenet news. Communications of the ACM 40(3) (1997)
7. Michinov, N., Primois, C.: Improving productivity and creativity in online groups through social comparison process: new evidence for asynchronous electronic brainstorming. Computers in Human Behavior 21(1) (2005)
8. Noakes, M., Clifton, P.: The CSIRO Total Wellbeing Diet. Penguin Publ., Australia (2005)
9. van Pinxteren, Y., Geleijnse, G., Kamsteeg, P.: Deriving a recipe similarity measure for recommending healthful meals. In: Proceedings of IUI (2011)
10. Svensson, M., Hook, K., Laaksolahti, J., Waern, A.: Social navigation of food recipes. In: Proceedings of CHI (2001)
11. Vassileva, J., Sun, L.: An improved design and a case study of a social visualization encouraging participation in online communities. In: Haake, J.M., Ochoa, S.F., Cechich, A. (eds.) CRIWG 2007. LNCS, vol. 4715, pp. 72–86. Springer, Heidelberg (2007)
12. Weiksner, G.M., Fogg, B.J., Liu, X.: Six patterns for persuasion in online social networks. In: Oinas-Kukkonen, H., Hasle, P., Harjumaa, M., Segerståhl, K., Øhrstrøm, P. (eds.) PERSUASIVE 2008. LNCS, vol. 5033, pp. 151–163. Springer, Heidelberg (2008)
13. World Health Organisation Chronic disease information sheet, `http://www.who.int/mediacentre/factsheets/fs311/en/index.html` (accessed January 2011)
14. Wu, A., DiMicco, J.M., Millen, D.R.: Detecting Professional versus Personal Closeness using an Enterprise Social Network Site. In: Proceedings of CHI (2010)

The Intelligent Ventilator Project: Application of Physiological Models in Decision Support

Stephen E. Rees[1], Dan S. Karbing[1], Charlotte Allerød[1,2], Marianne Toftegaard[2], Per Thorgaard[2], Egon Toft[3], Søren Kjærgaard[2], and Steen Andreassen[1]

[1] Center for Model-based Medical Decision Support (MMDS), Instiutute of Health Science and Technology, Aalborg University, Aalborg, Denmark
[2] Department of Anaesthesia, Aalborg Hospital, Denmark
[3] The Faculty of Medicine, Aalborg University, Denmark
MMDS, Aalborg University, Fredrik Bajers vej 7E, 9220 Aalborg, Denmark
sr@hst.aau.dk

Abstract. This paper describes progress in a model-based approach to building a decision support system for mechanical ventilation. It highlights that the process of building models promotes generation of ideas and describes three systems resulting from this process, i.e. for assessing pulmonary gas exchange, calculating arterial acid-base status; and optimizing mechanical ventilation. Each system is presented and its current status and impact reviewed.

Keywords: Mechanical ventilation, decision support, acid-base, gas exchange.

1 Introduction

This paper summarizes progress in the Intelligent Ventilator (INVENT) project over the past decade. The philosophy of this work is that building decision support systems based upon physiological models is a good thing to do. Physiological models provide a natural division between describing the patient and our preference towards clinical outcome using decision theory. Perhaps equally as important, is that the models tend to raise interesting questions and lead to new ideas for research, and for clinical and commercial applications.

Our application of this philosophy in the field of mechanical ventilation has led to the development of a number of systems under the umbrella of the INVENT project, illustrated in figure 1. The original, and existing, goal of this project is to build a model based decision support system (DSS) to suggest appropriate settings for mechanical ventilation. To do so has required building several physiological models (layer 1, figure 1). These include: pulmonary gas exchange focusing on oxygen transport and acid-base and oxygenation status of the blood, interstitial fluid and tissues focusing on carbon dioxide transport. Models require validation (layer 2, figure 1), and studies have compared the model of pulmonary gas exchange against the reference technique [1]; and the model of acid-base chemistry with literature and experimental data. These models have raised interesting scientific and clinical questions requiring close clinical collaboration (layer 3, figure 1). Addressing these questions has led to the development of two further systems, the Automatic Lung Parameter Estimator (ALPE) system, and

M. Peleg, N. Lavrač, and C. Combi (Eds.): AIME 2011, LNAI 6747, pp. 149–158, 2011.

a system for arterialisation of venous blood (ARTY) (layer 4, figure 1). Development of these systems has led to patent writing, the formation of start-up companies and product development. This paper reviews the branches of the INVENT project illustrated in figure 1. The ALPE, ARTY and INVENT systems are described as is their impact and current state of integration into clinical practice.

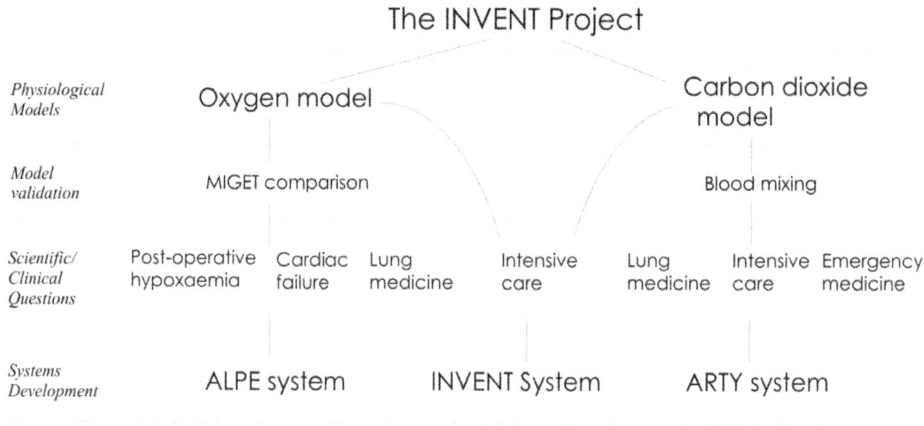

Fig. 1. The Intelligent Ventilator (INVENT) project

2 Systems

2.1 Pulmonary Gas Exchange and the Automatic Lung Parameter Estimator (ALPE) System

To simulate changes of mechanical ventilation strategy on patient state requires a model of pulmonary gas exchange. In the clinical setting, few techniques exist to appropriately assess pulmonary gas exchange in mechanically ventilated patients. Oxygenation problems are typically only assessed via arterial blood gas values or the ratio of arterial oxygen partial pressure to inspiratory oxygen fraction (PaO_2/FIO_2 ratio), a poor description of oxygenation problems [2]. In contrast, physiological understanding is much deeper, having been established by complex experimental techniques and mathematical models such as the Multiple Inert Gas Elimination Technique (MIGET), the reference technique in this field [1]. Given the large discrepancy between the clinical and experimental measurement of pulmonary gas exchange, this work has aimed at describing a mathematical model of gas exchange which is physiologically sound and identifiable from routine clinical data. The resulting model, figure 2 [3], represents steady state conditions of oxygen transport in the whole body. This model has recently been combined with those describing carbon dioxide and acid base [4] to form a model of the exchange of both O_2 and CO_2 in the lungs identifiable from clinical data.

Model parameters describing ventilation/perfusion matching in the lung can be identified from variation in FIO_2, and an automated system combining the model with a technique for varying FIO_2 has been developed [5] and is known as the Automated

Lung Parameter Estimator (ALPE). Figure 3 illustrates the research version of 2002 [5], and the current commercial form ALPEessential™ as developed by Mermaid Care A/S. ALPEessential™ is patented [6] and CE approved for medical use.

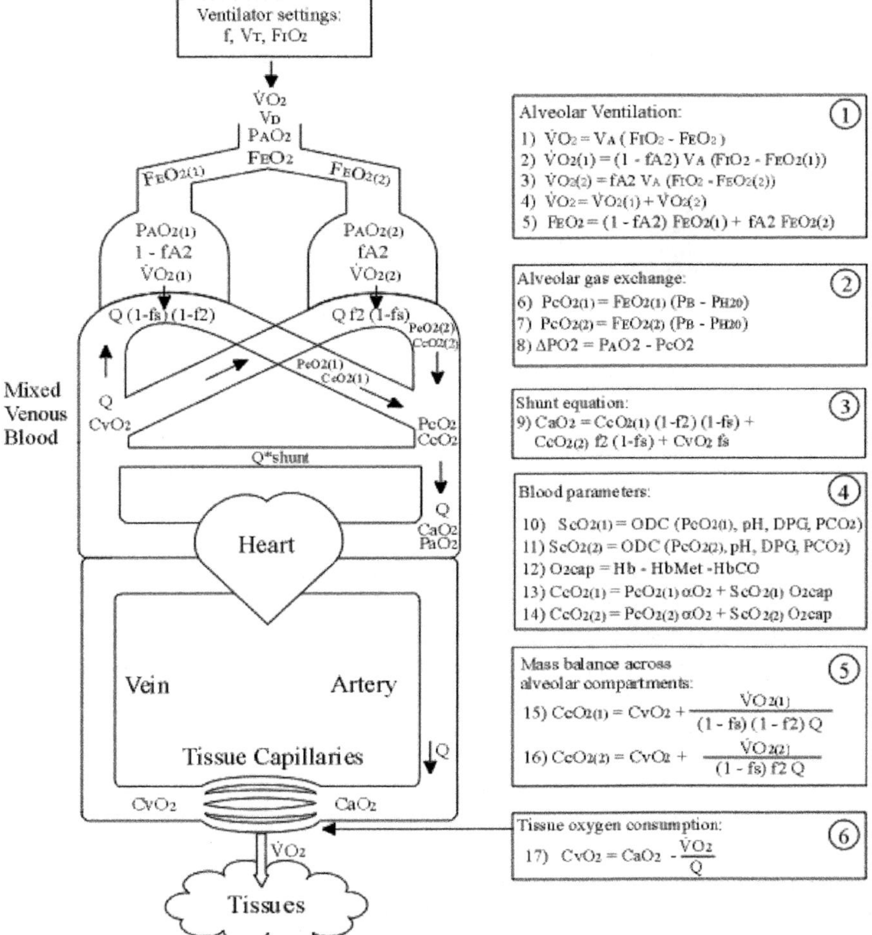

Fig. 2. The mathematical model of oxygen transport [3] (With kind permission from Springer Science+Business Media: Intensive Care Med., Non-invasive estimation of shunt and ventilation-perfusion mismatch, 29, 2003, electronic supplement, Kjærgaard S, Rees S, Malczynski J, Nielsen JA, Thorgaard P, Toft E, Andreassen S.)

2.2 Acid-Base Chemistry and a System for Arterialization of Peripheral Venous Blood (ARTY)

To simulate changes in mechanical ventilation strategy on patient state requires a model of the acid-base and oxygen status of the blood. Such a model requires functionality to simulate changes in gas partial pressure in the blood or the mixing of blood from

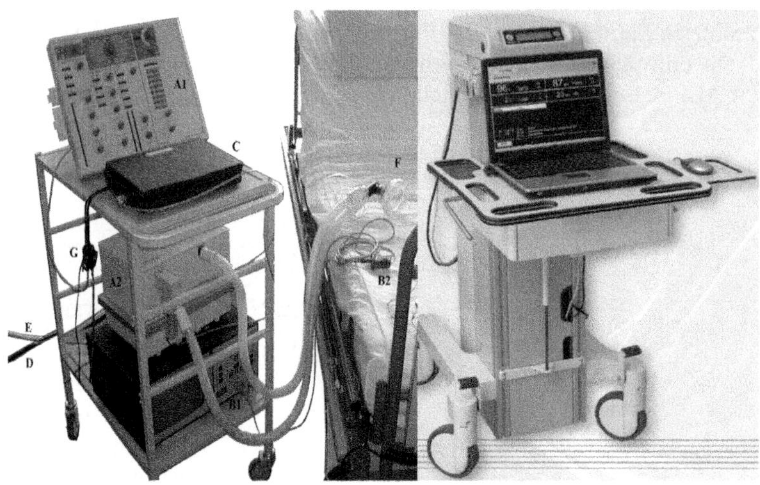

Fig. 3. The Automatic Lung Parameter Estimator (ALPE) system, in its research [5], and commercial (ALPEessential™) forms. (The research version is printed with kind permission from Springer Science+Business Media: J Clin Monit Comput, The Automatic Lung Parameter Estimator (ALPE) system: Non-invasive estimation of pulmonary gas exchange parameters in 10-15 minutes, 17, 2002, page 44, Rees SE, Kjærgaard S, Thorgaard P, Malczynski J, Toft E, Andreassen S, figure 1. The commercial picture is with kind permission of Mermaid Care A/S).

different regions of the body. In addition models need to represent all the relevant components of blood, and their relation to oxygen transport and acid-base chemistry. This includes the red blood cells and representation of Bohr-Haldane effects.

A model of this type has been formulated [7,8] and is illustrated in figure 4. Blood is described as 6 components i.e. non-bicarbonate buffers (Atot), strong ion difference or buffer base (SID/BB), carbon dioxide (CO_2), haemoglobin ($Hb(RH)_bNH_3^+$), oxygen (O_2) and 2,3-diphospohoglycerate (DPG). Mass balance, mass action and physico-chemical equations describe the interaction of these components, enabling simulation of addition or removal of each component. This model has been validated extensively using literature data [7] and in vitro mixing of blood [8]. Applying this model in a ventilator management system required its inclusion as part of a whole body model including circulation, respiration and other body stores, e.g. interstitial fluid [9].

The development of this model has led to a further idea for useful clinical application, this being that blood taken from peripheral venous measurements and analysed for acid-base and oxygenation status can be mathematically arterialized to calculate the equivalent variables in arterial blood. The method is illustrated in figure 5. Details of the steps are given in Rees et al. [10], however the principle is that O_2 is mathematically added and CO_2 removed in a predefined ratio (RQ), until the simulated arterial oxygen saturation matches that measured by a pulse oximeter. At that condition calculated values of all variables describing arterialised blood (pHa, PCO_2,a, PO_2,a, and SO_2,a) should be equal to measured arterial values. This idea, and the associated method, has been patented [11] and hopefully will be available commercially in the near future.

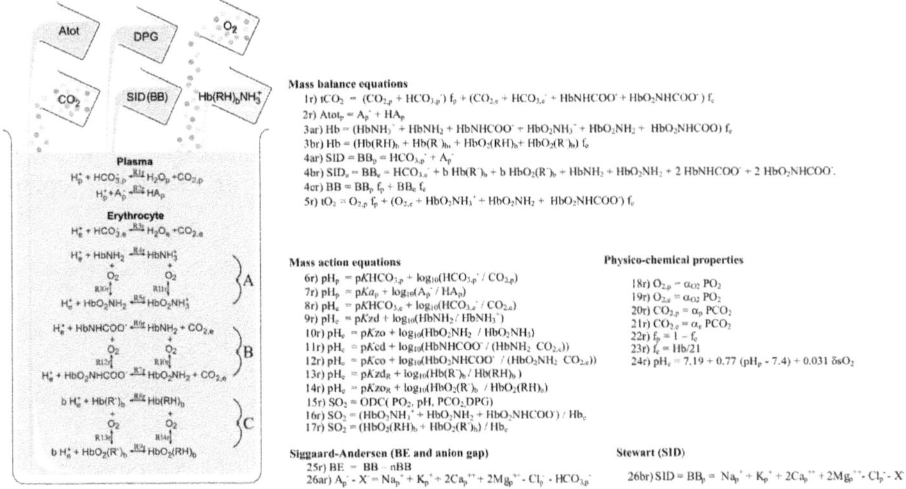

Fig. 4. A mathematical model of the acid-base chemistry in blood [8]. (With kind permission from Springer Science+Business Media: Eur J Appl Physiol, Mathematical modelling of the acid-base chemistry and oxygenation of blood – A mass balance, mass action approach including plasma and red blood cells, 108, 2010, page 485, S.E Rees, E.Klæstrup, J. Handy, S. Andreassen, S.R. Kristensen, Figure 1B).

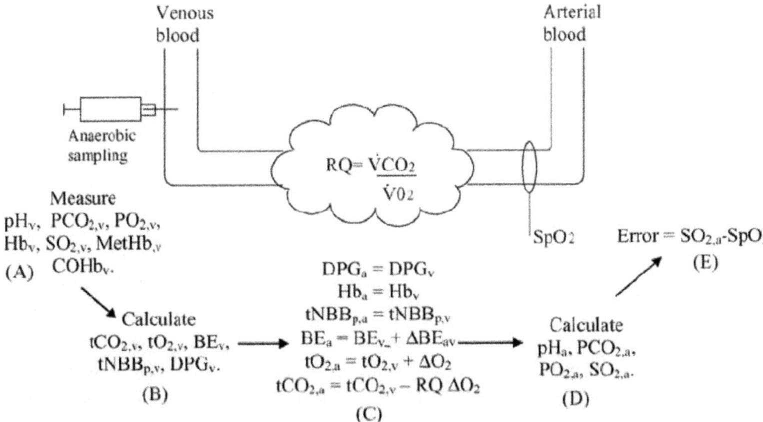

Fig. 5. – Mathematical arterialisation [10]. (Reprinted from: Comput Methods Programs Biomed., 81(1), Rees S.E, Toftegaard M, Andreassen S., A method for calculation of arterial acid-base and blood gas status from measurements in the peripheral venous blood, page 19, 2006, with kind permission from Elsevier.

2.3 The Intelligent Ventilator (INVENT) System

Figure 6 illustrates the structure of INVENT [12] which includes models of pulmonary gas exchange, acid-base, whole body O_2 and CO_2 transport, and lung mechanics. These models are tuned to the individual via parameter estimation and can simulate the effects of changes in ventilator settings on both pressures and volumes in the lung, and the oxygenation and acid–base status of the blood. Also represented in the system are mathematical penalty functions which quantify clinical preference to the goals and side effects of ventilator therapy including: sufficient oxygenation; minimizing the risk of acidosis and alkalosis, and minimizing the risk of ventilator induced lung injury. An optimization algorithm is included to automate the process of finding the optimal ventilator strategy, i.e. that which minimizes the total penalty.

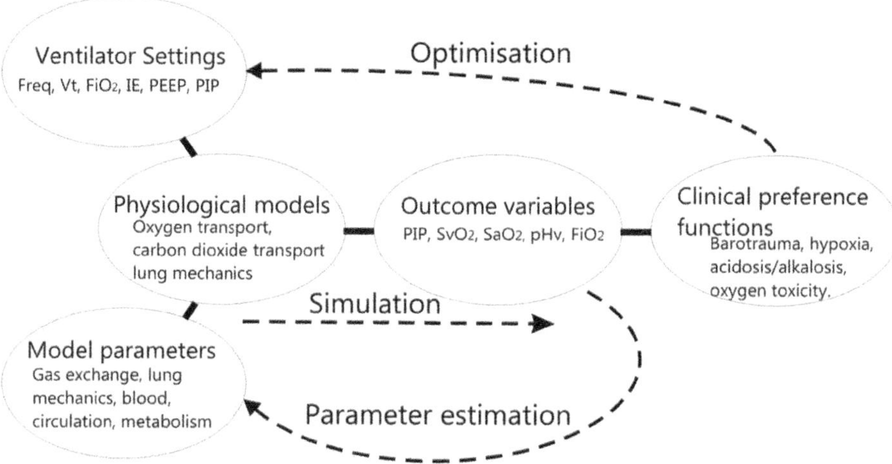

Fig. 6. - The structure of the decision support system, illustrating the components of the system (ovals), and the functionality (dashed lines) [12]. (With kind permission from Springer Science+Business Media: J Clin Monit Comput, Using physiological models and decision theory for selecting appropriate ventilator settings, 20, 2006, page 423, Rees S.E, Allerød C, Murley D, Zhao Y, Smith B.W, Kjærgaard S, Thorgaard P, Andreassen S, figure 1).

Figure 7 illustrates the user interface for INVENT III including a patient. As described in [12], the left hand side (LHS) and right hand side (RHS) have three different values in 3 columns, representing respectively the measured (Current), inputs or outputs from model simulations (Simulated), and the results of optimisation (Optimal). The LHS contains ventilator settings, penalties and function buttons of the system. The RHS contains data describing the lung, arterial blood and venous blood. The bottom of the screen includes patient specific parameters. These are organized according to organ system and include lung gas exchange and mechanics (shunt, fA2, Vd, compliance); blood (2,3 diphosphoglycerate (DPG), haemoglobin (Hb), carboxyhaemoglobin(COHb), methaemoglobin (MetHb), temperature(Temp)); circulatory status (cardiac output(Q); and metabolic status (oxygen consumption (VO_2), carbon dioxide production (VCO_2)). The system is used in three steps [12]. First, the physiological models are fitted to the patient data, estimating patient specific physiological models' parameters. The quality of the model fit to the data can be evaluated. Third the clinician can perform simulations, or ask INVENT for the optimal ventilator settings. To enable integration of INVENT into the ICU a system has been developed (ICARE) [13], which includes software for communication with standard ICU devices and a database

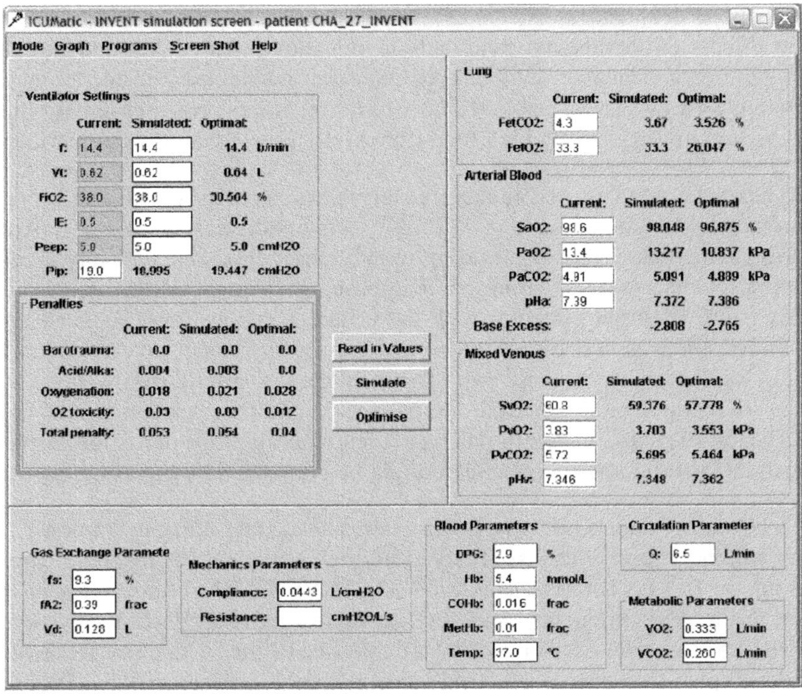

Fig. 7. The user interface for INVENT III. Reproduced from [12] with permission. ("With kind permission from Springer Science+Business Media: J Clin Monit Comput, Using physiological models and decision theory for selecting appropriate ventilator settings, 20, 2006, page 426, Rees S.E, Allerød C, Murley D, Zhao Y, Smith B.W, Kjærgaard S, Thorgaard P, Andreassen S, figure 4).

3 Impact/Lessons Learned

A number of general lessons can be learnt from this work: That DSS based on physiological models provides a natural separation between physiology and clinical preference, as expressed by utility functions. That model building should be at an abstraction level appropriate for the task at hand, enabling tuning of models to an individual from clinically available data. That model building is expensive, but that well validated models lead to the generation of ideas for further applications. For the specific systems developed here, the following impact has been obtained.

ALPE: Studies have been performed to evaluate whether ALPE compares with the MIGET, with positive results [14,15]. ALPE has been applied in a large number of patients, describing changes in pulmonary status in the clinic, focusing upon the post-operative effects and time course of surgical interventions on gas exchange [16-20].

The major finding of these studies has been the peak in gas exchange abnormalities seen in the late post-operative period, i.e. 2-3 days, consistent with episodic nighttime hypoxaemia during this period [21]. ALPE has been used to characterize gas exchange in a range of ICU patients [2, 22], and in those presenting at cardiology departments [23,24]. In the latter ALPE was used to evaluating the degree of edema and the effects of therapeutic intervention in patients with left sided heart failure resulting in decompensation [24]. The commercial development of the system means that the technology can be applied outside the inventors' research environment, an important step toward the potential for its broad use in evaluating pulmonary function.

ARTY has been shown to calculate arterial values accurately and precisely in ICU and pulmonary medicine patients [25,26]. This indicates a role for ARTY in improving patient care: Patients residing in pulmonary medicine typically do not have indwelling catheters. Evaluation of acid-base and oxygenation status therefore involves painful arterial puncture with associated complications. Typically patients are admitted for a period of 4-5 days, and during that time have repeated arterial samples. Replacement of these with mathematically arterialized venous samples represents a real potential benefit to the patient. In addition, patients acutely admitted to emergency medicine have arterial punctures made if suffering from dyspnea. For these patients painful arterial punctures might be eliminated by the technique.

INVENT's utility functions have been evaluated against clinical opinion [27], and behave similarly to clinicians. Three different versions of INVENT are under development: INVENT I optimizes for FIO_2; INVENT III optimizes for inspiratory oxygen, respiratory frequency and tidal volume, and INVENT V, is planned to optimize over the settings of INVENT III plus PEEP and I:E ratio. INVENT I has been developed, retrospectively and prospectively evaluated [28, 29] showing standardized, effective and responsive use of FIO_2 compared to clinical practice. INVENT III has been retrospectively evaluated in patients following surgery [30]. INVENT's models fit well to patient data and the system suggested ventilator settings which could be considered clinically reasonable: lowering or increasing FIO_2 in situations of high and low SpO_2 respectively, while maintaining simulated SpO_2 in the range 94.6 – 97.4 %; and suggesting lowering ventilation in situations of high pHa and increasing ventilation in situations of low pHa, while maintaining simulated pH in the range 7.368-7.404, simulated values of PIP $\leq$ 22.9cmH_2O, and f $\leq$ 18 breaths min^{-1}. The further success of INVENT depends upon a number of factors. INVENT III requires prospective evaluation. For INVENT V, models are required to describe effects of PEEP and I:E ratio. Probably the most important factor is collaboration with industry, enabling integration with ventilators and investigation of clinical impact.

References

1. Wagner, P.D., Saltzman, H.A., West, J.B.: Measurement of continuous distributions of ventilation perfusion ratios: theory. J. Appl. Physiol. 36, 588–599 (1974)
2. Karbing, D.S., Kjaergaard, S., Smith, B.W., Espersen, K., Allerod, C., Andreassen, S., Rees, S.E.: Variation in the PaO2/FiO2 ratio with FiO2: Mathematical and experimental description, and clinical relevance. Critical Care 11(6), R118 (2007)

3. Kjærgaard, S., Rees, S., Malczynski, J., Nielsen, J.A., Thorgaard, P., Toft, E., Andreassen, S.: Non-invasive estimation of shunt and ventilation-perfusion mismatch. Intensive Care Med. 29(5), 727–734 (2003)
4. Karbing, D.S., Kjærgaard, S., Andreassen, S., Espersen, K., Rees, S.: Minimal model quantification of pulmonary gas exchange in intensive care patients. Med. Eng. Phys., (Epub. ahead of print) (2010)
5. Rees, S.E., Kjærgaard, S., Thorgaard, P., Malczynski, J., Toft, E., Andreassen, S.: The Automatic Lung Parameter Estimator (ALPE) system: Non-invasive estimation of pulmonary gas exchange parameters in 10-15 minutes. J. Clin. Monit. Comput. 17, 43–52 (2002)
6. Rees, S.E., Toft, E.S., Thorgaard, P., Kjærgaard, S.C., Andreassen, S.: Automatic lung parameter estimator. US Patent 7008380, European Patent EP1152690
7. Rees, S.E., Andreassen, S.: Mathematical models of oxygen and carbon dioxide storage and transport: The acid-base chemistry of blood. Crit. Rev. Biomed. Eng. 33(3), 209–264 (2005)
8. Rees, S.E., Klæstrup, E., Handy, J., Andreassen, S., Kristensen, S.R.: Mathematical modelling of the acid-base chemistry and oxygenation of blood – A mass balance, mass action approach including plasma and red blood cells. Eur. J. Appl. Physiol. 108, 483–494 (2010)
9. Andreassen, S., Rees, S.E.: Mathematical models of oxygen and carbon dioxide storage and transport: Interstitial fluid and tissue stores and whole body transport. Crit. Rev. Biomed. Eng. 33(3), 265–298 (2005)
10. Rees, S.E., Toftegaard, M., Andreassen, S.: A method for calculation of arterial acid-base and blood gas status from measurements in the peripheral venous blood. Comput. Methods Programs Biomed. 81(1), 18–25 (2006)
11. Rees, S.E., Andreassen, S.: Method for converting venous blood values to arterial blood values, system for utilising said method and devices for such system. US patent US2006105319
12. Rees, S.E., Allerød, C., Murley, D., Zhao, Y., Smith, B.W., Kjærgaard, S., Thorgaard, P., Andreassen, S.: Using physiological models and decision theory for selecting appropriate ventilator settings. J. Clin. Monit. Comput. 20, 421–429 (2006)
13. Smith, B.W., Rees, S.E., Christensen, T.F., Karbing, D.S., Andreassen, S.: Getting the most from clinical data through physiological modeling and medical decision support. In: ESCTAIC, Aalborg (Denmark), September 7-10 (2005); J. Clin. Monit. Comput. 20, 117–144 (2006)
14. Rees, S.E., Kjærgaard, S., Andreassen, S., Hedenstierna, G.: Reproduction of MIGET retention and excretion data using a simple model of gas exchange in lung damage caused by oleic acid infusion. J. Appl. Physiol. 101(3), 826–832 (2006)
15. Rees, S.E., Kjaergaard, S., Andreassen, S., Hedenstierna, G.: Reproduction of inert gas and oxygenation data: a comparison of the MIGET and a simple model of pulmonary gas exchange. Intensive Care Med. 36(12), 2117–2124 (2010)
16. Andreassen, S., Rees, S.E., Kjærgaard, S., Thorgaard, P., Winter, S.M., Morgan, C.J., Alstrup, P., Toft, E.: Hypoxemia after coronary bypass surgery modeled by resistance to oxygen diffusion. Crit. Care Med. 27(1), 2445–2453 (1999)
17. Kjærgaard, S., Rees, S.E., Grønlund, J.S., Malte, E.M., Lambert, P., Thorgaard, P., Toft, E., Andreassen, S.: Hypoxaemia after cardiac surgery: Clinical application of a model of pulmonary gas exchange. Eur. J. Anaesthesiol. 21(4), 296–301 (2004)
18. Kjærgaard, S., Rees, S.E., Nielsen, J.A., Freundlich, M., Thorgaard, P., Andreassen, S.: Modelling of hypoxaemia after gynaecological laparotomy. Acta Anaesthesiol. Scand. 45(3), 349–356 (2001)

19. Rasmussen, B.S., Laugesen, H., Sollid, J., Grønlund, J., Rees, S.E., Toft, E., Gjedsted, J., Dethlefsen, C., Tønnesen, E.: Oxygenation and release of inflammatory mediators after off-pump compared to after on-pump coronary artery bypass surgery. Acta Anaesthesiol. Scand. 51(9), 1202–1210 (2007)
20. Rasmussen, B.S., Sollid, J., Rees, S.E., Kjærgaard, S., Murley, D., Toft, E.: Oxygenation within the first 120 h following coronary artery bypass grafting. Influence of systemic hypothermia (32 degrees C) or normothermia (36 degrees C) during the cardiopulmonary bypass: a randomized clinical trial. Acta Anaesthesiol. Scand. 50(1), 64–71 (2006)
21. Rosenberg, J., Ullstad, T., Rasmussen, J., Hjørne, F.P., Poulsen, N.J., Goldman, M.D.: Time course of postoperative hypoxaemia. Eur. J. Surg. 160(3), 137–143 (1994)
22. Kjærgaard, S., Rees, S., Malczynski, J., Nielsen, J.A., Thorgaard, P., Toft, E., Andreassen, S.: Non-invasive estimation of shunt and ventilation-perfusion mismatch. Intensive Care Med. 29(5), 727–734 (2003)
23. Rees, S.E., Malczynski, J., Korup, E., Kjærgaard, S., Thorgaard, P., Andersen, S., Toft, E.: Assessing pulmonary congestion in left sided heart failure using pulmonary gas exchange parameters. In: 25th Conference of the IEEE Engineering in Medicine and Biology Society (EMBS), pp. 435–438 (2003)
24. Moesgaard, J., Kristensen, J.H., Malczynski, J., Holst-Hansen, C., Rees, S.E., Murley, D., Andreassen, S., Frokjaer, J.B., Toft, E.: Can new pulmonary gas exchange parameters contribute to evaluation of pulmonary congestion in left-sided heart failure? Can. J. Cardiol. 25(3), 149–155 (2009)
25. Toftegaard, M., Rees, S.E., Andreassen, S.: Evaluation of a method for converting venous values of acid-base and oxygenation status to arterial values. Emerg. Med. J. 26(4), 268–272 (2009)
26. Rees, S.E., Hansen, A., Toftegaard, M., Pedersen, J., Kristiensen, S.R., Harving, H.: Converting venous acid-base and oxygen status to arterial in patients with lung disease. Eur. Respir. J. 33(5), 1141–1147 (2009)
27. Allerød, C., Karbing, D.S., Thorgaard, P., Andreassen, S., Kjærgaard, S., Rees, S.E.: Variability of preference towards mechanical ventilator settings: a model based behavioral analysis. Journal of Critical Care (in press, 2011)
28. Karbing, D.S., Kjærgaard, S., Smith, B.W., Allerød, C., Espersen, K., Andreassen, S., Rees, S.E.: Decision support of inspired oxygen fraction using a model of oxygen transport. In: IFAC PapersOnLine, Proceedings of the 2008 Congress of the International Federation of Automatic Control, Seoul, Korea, July 6-11, vol. 17(1) (2008)
29. Karbing, D.S., Allerød, C., Thorgaard, P., Carius, A., Frilev, L., Andreassen, S., Kjærgaard, S., Rees, S.: Prospective evaluation of a decision support system for setting inspired oxygen fraction in intensive care patients. J. Crit. Care 25(3), 367–374 (2010)
30. Allerød, C., Rees, S.E., Rasmussen, B.S., Karbing, D.S., Kjærgaard, S., Thorgaard, P., Andreassen, S.: A decision support system for suggesting ventilator settings: Retrospective evaluation in cardiac surgery patients ventilated in the ICU. Comput. Methods Programs Biomed. 92, 205–212 (2008)

Clinical Time Series Data Analysis Using Mathematical Models and DBNs

Catherine G. Enright[1], Michael G. Madden[1], Niall Madden[1], and John G. Laffey[1,2]

[1] National University of Ireland, Galway
[2] Galway University Hospitals, Ireland
{c.enright2,michael.madden,niall.madden,john.laffey}@nuigalway.ie

Abstract. Much knowledge of human physiology is formalised as systems of differential equations. For example, standard models of pharmacokinetics and pharmacodynamics use systems of differential equations to describe a drug's movement through the body and its effects. Here, we propose a method for automatically incorporating this existing knowledge into a Dynamic Bayesian Network (DBN) framework. A benefit of recasting a differential equation model as a DBN is that the DBN can be used to individualise the model parameters dynamically, based on real-time evidence. Our approach provides principled handling of data and model uncertainty, and facilitates integration of multiple strands of temporal evidence. We demonstrate our approach with an abstract example and evaluate it in a real-world medical problem, tracking the interaction of insulin and glucose in critically ill patients. We show that it is better able to reason with the data, which is sporadic and has measurement uncertainties.

Keywords: Dynamic Bayesian Networks, Model Individualization.

1 Introduction

Systems of ordinary differential equations (ODEs) play a prominent role in medical settings, modelling for example, physiological systems and drug dynamics. The vast majority of models found in standard textbooks, e.g., [1,2], are based on ODEs. In Section 2, we describe how systems of ODEs can be automatically mapped to a Dynamic Bayesian Network (DBN), thus taking advantage of an existing body of knowledge to reason more effectively with the real-time data available at the bedside. (Discussions of DBNs can be found in [3,4].)

The motivation for moving from an ODE formulation to a DBN formulation is that the DBN offers an efficient framework for re-estimating model parameters dynamically over time, based on accumulated evidence. Specifically we are concerned with non-linear systems where evidence may be sparse and have measurement uncertainties.

To evaluate these hypotheses and demonstrate the methodology, it is applied to an abstract example involving a system of two ODEs, for which the exact

M. Peleg, N. Lavrač, and C. Combi (Eds.): AIME 2011, LNAI 6747, pp. 159–168, 2011.

solution is known (Section 3). To further demonstrate its value, it is applied to the problem of regulating plasma (blood) glucose levels in critically ill patients using insulin infusions (Sections 4 and 5). By using the DBN framework we account for uncertainty in the reactions of unstable patients, and uncertainty in measurement errors. Our results and related research are discussed in Section 6

The methodology described here can be applied to any system of ODEs where model terms vary over time, good population values do not exist and data is both sparse and uncertain. Although the examples presented are for systems of first-order equations, the method can be applied any high-order initial value problem that can be reframed as a system of first-order ODEs, and so is widely applicable.

2 Mapping ODEs to a DBN

2.1 Construction of DBN Structure

It is rarely possible to write down the exact solution to a system of ODEs that models any nontrivial real-world situation, and so numerical methods must be used. These methods yield an estimate for the solution at discrete points in time. The simplest technique for initial value problems (IVPs) is Euler's method, see e.g., [5]. Consider the following IVP: find $N(t)$ such that $N(t_0)$ is given, and

$$\frac{dN}{dt} = f(N,t) = f(N,t;A,P_1,P_2,...,P_3), \qquad \text{for all } t > t_0,$$

where N may be scalar-valued (for a single equation) or vector-valued (for a coupled system). Other terms in f are a time-varying coefficient A, and constant parameters $P_1,\dots,P_m$. Denote by N_k an approximation for N at $t = t_k : N_k \approx N(t_k)$. Euler's method is:

$$N_{k+1} = N_k + (t_{k+1} - t_k)f(N_k,t_k), \qquad \text{for } k = 1,2,\dots. \tag{1}$$

Thus, the change in N at each time step is

$$\Delta N_k := N_{k+1} - N_k = (t_{k+1} - t_k)f(N_k,t_k). \tag{2}$$

This approximation is first-order accurate in the sense that the error is proportional to $\Delta t = t_{k+1} - t_k$. As the DBN uses discrete time steps also of duration Δt, (1)–(2) are mapped directly to two deterministic nodes in the DBN, as illustrated in Fig. 1 (left). This procedure may be applied to a system of ODEs, by creating a sub-net for each equation and adding dependencies between them, as dictated by terms appearing in the equations. We have carried out studies incorporating ODE solvers of orders higher than the first-order Euler method, in the DBN. However, we found that, in the systems we are modelling, the data error dominates the numerical error. Therefore, once the first-order method is stable, no benefit is gained by using a higher-order method to increase the numerical accuracy.

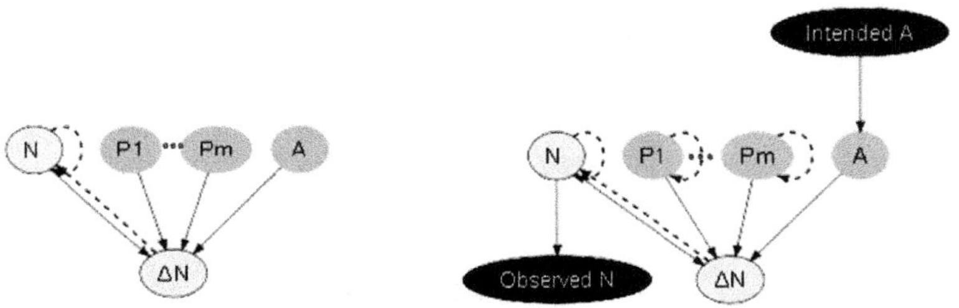

Fig. 1. Nodes N and ΔN are deterministic nodes implementing (1)–(2) respectively. Solid arrows connect nodes within a time slice; dashed arrows connect nodes between time slices. On the right, extra evidence nodes (black) are added to model the relationship between observed and true values, and extra inter-slice arcs on nodes $P_1, \ldots, P_m$ to allow parameters to be tuned to the evidence over time.

2.2 Expanding the DBN to Represent Measurement Uncertainty and Re-estimate Parameters

The DBN provides a natural framework to handle instrument measurement uncertainty. The observed value for the variable to be approximated is assumed to contain a certain amount of measurement error. As can be seen in Fig. 1 (right) observed measurements can be modelled as a continuous distribution whose mean is its parent node, the true variable value. Similarly, the actual inputs to a system differ from the intended input, which is observed, and so a clear distinction is created in the DBN.

In Fig. 1 (right), model parameters are represented as continuous nodes. Distributions on the sensor model can be viewed as the distribution of the population values. These population values can be learned but in our case are obtained from the published literature. All model parameters are allowed to vary in each Δt by including a conditional dependency on its value in the previous time; they can therefore converge to values appropriate to the individual case over time, based on evidence.

3 Abstract Example

This methodology is validated in a setting that is independent of model and data errors, by choosing a system of ODEs for which the exact solution is available:

$$\frac{dG}{dt}(t) = G(t)\,X(t) - P_1, \qquad \frac{dX}{dt}(t) = P_2 X(t) + A(t)G(t), \tag{3}$$

subject to the initial conditions $G(0) = 1, X(0) = 0$. If we take $P_1 = P_2 = 1$, and the time varying term as $A(t) = e^t$, then the solution is $G(t) = e^{-t}, X(t) = e^t - 1$.

Suppose that we wish to simulate the solution from time $t = 0$ to $t = 120$, and there is an error in the observations of P_1 and P_2, but the true solution of G is observed at time points $t = 10, 20, 40, 60, 90$ and 100. Computing the solution

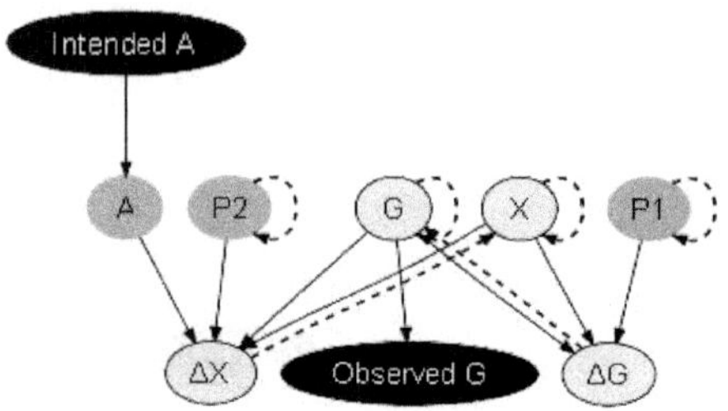

Fig. 2. DBN for abstract example

using Euler's method, but the incorrect values of $P_1 = 1.2$ and $P_2 = 0.8$, and updating the value of G to the correct value, at the given time points, the difference between the true and estimated solution, measured as the *root mean squared error* (i.e., the Euclidean norm) is found to be

$$RMSE_G = \sqrt{\sum_{k=0}^{120} (G(t_k) - G_k)^2} = 0.277,$$

compared to 5.74×10^{-3} (which is the pure numerical error) when the correct values of P_1 and P_2 are used. The corresponding values for $RMSE_X$ are 1.11 and 6.28×10^{-2}, respectively. Clearly data error dominates.

Using the methodology of Section 2.1, a DBN structure is derived from (3), and is expanded as described in Section 2.2 to produce the structure shown in Fig. 2. We repeat the numerical experiment using this DBN, again with inaccurate starting values of $P_1 = 1.2$ and $P_2 = 0.8$ and with correction observations for G at $t = 10, 20, 40, 60, 90$ and 100. As shown in Table 3, this yields much smaller errors than those obtained using Euler's method above.

Table 1. RMSE relative to the true solution

	G Error	X Error
Euler Solution	0.277	1.11
DBN Solution	0.0294	0.642

The results show that the DBN-based solution produces a closer approximation of the true solution. This is because in the standard ODE solution, updated values of G (the evidence) are used only to correct G at that point in time; no changes are made to P_1, P_2 or A. Conversely, the DBN solution not only corrects G, it also seeks to infer from this new evidence what P_1 and P_2 should be.

4 Application to Modelling Glycaemia in ICU Patients

4.1 Background

In an intensive care unit (ICU), patients often experience stress-induced hyperglycaemia [6]. The occurrence of hyperglycaemia is associated with increased morbidity and mortality. To regulate glycaemia in the ICU, glucose and insulin are administered intravenously. This is a complex system; some of the most important considerations are listed here.

Inter-Patient Variability: Substantial variability is seen in the responses of different patients to insulin and glucose infusions. This is due to a variety of reasons, e.g., interactions with other medications or pre-existing conditions.

Patient Instability: Patients in an ICU tend to be unstable: their individual insulin sensitivity can fluctuate. Patient parameters must therefore be continually re-estimated in real-time to account for both sudden and slow changes.

Inaccurate and Incomplete Data: Plasma glucose measurements are subject to instrumentation error. There may also be inaccuracies in the recording of data or data may be missing; e.g., medications administered in a glucose solution may not be recorded.

Sparse and Sporadic Evidence: The plasma glucose measurements provide evidence for the DBN framework to infer values for hidden nodes in the network. These measurements are both sparse and sporadic. Typically they are made only every 4 hours.

4.2 The System of ODEs

The starting point for constructing the DBN is the ICU-Minimal Model (ICU-MM) of Van Herpe et al. [7], which is a model for predicting plasma glucose levels in critically ill patients who are in receipt of a glucose and insulin infusion. It is described by a system of four differential equations:

$$\frac{dG}{dt}(t) = \big(P_1 - X(t)\big)G(t) - P_1 G_b + \frac{F_G}{V_G}, \tag{4a}$$

$$\frac{dX}{dt}(t) = P_2 X(t) + P_3\big(I_1(t) - I_b\big), \tag{4b}$$

$$\frac{dI_1}{dt}(t) = \alpha \max\big(0, I_2(t)\big) - n\big(I_1(t) - I_b\big) + \frac{F_I}{V_I}, \tag{4c}$$

$$\frac{dI_2}{dt}(t) = \beta\gamma\big(G(t) - h\big) - nI_2(t). \tag{4d}$$

Here, G is the plasma glucose level, X is the effect insulin has on the plasma glucose, I_1 is the plasma insulin level and I_2 the endogenous insulin produced by the pancreas.

4.3 The DBN Derived from the ODEs

Using the procedure that was described in Section 2, the DBN structure shown in Fig. 3, is derived from the ICU-MM. As can be seen, each equation is mapped to a subnet in the DBN. The DBN contains both hidden and observed nodes. Hidden (continuous or discrete) random nodes are dark grey, observed nodes are black and deterministic nodes are light grey.

The DBN is expanded as described in Section 2.2. Model parameters are represented as truncated Gaussian nodes and allowed to vary over time. Their

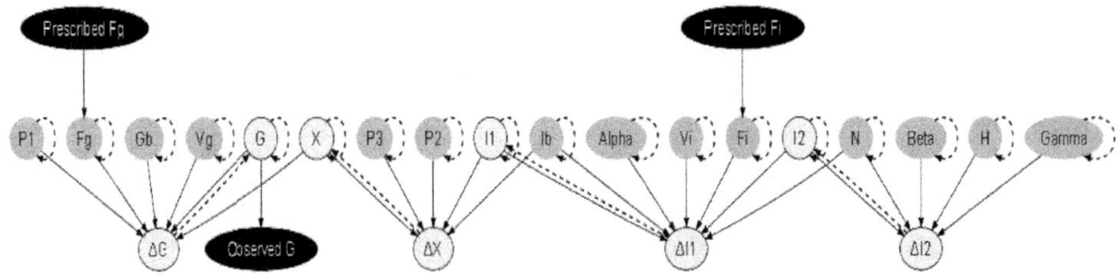

Fig. 3. The ICU-MM system of differential equations mapped to a DBN

initial mean values are based on the literature. The observed value for plasma glucose (Observed G in the DBN) is assumed to contain a certain amount of measurement error. It is therefore modelled with a Gaussian distribution whose mean is its parent node, the actual plasma glucose level, G. Likewise, the data from the ICU reflects the prescribed intravenous infusion rates for insulin and glucose; the actual administered rates may be different. Therefore, the actual rates are modelled with Gaussian distributions whose means are the prescribed rates. In this way, data uncertainty is handled. Note that where we use Gaussian distributions in this model, other distributions can be used where suitable.

The delta nodes capture changes in quantities over time. These changes are calculated using the differential equations of the ICU-MM. Each delta node has, as parent nodes, the various terms needed to solve the appropriate differential equation. A standard particle filtering algorithm by Gordon et al. [8] is used to determine the most probable states of the DBN nodes.

5 Evaluation

5.1 Description of the Data

For comparative evaluation of the methods, data was used from historical patient records from the ICU of University College Hospital, Galway. The patients are not on specific insulin therapy trials, so the dataset only contains routine measurements. Accordingly, plasma glucose measurements are infrequent and sporadic. At times, changes in the plasma glucose cannot be explained with the data available; this may be because either information is incomplete (e.g., the patient was administered glucose that was not recorded) or measurements are inaccurate (e.g., due to data-entry errors or measurement assay).

However, this dataset provides a realistic sample of the routine data available in a busy ICU where a system such as the one described here could eventually be deployed for patient monitoring and simulations of the effects of therapies.

5.2 DBN Results for a Sample Patient

For the purposes of this discussion, a reasonably stable patient is selected. As can be seen in Fig. 4, the observations for plasma glucose are intermittent;

the DBN therefore makes internal predictions of plasma glucose levels in between observations. The accuracy of the predictions can be evaluated by comparing the predicted value at the time of a measurement to the actual value. In Fig. 4, the dark lines are the mean values inferred by the DBN at each minute, and the lighter shaded areas show their standard deviations, to give a sense of the uncertainty associated with each prediction. One can observe that the mean

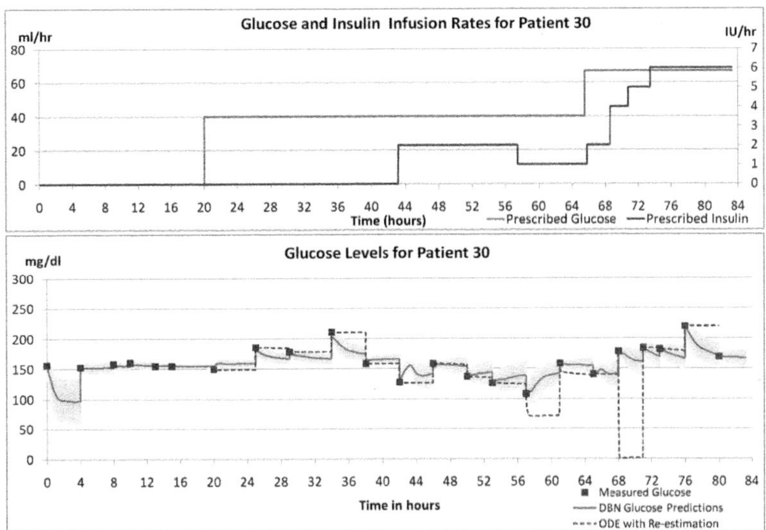

Fig. 4. The top graph shows the prescribed insulin and glucose infusion rates. The lower graph shows the measured glucose levels as boxes and the predicted mean plasma glucose level in blue along with a shaded area showing the predicted standard deviation.The dashed line shows the Euler approximation of the ODEs with an optimisation algorithm for parameter re-estimation.

value often jumps when a new observation becomes available. There are factors that are unknown to the model that influence plasma glucose levels. Because of these, mean values predicted by the model can drift from reality in between observations. When a new observation is available, the model tends to realign with it. It is informative to consider how the standard deviations vary over time. Because the DBN always assumes variability of values over time, and because observations of plasma glucose levels are available only intermittently, as the time since the last observation increases, the range of possible values increases, so the uncertainty of the predictions also increases. Whenever an observation is provided, the DBN's plasma glucose prediction realigns to a value close to this, and its uncertainty collapses.

It should be noted that glucose measurements (evidence) are very infrequent relative to the time step (1 minute) used in the DBN. This time step is determined by the system dynamics.

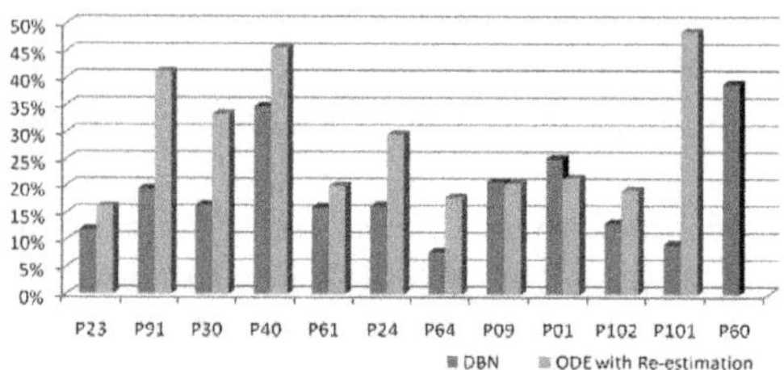

Fig. 5. Average RMSPE (lower is better) for 12 patients, comparing results using our DBN approach and an Euler approximation with parameter re-estimation

5.3 Comparison to ODEs With Parameter Re-estimation

Van Herpe et al. re-estimate the model parameters by using an unconstrained nonlinear optimization algorithm [9]. Attempts to apply that specific approach on our dataset, which has less frequent evidence, were unsuccessful; the optimisation algorithm frequently failed to converge. Therefore, a variant on the method is used [10], which allows bounds to be placed on the parameters to be re-estimated. As our glucose measurements are less frequent, all measurements within the previous 24 hours are used each time parameters are re-estimated. The dashed line in Fig. 4 shows the trajectory for the ODEs with re-estimation.

5.4 DBN Results for Twelve Patients

Fig. 5 shows a comparison of the average root mean squared percentage error (RMSPE) calculated using the difference between the actual glucose measurements and glucose predictions for twelve ICU patients, chosen at random according to the criteria in Section 5.1. In 10 out of 12 cases the DBN method out-performs the other method, very substantially so in some cases, such as Patient 101, where the ODE solution gives an error of 48.57% but the DBN framework produces a much lower error of 9.28%. In the case of patient (P60), the optimisation algorithm could not find appropriate parameters, whereas the DBN framework was able to make predictions, albeit with a high RMSPE of 38.98%. Hence the ODE result is not plotted in Fig. 5. It should be noted that while we are comparing the RMSPE of predictions relative to measured values, the measured values are not always perfectly accurate.

6 Discussion and Related Research

In the evaluation presented on the abstract and real-world examples, the DBN out-performed the traditional analysis method. We believe similar results would be obtained for systems with similar characteristics: large inter- and intra-individual variability; model uncertainty; data uncertainty; sparse, sporadic data.

For the comparisons presented in Section 5, only predictions made after the first 24 hours are used, since the ODE approach requires this time for its initial calibration. However, the DBN does not require a large parameter estimation window; as can be seen in Fig. 4, it starts to adjust to the individual patient once it gets the first glucose measurement after t_0. The DBN also predicts means and standard deviations rather than a single glucose value. In a system which contains such high levels of uncertainty, this can be more useful.

We have described a methodolgy for building DBNs from systems of ODEs and demonstrated its effectiveness on a non-linear system where evidence is sparse and infrequent. We have shown how it can individualize model parameters in real-time based on accumulated evidence while handling data uncertainty.

Work somewhat similar to ours was carried out by Andersen and Højbjerre [11]. They reworked Bergman's Minimal Model [12], which is a system of DEs to assist in the diagnoses of diabetes, into a DBN model. Their approach is, however, significantly different. They first derive a system of stochastic differential equations from the Minimal Model and then encode these equations in a DBN. Our approach is a more direct mapping and does not require any such transformation of a system of DEs prior to constructing the DBN.

Indeed much work has previously been carried out to represent dynamic systems in both Bayesian Networks and DBNs. Bellazzi et al. [13] provide a good comparison of some of these methods. While some focus on predicting the patient specific model parameters which are then used offline [14], others discretise the state-space [15] and so do not explicitly incorporate the model equations. Voortman et al. [16] propose building causal graphs from time-series data and exploiting the ODEs to impose constraints on the model structure.

7 Future Work and Conclusions

Much knowledge of human physiology is formalised as systems of differential equations. This paper has presented a methodology for incorporating this knowledge in a DBN framework. The methodology is used to predict a critically ill patient's plasma glucose levels in response to insulin and glucose infusions. With the data available, which is sporadic and may be inaccurate and incomplete, the DBN approach out-performs a previous approach demonstrating that the DBN method is effective at re-estimating model parameters and reasoning with sparse and potentially unreliable data.

While the methodology described in this paper concerns building the DBN structure using an existing body of knowledge in the form of ODEs, future work will exploit the knowledge in the ICU database to learn the conditional probability tables. By combining the knowledge available in the data with the expert knowledge available in the form of differential equations we believe we will have a powerful tool for reasoning with uncertain and sparse data.

Acknowledgements. We are grateful to the UHG Research Ethics Committee for granting permission to extract historical records from the database in the ICU of University Hospital Galway and to Brian Harte, Anne Mulvey and

Conor Lane for their assistance in extracting and interpreting the data. This material is based upon works supported by the Science Foundation Ireland under Grant No. 08/RFP/CMS1254.

References

1. Ottesen, J.T., Olufsen, M.S., Larsen, J.K.: Applied Mathematical Models in Human Physiology. SIAM: Society for Industrial and Applied Mathematics, Philadelphia (2004)
2. Berg, H.V.D.: Mathematical Models of Biological Systems. Oxford University Press, Oxford (2011)
3. Russell, S., Norvig, P.: Artificial Intelligence: A Modern Approach, 2nd edn. Prentice Hall, Englewood Cliffs (2002)
4. Murphy, K.: Dynamic Bayesian Networks: Representation, Inference and Learning. PhD thesis, Dept. Computer Science, UC Berkeley (2002)
5. Iserles, A.: A First Course in the Numerical Analysis of Differential Equations. Cambridge University Press, Cambridge (2008)
6. Krinsley, J.S., Grover, A.: Severe Hypoglycemia in Critically Ill Patients: Risk Factors and Outcomes. Crit. Care Med. 35, 2262–2267 (2007)
7. Van Herpe, T., Pluymers, B., Espinoza, M., Van den Berghe, G., De Moor, B.: A Minimal Model for Glycemia Control in Critically Ill Patients. In: 28th IEEE EMBS Annual International Conference, pp. 5432–5435 (2006)
8. Gordon, N.J., Salmond, D.J., Smith, A.F.M.: Novel Approach to Nonlinear/Non-Gaussian Bayesian State Estimation. In: IEE Proceedings F, Radar and Signal Processing, pp. 107–113 (1993)
9. Lagarias, J.C., Reeds, J.A., Wright, M.H., Wright, P.E.: Convergence Properties of the Nelder-Mead Simplex Method in Low Dimensions. SIAM J. Optimiz. 9, 112–147 (1998)
10. D'Errico, J.: Matlab Function fminsearchbnd, `http://www.mathworks.com/matlabcentral/fileexchange/8277-fminsearchbnd`
11. Andersen, K.E., Højbjerre, M.: A Bayesian Approach to Bergman's Minimal Model. In: The Ninth International Workshop on Artificial Intelligence and Statistics, pp. 236–243 (2003)
12. Bergman, R.N., Phillips, L.S., Cobelli, C.: Physiologic Evaluation of Factors Controlling Glucose Tolerance in Man: Measurement of Insulin Sensitivity and Beta-Cell Glucose Sensitivity from the Response to Intravenous Glucose. J. Clin. Invest. 68, 1456–1467 (1981)
13. Bellazzi, R., Magni, P., De Nicolao, G.: Dynamic Probabilistic Networks for Modelling and Identifying Dynamic Systems: A MCMC Approach. Intelligent Data Analysis 1, 245–262 (1997)
14. Bellazzi, R.: Drug Delivery Optimization through Bayesian Networks. In: Annual Symposium on Computer Application in Medical Care, pp. 572–578 (1992)
15. Hejlesen, O.K., Andreassen, S., Hovorka, R., Cavan, D.A.: DIAS-The Diabetes Advisory System: An Outline of the System and the Evaluation Results Obtained So Far. Computer Methods and Programs in Biomedicine 54, 49–58 (1997)
16. Voortman, M., Dash, D., Druzdzel, M.J.: Learning Why Things Change: The Difference-based Causality Learner. In: 26th Conference on Uncertainty in Artificial Intelligence (2010)

Managing COPD Exacerbations with Telemedicine

Maarten van der Heijden[1,2], Bas Lijnse[1], Peter J.F. Lucas[1], Yvonne F. Heijdra[3], and Tjard R.J. Schermer[2]

[1] Institute for Computing and Information Sciences, Radboud University Nijmegen, The Netherlands
[2] Department of Primary and Community Care, Radboud University Nijmegen Medical Centre, The Netherlands
[3] Department of Pulmonary Diseases, Radboud University Nijmegen Medical Centre, The Netherlands

Abstract. Managing chronic disease through automated systems has the potential to both benefit the patient and reduce health-care costs. We are developing and evaluating a monitoring system for patients with chronic obstructive pulmonary disease which aims to detect exacerbations and thus help patients manage their disease and prevent hospitalisation. We have carefully drafted a system design consisting of an intelligent device that is able to alert the patient, collect case-specific, subjective and objective, physiological data, offer a patient-specific interpretation of the collected data by means of probabilistic reasoning, and send data to a central server for inspection by health-care professionals. A first pilot with actual COPD patients suggests that an intervention based on this system could be successful.

1 Introduction

Increasing demands on health-care and continuous pressure from health-care authorities and insurance companies to reduce costs has created a situation in which automated patient assistance by telemedicine has become an attractive idea. Specifically in the context of chronic disease management, where patients are continuously at risk of deteriorating health, automated monitoring can relieve work-load of health-care workers, while helping patients self-manage their disease. These possible benefits are worth to be investigated, to establish whether or not telemedicine can effectively help.

Chronic obstructive pulmonary disease, or COPD for short, is a chronic lung disease with high impact on patient well-being and with considerable health-care related costs [1]. Exacerbations – acute events of worsening of symptoms – are important events in the progression of COPD, such that monitoring patients in a home setting to detect exacerbation onset may be warranted [2]. In this paper we describe a research project on detecting and managing the occurrence of exacerbations of COPD at an early stage. We aim to decrease the impact of chronic obstructive pulmonary disease on the patient's quality of life by means of a monitoring system that collects and interprets data by a probabilistic model to assess the exacerbation risks. This should help patients with self-management and prevent unscheduled doctor visits and hospitalisation due to exacerbations, as the monitoring system enables a faster response to their occurrence. In

M. Peleg, N. Lavrač, and C. Combi (Eds.): AIME 2011, LNAI 6747, pp. 169–178, 2011.

the research described here, we report on work on the construction of such a system and a study of its technical and clinical feasibility with a number of COPD patients.

An important feature of the system is that we use smartphones for the monitoring, thereby foregoing the need for a personal computer (PC) with internet connectivity. This has the advantage that whereas most people are used to responding to phone alerts, sending reminders via a PC may have little effect on the patient's behaviour. Most important, perhaps, is that data interpretation is performed directly on the smartphone enabling instant feedback to the patient. This is different from earlier work (e.g. [3]) in which telemonitoring data was analysed remotely by hand.

From a clinical point of view the importance of the research lies in empowering patients to monitor their disease and in providing timely intervention if needed. It also provides the nurse or physician with a means to stay informed on the patient's COPD-related health status. There exists some work on telemonitoring for COPD [4,5], however these systems are not as extensive as the support system we are developing now, including automated intelligent interpretation of questionnaire answers and sensor readings.

The rest of this paper is structured as follows: first in Section 2 we describe in more detail our current application domain COPD, followed by a description of the monitoring system being developed in Section 3; then in Section 4 we describe the model used to estimate exacerbation risk; Section 5 presents some initial pilot results; finally we conclude and note some future work that remains.

2 Chronic Obstructive Pulmonary Disease

Chronic obstructive pulmonary disease currently affects some 210 million people worldwide[1] and is one of the major chronic diseases in terms of both morbidity and mortality. COPD affects airways and lungs, decreasing lung capacity and obstructing airways, thus interfering with normal breathing. Patients often suffer from a combination of emphysema and chronic bronchitis, causing shortness of breath and therefore reducing their capability of performing day-to-day activities. The main cause of COPD is exposure to tobacco smoke, followed by severe air pollution. COPD is currently not curable, but treatment does reduce the burden considerably (for further information on COPD see e.g. the Global Initiative for Chronic Obstructive Lung Disease (GOLD)[2]).

An important aspect of COPD which is particularly relevant in the present context is the progressive nature of the disease. Specifically acute deterioration has a profound impact on patient well-being and on health-care cost [1]. These exacerbations are mainly caused by infections resulting in symptom worsening [6]. Important to note is also that patients with frequent exacerbations usually have faster disease progression, which makes exacerbation prevention a particularly interesting goal. Additionally, a faster treatment response to exacerbations leads to better recovery [7].

The state of the respiratory system is observable via symptoms including dyspnea, productive cough, wheezing breath and decreased activity due to breathlessness.

[1] World Health Organization http://www.who.int/mediacentre/factsheets/fs315/en/index.html Accessed: January 2011.

[2] www.goldcopd.com

Besides these symptoms a number of physiological signs are relevant, in particular the forced expiratory volume in 1 second (FEV_1) and blood oxygen saturation. FEV_1 measures airway obstruction by testing whether the patient can overcome obstructive and restrictive resistance during forced exhalation. A number of other indicators of deterioration exist, like blood-gas pressure, inflammatory proteins and white blood-cell count, however, measuring these factors requires hospital-grade equipment and incurs considerable inconvenience for the patient. Blood oxygen pressure can be observed by proxy, with a pulse-oximeter that measures blood oxygen saturation.

3 Patient Monitoring at Home

The long term nature of COPD and associated exacerbation risk requires that a monitoring system can easily be deployed in a home-care setting. Not only efficacy, but also usability is an important factor in the design. This section describes the current system design and some of the issues that arise.

3.1 System Description

In Fig. 1 a graphical representation of the exacerbation monitoring system-setup is shown. The monitoring system consists of a smartphone, a sensor interface (Mobi) to which a micro-spirometer and pulse-oximeter are connected, and a web-centre. Data is collected from the patient through the smartphone, which also communicates wirelessly with the sensor interface. The web-centre receives the data from the smartphone and provides data access for health-care workers.

Before going into more detail on the various components let us first describe the monitoring process. At regular intervals, adjustable in frequency and in time of the day, the patient gets an automatic reminder for data entry from the smartphone. The patient is presented with a simple touch-interface to answer a set of questions about COPD symptoms and is subsequently asked to perform a spirometry test and pulse-oximeter measurement. The results of the measurements are transmitted to the phone,

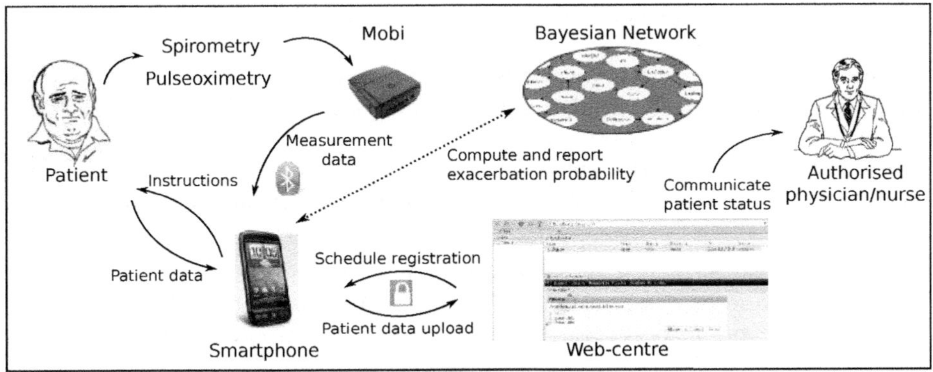

Fig. 1. Schematic of the system setup for COPD exacerbation detection and monitoring

and entered in a Bayesian network model (described in more detail in the next section) to obtain a probability of exacerbation. In addition, the data is synchronised with the web-centre, which allows the responsible health-care workers to examine the patient data; depending on the situation this may be a nurse specialised in lung diseases, general practitioner or pulmonologist. If necessary, the patient can be advised to take action, based on the model's prediction.

Technical Details

Smartphone. Currently our monitoring system runs on an HTC Desire smartphone as an application in the Android OS. In principle any Android phone with Bluetooth capability should suffice, which makes the platform fairly general. The application has been custom-made to provide the questionnaire functionality; manage communication with the sensors and web-centre; and compute the model predictions.

Model Implementation. The Bayesian network has been developed using SamIam[3], and ProBT[4], which provides an implementation of the expectation-maximisation algorithm used for learning probabilities from data. For the monitoring application we used the lightweight reasoning engine EBayes[5], in combination with a custom Perl script to perform the necessary conversion in network representation. Since EBayes is written in Java the model inference could easily be integrated in the Android application. Due to the relatively small size of the Bayesian network and the processing power of modern smartphones it turns out that the inference does not have to be deferred to a server but can be performed on site. This has the advantage that even when mobile phone network coverage is suboptimal the application can still provide a probability estimate.

Sensor Interface. The phone communicates with the sensors via a Mobi, a Bluetooth-capable multichannel sensor-interface, from Twente Medical Systems International. In our case a Nonin pulse-oximeter and a custom micro-spirometer were connected to the Mobi. An important advantage of using the Mobi sensor interface is the availability of the communication-protocol specification, enabling us to integrate the sensor readings seamlessly into the Android application. Most of the other micro-spirometers on the market do not allow this, which makes them unsuitable for easy deployment in a home setting. The monitoring kit is shown in Fig. 2.

Pulse-Oximeter. The pulse-oximeter used in this study was a Nonin Medical 8000AA, which is an industry standard pulse-oximeter. SpO_2 accuracy is 70-100% ± 2 digits.

Spirometer. We used custom-made pneumotachograph micro-spirometer prototypes by Twente Medical Systems International. These spirometers are newly developed to

---

[3] Automated Reasoning Group, University of California, Los Angeles. `http://reasoning.cs.ucla.edu/samiam/` Accessed: April 2011.

[4] Probayes `http://www.probayes.com/index.php/en/products/sdk/probt` Accessed: April 2011.

[5] F.G. Cozman, `http://www.cs.cmu.edu/~javabayes/EBayes/index.html/` Accessed: April 2011.

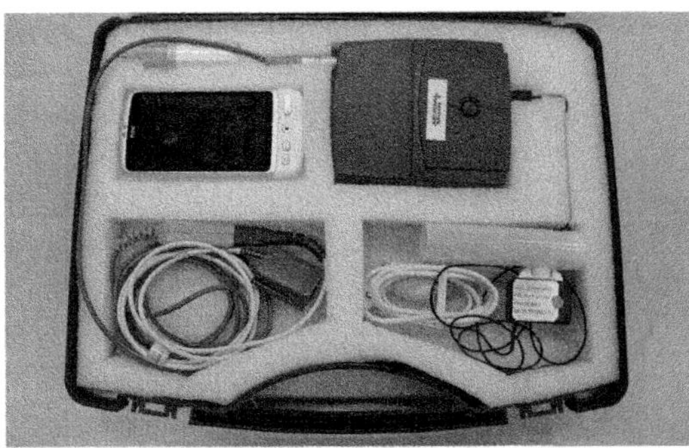

Fig. 2. The monitoring kit consisting of a smartphone, sensor interface and sensors

interact with the Mobi sensor interface and have the advantage of providing raw data such that analysing the spirometer readings is possible without requiring external software. This enables tight integration with our application, which is difficult or impossible with most commercial spirometers on the market.

Web-Centre. The web-centre provides an interface to the gathered data and is used to enrol patients, schedule registrations and similar practical issues. It is built using the workflow management system iTasks [8], which implements advanced features to generate and coordinate tasks and provides a generic (web)interface. Since the data management involved with patient monitoring is suitable to be represented as a workflow, iTasks provides a simple and effective way to construct the web-centre.

3.2 Design Considerations

Monitoring patients over longer periods of time requires a careful balance between costs and benefits. Specifically the intrusiveness of monitoring systems and costs both monetary and in terms of patient time investment result in a target population of patients with moderate to severe COPD and frequent exacerbations. These patients suffer greatly from the consequences of exacerbations, hence providing regular data to detect exacerbations in an early stage will in general be more acceptable. The most appropriate time to start the intervention would be directly after hospitalisation due to COPD, because then the goal of preventing hospitalisation is clearly relevant for the patient.

Due to the privacy sensitive nature of the data, all data transmission is encrypted (HTTPS). Also access-rights to the data in the web-centre have to be controlled and patients should give prior consent. Since these are general issues when working with patient data, we will not focus on them here, but they remain important.

Ease of use is a critical requirement for any system that has to be used on a regular basis for a prolonged period of time. Since the interval between exacerbations is usually in the order of months, one should take care to reduce patient effort to a minimum, lest patients would stop entering data due to it being inconvenient. The patient population is relatively old on average – possibly not very experienced with technology – hence to facilitate understanding the web-centre provides the ability to do practice runs. The nurse will have a supportive role in training patients.

Depending on the health status of the individual patient the rate of data acquisition can be varied, which can be automated based on the acquired data and the model. As long as a patient has low risk of an exacerbation, monitoring can take place on a weekly basis, keeping the time investment at a minimum. If a patient is at risk according to model predictions, the system check-in can be scheduled daily to ensure the possible exacerbation is detected and acted upon appropriately. Unscheduled, patient initiated registrations are being implemented for the next pilot, facilitating self-management. Currently the system only advises to contact a physician, but further self-management supporting advice could be implemented. Advising to see a clinician does not interfere with current clinical practice guidelines, other advice will have to be implemented in accordance with the guidelines.

4 A Model for COPD Exacerbation Detection

4.1 Bayesian Network Structure

Data interpretation for exacerbation detection is performed by a Bayesian network, which is a probabilistic graphical model consisting of vertices representing random variables of interest and arcs representing dependencies between variables [9]. Each random variable has a quantitative part, denoting conditional probabilities of the type $P(X \mid pa(X))$, that is the probability that X takes on a specific value given the values of its parent variables. Probabilities of interest can be computed from the joint probability of all variables: in this case the probability of exacerbation given the evidence obtained from monitoring. An important observation is that although the model describes general relations between the variables of interest, all predictions are personalised by entering patient specific data. The model is thus capable of making predictions for individual situations, and can provide 'what-if'-predictions by entering virtual evidence.

The current COPD-exacerbation prediction model is depicted in Fig. 3. The main outcome variable is 'exacerbation', but the nature of a Bayesian network allows us to easily inspect probabilities for any variable. The network contains two 'hidden' variables, namely 'infection' and 'lung function' which cannot be observed directly, but whose values can be derived based on indirect measures, such as body temperature for infection and the forced expiratory volume in 1 second (FEV_1) for lung function. Other important variables are the symptoms that one might expect a patient to report, such as dyspnea (breathlessness), sputum volume and purulence, cough, wheeze and whether performing daily activities is difficult due to COPD. Additionally some clinical signs have been included such as the aforementioned FEV_1, blood oxygen saturation (SpO_2), CRP concentration, leukocytosis and blood gas and pH levels. Except for FEV_1 and SpO_2, these variables are mostly included for the sake of completeness, as they will not be observable in a home-care setting, which is the application's target.

4.2 Model Construction

The Bayesian network has been constructed in close cooperation with specialists of the Radboud University Nijmegen Medical Centre. A set of relevant variables that are

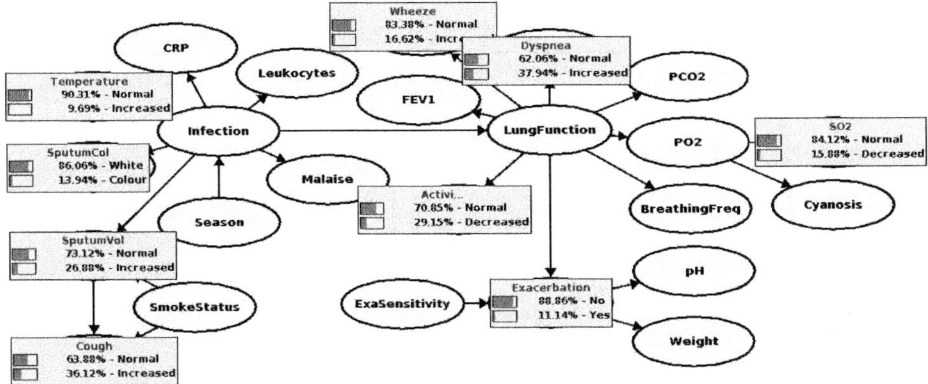

Fig. 3. Bayesian network for prediction of COPD exacerbations (probabilities partially shown)

related to exacerbations has been identified by domain experts – in this case two pulmonologists – supported with findings from current medical literature (e.g. [6]). As a second step the dependence relations between the variables have been elicited from the domain experts, resulting in the qualitative part of the model. Subsequently, probabilities have been estimated: starting from qualitative constraints we elicited probabilities from expert opinion and secondly, using a data set from an earlier project at the Radboud University Nijmegen Medical Centre, we estimated probabilities using the expectation-maximisation algorithm. Unfortunately, the data set does not include all variables of interest, therefore additional data (i.a. from [10]) will be used in a later stage for further evaluation of the probabilities. The expert opinion serves as an important comparison to make sure learned parameters are plausible.

4.3 Model Test

To get some feeling for the efficacy of the model we performed a preliminary evaluation with the available data consisting of questionnaire answers of 86 Dutch COPD patients, 54 of which had an exacerbation during the study. The data has been acquired biweekly during 2006-2007 via automatic telephone interviews, resulting in time series data with a total of 1922 data entries, of which 162 entries provided exacerbation data. It should therefore be noted that data correlation may influence the analysis result, as these temporal correlations were not taken into account. Data is only available for a subset of the variables in the model, specifically: exacerbation, dyspnea, sputum volume and colour, wheeze, cough, activity and season. We performed an ROC-analysis on this sub-model with expert opinion probabilities and with learned probabilities, using 10-fold cross-validation. In Fig. 4 the curves are shown for both the data and expert model, conveying that the predictions can indeed distinguish the exacerbation cases. For the data model we find a mean area under the curve (AUC) of 0.93; and for expert model a mean AUC of 0.97. It should be noted however that these results are based on cross-validation only and not on an independent test set; also the limited number of positive examples results in a rather large increase in true positive rate for each case classified correctly.

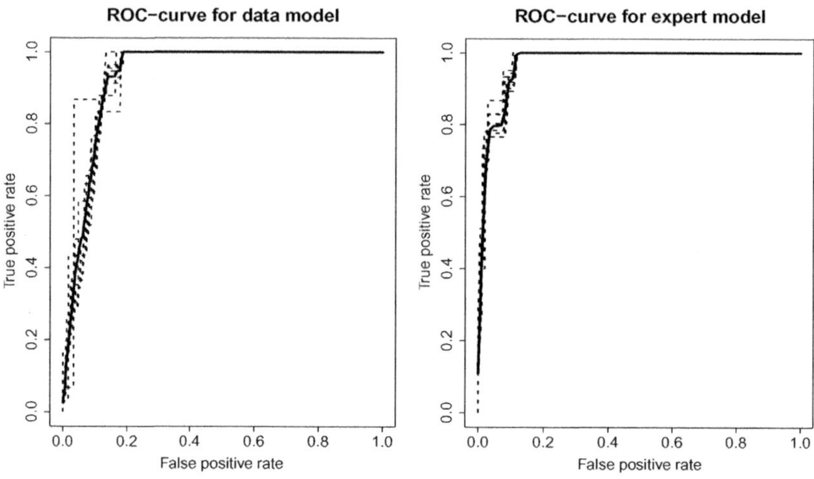

Fig. 4. ROC-curves, cross-validation results (dashed lines) and average (bold)

These first results indicate that we can at least detect exacerbations as they are happening, which is already useful. However, the more interesting task of actually predicting exacerbations still lies ahead, as currently we lack sufficient data to model the temporal progression. In further testing of the system we also plan to gather the necessary data to construct a temporal model, which requires trend analysis of time courses of symptoms and signs leading up to an exacerbation.

5 Evaluation

5.1 Pilot Study

Careful evaluation of a number of different aspects is needed to assess the system's efficacy, ranging from usability to the accuracy of probabilities, overall effectiveness of predicting exacerbations and finally influence on disease management and health-care utilisation. We have carried out a initial feasibility study with COPD patients.

We performed a technical evaluation with a limited number of stable COPD patients, testing the monitoring equipment and data entry procedures to make sure they are bug-free, and usable from a patient perspective. This stage is described in more detail below. The second stage of evaluation consists of a small scale test in a home setting, supported by a nurse, to assess the full system and specifically obtain data to check the accuracy of the model and to construct a temporal model. The model accuracy testing will entail a side-by-side comparison of pulmonologists' assessment of exacerbations with model predictions, as well as a comparison with a data set with relevant measurements and exacerbation outcomes. If this stage turns out to be favourable, a follow-up project will have to test clinical validity.

5.2 Methods and Results

In order to test the technical feasibility and usability we conducted a pilot study with COPD patients recruited from the University Centre for Chronic Disease Dekkerswald in Groesbeek, the Netherlands.

Methods. For this study 5 stable patients were recruited by convenience sample from the lung rehabilitation program who gave informed consent to participate in the study. Using three exacerbation monitoring kits (as described in Section 3) patients were monitored for a duration of 9 days, starting in January 2011. Patients were contacted daily during this time to answer a set of questions and perform spirometry and oximetry measurement. The answers were entered as evidence into the Bayesian network model to determine the probability of occurrence of an exacerbation. These predictions have not been used for patient advice yet, as further model validation is required. Patients were asked to report malfunctioning which together with the received data and server-logs could be used to verify system performance. At the end of the monitoring period a semi-structured evaluation interview was held – both with the patient and with the health-care staff involved – to obtain qualitative feedback on the usability of the system. In the interview we established whether or not the patients understood the procedure and the questions and whether they found the phone-interface sufficiently usable. Also, we checked anomalous data we received (if any) and asked for suggestions for improvement. The evaluation results of the first 2 patients were used to improve the system before starting with the second group. As this was a technical feasibility test, the clinical data obtained were only used to check for errors in the application or obvious model inaccuracies, and checking the clinical accuracy of the model predictions is deferred to the next stage of experimental testing.

Results. The goal of the pilot test was twofold, first, to ascertain the technical feasibility of the system in a real but controlled test environment; and second, to obtain early feedback from end users on usability. As for the first goal, the pilot resulted in finding some inaccuracies in the server-side software specifically with respect to adequately recovering from connection errors, which could be amended and retested relatively easily. We can conclude that the system functions as designed at the technical level. With respect to the usability goal, some improvements became apparent at an early stage, such as response buttons being placed too close together for comfortable use and an unclearly worded question resulting in confusion. In the evaluation interview with the patients the consensus was that the system could be useful to gain insight in the disease, was easy to use and not found to be intrusive. In particular patients indicated that they would be willing to use such a system in a home-care setting, which will need to be verified more rigorously in the next pilot stage. It thus turns out that the patients' impression of the system after using it, is quite positive. Although the generalisability of these findings is limited (due to convenience sampling) it did provide us with early feedback from actual COPD patients, which we think is especially important because acceptance of this kind of systems is often a concern.

6 Conclusion

We have described the results of a feasibility study of the development of a smartphone-based home-monitoring system for COPD. The COPD exacerbation detection and monitoring system described in this paper uses probabilistic reasoning to automatically interpret patient specific data. Initial testing shows that applying the system is technically feasible and patients are capable and willing to use the system. The model is well-founded on expert knowledge, literature and data, providing exacerbation risk predictions that seem usable. We have thus produced and evaluated on a pilot scale an advanced system architecture for home monitoring of COPD exacerbations, with promising results. Future work will involve a more extensive test in a home-care setting, finally leading to a system capable of exacerbation detection in an early stage such that COPD exacerbation impact can be reduced.

Acknowledgements

This work is supported by the Netherlands organisation for health research and development, ZonMw project 300050003.

References

1. Viegi, G., Pistelli, F., Sherrill, D., Maio, S., Baldacci, S., Carrozzi, L.: Definition, epidemiology and natural history of COPD. Eur. Respir. J. (2007)
2. McKinstry, B., Pinnock, H., Sheikh, A.: Telemedicine for management of patients with COPD? The Lancet (2009)
3. Maiolo, C., Mohamed, E., Fiorani, C., Lorenzo, A.D.: Home telemonitoring for patients with severe respiratory illness: the Italian experience. J. Telemed. Telecare (2003)
4. Paré, G., Sicotte, C., St Jules, D., Gauthier, R.: Cost-minimization analysis of a telehomecare program for patients with chronic obstructive pulmonary disease. Telemed. J. e-Health (2006)
5. Trappenburg, J., Niesink, A., de Weert-van Oene, G., van der Zeijden, H., van Snippenburg, R., Peters, A., Lammers, J., Schrijvers, A.: Effects of telemonitoring in patients with chronic obstructive pulmonary disease. Telemed. J. e-Health (2008)
6. Wedzicha, J., Seemungal, T.: COPD exacerbations: defining their cause and prevention. The Lancet (2007)
7. Wilkinson, T., Donaldson, G., Hurst, J., Seemungal, T., Wedzicha, J.: Early therapy improves outcomes of exacerbations of chronic obstructive pulmonary disease. Am. J. Respir. Crit. Care Med. (2004)
8. Lijnse, B., Plasmeijer, R.: iTasks 2: iTasks for end-users. In: Morazán, M.T., Scholz, S.-B. (eds.) IFL 2009. LNCS, vol. 6041, pp. 36–54. Springer, Heidelberg (2010)
9. Pearl, J.: Probabilistic reasoning in intelligent systems: networks of plausible inference. Morgan Kaufmann, San Francisco (1988)
10. Hurst, J., Donaldson, G., Quint, J., Goldring, J., Patel, A., Wedzicha, J.: Domiciliary pulse-oximetry at exacerbation of chronic obstructive pulmonary disease: prospective pilot study. BMC Pulm. Med. (2010)

A Predictive Bayesian Network Model for Home Management of Preeclampsia

Marina Velikova[1], Peter J.F. Lucas[1], and Marc Spaanderman[2]

[1] Radboud University Nijmegen,
Institute for Computing and Information Sciences, The Netherlands
{marinav,peterl}@cs.ru.nl
[2] Maastricht University Medical Center,
Department of Obstetrics and Gynecology, The Netherlands
marc.spaanderman@mumc.nl

Abstract. There is increasing consensus among health-care professionals and patients alike that many disorders can be managed, in principle, much better at home than in an out-patient clinic or hospital. In the paper, we describe a novel temporal Bayesian network model for the at home time-related development of preeclampsia, a common pregnancy-related disorder. The network model drives an android-based smartphone application that offers patients and their doctor insight into whether or not the disorder is developing positively—no clinical intervention required—or negatively—clinical intervention is definitely required. We discuss design considerations of the model and system, and review results obtained with actual patients.

1 Introduction

In contrast to earlier telephone-based telemedicine solutions, where a cell phone was merely use as a device to transmit patient data to a central information service [1,2], available smartphones provide sufficient computing power for offline decision-making support, while offering at the same time more communication facilities. Therefore, the new big research challenge in telemedicine is to move part of the clinical decision-making process from the clinic to the home environment. This may also pave the way for *patient empowerment*, a promising health-care concept that assumes that patients themselves should be responsible for their own health.

In this paper, we describe research that aims at providing decision support to women with pregnancy-related disorders. These women are unique as: (i) their disorder is pregnancy related, the disorder will be 'cured' automatically after child birth; (ii) they are relative young and have more interest in applying modern technology such as smartphones to the management of their disease; (iii) they have a strong wish to be actively involved in improving the health of both their child and their own. The system we are developing for this purpose is called the *e-MomCare* system [3] and here, we describe a research part of it aimed at the development and evaluation of the decision-making technology. As the field of pregnancy-related disorders is a very practical clinical area, with limited time and money for clinical research, a major challenge lies in dealing with these important problems in the face of limited available data.

M. Peleg, N. Lavrač, and C. Combi (Eds.): AIME 2011, LNAI 6747, pp. 179–183, 2011.

2 Pregnancy-Related Disorders and Preeclampsia

The first pregnancy-related disorder we deal with in our research is the syndrome called *preeclampsia*: approximately 15% of first-time pregnant women develop part of this syndrome, characterised by high blood pressure and kidney damage with associated proteinuria (leakage of serum protein into the urine). It is the most important cause of death among pregnant women and a leading cause of foetal complications. As a pregnancy-related condition the only way to cure preeclampsia is to deliver the baby. However, early anti-hypertensive treatment in the subclinical, mostly moderately hypertensive phase, reduces the risk of getting preeclampsia.

Timely detection allows closer monitoring of those patients at risk and gives the opportunity to start with preventive medication. Common risk factors include [4]: age, a family or personal history of preeclampsia, chronic hypertension or kidney disease. For parous women (women who have given birth) without a history of preeclampsia the risk of developing preeclampsia is low. The stage in pregnancy where high blood pressure develops is variable and associated problems can appear within days. This requires frequent outpatient checks for taking measurements, increasing the workload for the second- and third-line health-care centres.

3 A Temporal Bayesian Network Model for Preeclampsia

Description. A Bayesian network $\mathcal{B}$ is a pair $\mathcal{B} = (G, P)$, where $G = (V, A)$ is an acyclic directed graph with vertices V and arcs $A \subseteq V \times V$ representing conditional independences that are respected by the associated joint probability distribution P [5]. This probability distribution is specified according to the factorisation structure of the graph by $P(X_V) = \prod_{v \in V} P(X_v \mid X_{\pi(v)})$, where $P(X_v \mid X_{\pi(v)})$ is a set of conditional probability distributions associated with variable X_v with corresponding vertex $v \in V$, also called conditional probability tables (CPTs) in the discrete case.

Preeclampsia is a *syndrome* that summarises the physiological changes of the cardiovascular and renal systems. These changes are partly an effect of risk factors and of treatments such as taking drugs, which may reduce the effect of particular risk factors. To make plausible predictions about the evolution of a syndrome, observing the organs' functioning over time is a necessity. The functioning of a particular organ X at a specific moment t, which is influenced by the drugs taken, affects the outcomes of laboratory tests. However, taking into account the functioning of X at the previous checkup $t - 1$, allows the medical doctor to conclude whether or not big changes in the functioning occur. The presence of a particular temporal pattern may then act as the basis (i) for a diagnosis at time t, which in turn may trigger the start of a treatment, and (ii) for predicting the future development of the syndrome.

The design of the Bayesian network model for preeclampsia was guided by this temporal conceptualisation. The model includes the risk factors and laboratory measurements taken during 10 checkups at 12, 16, 20, 24, 28, 32, 36, 38, 40 and 42 weeks of pregnancy and contains 112 variables; part of its structure is depicted in Fig. 1. The set of risk factors, as defined here, have an impact on the functioning of the vascular system and hence, they determine the risk for vascular dysfunction, which for brevity we referred as to *vascular risk* (VASCRISK). The cause-effect relationships are represented by RISKFACTOR $\rightarrow$ VASCRISK structures. To define the CPT of VASCRISK given all possible combinations of risk factor values, we need to fill in a table with 20736 entries, which is practically impossible. To represent in a compact fashion this CPT, we use causal independence modelling [6], where the non-observed variables C_i, $i = 1, \ldots, 9$ were added to model the interaction between the risk factors and the vascular risk.

The renal and vascular functions are major conditions determining the syndrome of preeclampsia. In our model these functions are represented as two binary variables with values of *ok* and *nok* (not ok), indicating the respective functional status. These variables cannot be directly measured but several laboratory tests are performed to determine their status such as blood pressure and protein to creatinine ratio. In the current e-MomCare system, the blood pressure is obtained via Bluetooth using a digital blood pressure device. We are also developing a module for automatic analysis of urine reagent test strips to determine the level of protein and creatinine, using the phone's camera and colour imaging techniques. The values of the measurements are explained by the presence of certain risk factors; for example chronic hypertension affects the blood pressure values, and smoking usually increases the level of hemoglobin. Any treatment taken by the patient at the time of the checkup has an impact on the status of the renal and vascular function as well, which is captured by the TREATMENT $\rightarrow$ FUNCTION graph structure. To capture the temporal development of both renal and vascular functions, we created a temporal model by adding links between the respective functional status at successive checkups. As a result, the combined status of the renal and vascular function define the development of the syndrome of preeclampsia at each medical checkups.

We next estimated the conditional probability distributions for the variables concerned. For the risk factors we used incidence rates and the literature mentioned in Section 2, whereas for the measurements we used the estimates provided by one gynaecologist and research studies. The prior probabilities are shown in Fig. 1. Time invariance of the conditional probability distributions, i.e., $P(X_t \mid X_{t-1}) = P(X_u \mid X_{u-1})$, for each time point t, u, was *not* assumed given that the patient's physiology changes drastically as a function of time.

Preliminary Model Evaluation. We performed a preliminary analysis of the prediction performance of the model using data of actual patients. Table 1 includes clinical and laboratory data for up to 24 week checkups for one patient with and one patient without preeclampsia (PE), including the prediction for preeclampsia computed by the model. To facilitate the analysis of the results we added the relative change of the current risk $P_{CURR}(PE)$ with respect to the prior $P_{PRIOR}(PE)$ computed as $(P_{CURR}(PE) - P_{PRIOR}(PE))/P_{PRIOR}(PE)$, used also by the clinicians in evaluating the patient's status. It is clear that for the preeclamptic patient the risk increases almost up to 5 times with respect to her prior risk in very early pregnancy, whereas for the non-preeclamptic patient the risk remains comparable over the pregnancy duration.

We next used data of 417 pregnant patients, of whom 33 ($\pm 7.9\%$) were preeclamptic, to evaluate to what extent the model is capable of distinguishing between the two groups of patients. In particular, we looked at cases with an increased relative risk change ≥ 1

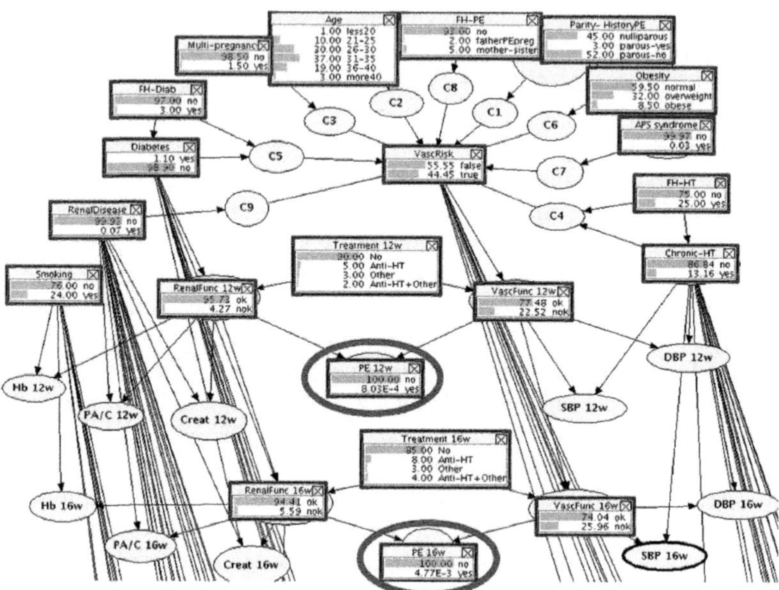

Fig. 1. Part of the temporal Bayesian network model for preeclampsia with prior probabilities

with respect to the prior at a particular time point; the results are reported in Table 2. We considered a relative risk change larger than 1 as suspicious patient's condition for the development of PE, requiring more regular monitoring.

At 12 weeks the model is able to detect 82% of the preeclamptic patients as suspicious, whereas almost half of the non-preeclamptic patients are judged as being non-suspicious. This is a desired result in patient monitoring where at an early stage a large part of the normal cases would not require intensive checkups thus reducing the workload of the physician and the number of visits to the out-patient clinic by patients. In addition, we considered the whole pregnancy duration as an alternative to the weekly selection period to allow future risk changes to be taken into account as well. Then the model is capable of detecting a higher number of preeclamptic patients but at the cost of increased inclusion of a number of normal cases as being preeclamptic. We note that these results are peliminary as the collected data was not fully representative—the clinical information and laboratory measurements were not consistently recorded. For example, we lacked proper treatment information and for some of the preeclamptic patients blood pressure measurements were missing. We are currently collecting more data, which will be used to gain further insight in the model's performance.

4 Discussion

We have described an intelligent model, first of its kind, for home-monitoring of pregnancy-related disorders. Early evaluation results indicate that the model structure are adequate, but that the probability distribution must be further refined. Getting access

Table 1. Input and output data for one patient with and one patient without preeclampsia

Risk factors	Patient A: Not-preeclamptic				Patient B: Preeclamptic			
Age	26-30				36-40			
Smoking	yes				yes			
Obese	obese				normal			
Chronic HT	yes				no			
Parity-HistoryPE	parous-yes				parous-yes			
Per control	**12 wk**	**16wk**	**20wk**	**24wk**	**12 wk**	**16wk**	**20wk**	**24wk**
Treatment	Other	Other	Other	Other	Other	Other	Other	n/a
Systolic BP	127-129	118-120	121-123	121-123	124-126	118-120	118-120	136-138
Diastolic BP	76-79	68-71	72-75	76-79	64-67	72-75	64-67	80-83
Hemoglobin	n/a	6.7	n/a	6.2	7.5	n/a	7.4	7.4
Creatinine	n/a	58-61	n/a	46-49	50-53	n/a	n/a	62-65
Protein/Creatinine	n/a	0	n/a	0	0	n/a	n/a	0.3-0.6
$P_{PRIOR}(PE)$	***0.0014***	***0.0076***	***0.05***	***0.16***	***0.0013***	***0.007***	***0.05***	***0.15***
$P_{CURR}(PE)$	***0.003***	***0.008***	***0.08***	***0.18***	***0.003***	***0.04***	***0.19***	***0.89***
Rel. change	*1.23*	*0.11*	*0.60*	*0.13*	*1.36*	*4.71*	*2.80*	*4.93*

Table 2. Number (%) of patients selected at a particular time with a relative change of risk ≥ 1

Time	PE patients	non-PE patients	Total
12 week	27 (82%)	207 (54%)	234 (56%)
16 week	24 (73%)	149 (39%)	173 (41%)
Whole pregnancy	31 (94%)	247 (64%)	278 (67%)

to clinical data in this area is not easy, and we have therefore set-up a data-collection process in the hospital. These data will be used to tune the probability distribution of the model such that it reflects current clinical practice in this area. Further field test will be carried out in close collaboration with a patient group.

References

1. Wu, W.H., Bui, A.A.T., Batalin, M.A., Au, L.K., Binney, J.D., Kaiser, W.J.: MEDIC: Medical embedded device for individualized care. AI Medicine 42(2), 137–152 (2008)
2. Rubel, P., Fayn, J., Simon-Chautemps, L., et al.: New paradigms in telemedicine: Ambient intelligence, wearable, pervasive and personalized. Wearable eHealth Systems for Personalised Health Management: State of the Art and Future Challenges 108, 123–132 (2004)
3. Velikova, M., Lucas, P., Spaanderman, M.: e-MomCare: a personalised home-monitoring system for pregnancy disorders. In: Proc. of the 5th Int. Workshop on Personalisation for e-Health (2010)
4. Duckitt, K., Harrington, D.: Risk factors for pre-eclampsia at antenatal booking: systematic review of controlled studies. BMJ 330(7491), 565–571 (2005)
5. Cowell, R., Dawid, A., Lauritzen, S., Spiegelhalter, D.: Probabilistic Networks and Expert Systems. Springer, New York (1999)
6. Heckerman, D., Breese, J.S.: Causal independence for probability assessment and inference using Bayesian networks. IEEE Trans. on SMC–A 26, 826–831 (1996)

Voting Techniques for a Multi-terminology Based Biomedical Information Retrieval

Duy Dinh and Lynda Tamine

University of Toulouse,
118 route de Narbonne, 31062 Toulouse, France
{dinh,lechani}@irit.fr

Abstract. We are interested in retrieving relevant information from biomedical documents according to healthcare professional's information needs. It is well known that biomedical documents are indexed using conceptual descriptors issued from terminologies for a better retrieval performance. Our attempt to develop a conceptual retrieval framework relies on the hypothesis that there are several broad categories of knowledge that could be captured from different terminologies and processed by retrieval algorithms. With this in mind, we propose a multi-terminology based indexing approach for selecting the best representative concepts for each document. We instantiate this general approach on four terminologies namely MeSH (Medical Subject Headings), SNOMED (Systematized Nomenclature of Medicine), ICD-10 (International Classification of Diseases) and GO (Gene Ontology). Experimental studies were conducted on large and official document test collections of real world clinical queries and associated judgments extracted from MEDLINE scientific collections, namely TREC Genomics 2004 & 2005. The obtained results demonstrate the advantages of our multi-terminology based biomedical information retrieval approach over state-of-the art approaches.

Keywords: Biomedical Information Retrieval, Voting Techniques, Controlled terminologies, Concept Extraction.

1 Introduction

With the rapid development of information technology, the innovation and advancement in healthcare, biomedical information from literature has been experienced an explosive growth in terms of size. In an attempt to facilitate the access to the vast amount of biomedical information, it is well known nowadays that the use of controlled terms through terminological systems is necessary. To cope with this need, several biomedical terminologies have been developed such as MeSH (Medical Subject Headings), SNOMED (Systematized Nomenclature of Medicine), ICD-10 (International Classification of Diseases), GO (Gene Ontology), UMLS[1] (Unified Medical Language System) and so on.

[1] The largest medical knowledge resource containing over 120 biomedical terminologies.

M. Peleg, N. Lavrač, and C. Combi (Eds.): AIME 2011, LNAI 6747, pp. 184–193, 2011.

In biomedical information retrieval (IR), concepts extracted from terminologies are used for normalizing the document or the query content and consequently lead to alleviate the term mismatch problem [1]. In this paper, the indexing using only one terminology is referred to as *mono-terminology indexing* and the one using several terminologies as *multi-terminology indexing*. While the former is usually based on MeSH, the latter is based on different terminologies. In general, indexing can be done manually or automatically. Manual indexing is undertaken by experienced human experts with specialized knowledge of terminologies. Automatic indexing is less likely to be expensive in terms of costs and time and thus could be an alternative for helping the manual task. It is mainly supported by the task of concept extraction, which is one of the important techniques in natural language processing for identifying concepts in controlled terminologies[2].

Although the MeSH thesaurus has been widely accepted as the main controlled vocabulary to index biomedical citations, it is so far unable to cover all medical terms in all the domains of medicine [3]. For instance, a growing interest has arisen in the use of SNOMED as a standard for the electronic health record and content coverage [4]. This problem has been faced so far by adopting two main approaches. The first one aims at building automatic or semi-automatic mappings between terminologies [5, 6]. The second main approach, most related to our work, attempts to extract concepts from different terminologies in order to better cover the subject matter(s) of the document and so to improve the recall of concept extraction in the latter task[7–9].

In this paper, we consider a different and novel multi-terminology based concept extraction approach for indexing and retrieving biomedical information. More specifically, our approach is inspired by the principle of poly-representation in IR [10] making simultaneous combination of evidences that are cognitively different in order to increase the information value of documents via concept extraction using several terminologies. In particular, we consider concept extraction as a voting problem taking into account both the scores and ranks of identified concepts predefined in different terminologies (viewed as sources of evidence). More specifically, using the list of concepts extracted from each document when applying an approximate concept extraction on each terminology, we propose first to weight concepts using a particular term weighting model. Second, we propose to merge the candidate concept lists by means of a voting process [11]. The remainder of this paper is structured as follows. Section 2 presents related work. Section 3 details our multi-terminology approach to biomedical IR. Experimental results are discussed in section 4. Section 5 concludes the paper.

2 Mono *vs.* Multi Terminology Biomedical Indexing

Document indexing or also document representation is the process of assigning the most representative terms to each document resulting in an inverted index structure for the retrieval purpose. In the general domain, indexes contain general keyword terms in the vocabulary. In a specific domain, the idea of using concepts from controlled vocabularies in IR comes from the fact that they are able to cover different instances related to a given idea in a domain such as synonyms, abbreviations, etc. In the biomedical domain, works on conceptual indexing have been extensively studied in literature [12–17]. Current conceptual indexing approaches, which focus on concept extraction using a mono terminology, can be categorized as (1) *dictionary-based* and (2) *statistical* approaches.

Dictionary-based approaches make use of existing terminologies to map free text to concept entries in a dictionary. For example, MTI [13] integrates several concept extraction methods for indexing MEDLINE citations. It provides first several lists of UMLS concepts and then restricts to MeSH concepts using the mappings between UMLS and MeSH. The work in [12] suggested a method based on an approximate string matching to recognize gene and protein names. In their approach, both protein dictionaries and target text are encoded using the nucleotide code (A, C, G, T). Then, the alignment techniques of DNA and protein sequences in databases are applied to the converted text in order to identify character sequences that are similar to existing gene and protein names. Authors in [15] proposed an approximate dictionary lookup to cope with term variations. The basic idea of their approach is to capture the significant words instead of all words of a particular concept. In a comparative study, their approximate extraction method reached a 71.60% precision and a 75.18% recall.

Statistical approaches have been proposed to address the recognition of general terms. For example, authors in [16] proposed the *C/NC* value method for recognizing technical terms used in Digital Libraries, which has been later used for recognizing biomedical terms [17]. The *C/NC* value is a domain-independent method combining statistical and linguistic information for extracting multi-word and nested terms. The work in [14] introduced a retrieval-based concept extraction where each MeSH concept (its synonyms and description) is indexed as a single document. A piece of text, the query to the retrieval system, is classified with the best ranked MeSH documents.

To the best of our knowledge, there is so far no work investigating the evaluation of the multi-terminology indexing for biomedical IR. However, there has been few works focusing on the use of multiple terminologies for indexing documents [8, 9]. The work in [8] proposed a multi-terminology indexing approach based on the bag-of-words concept extraction. In their approach, each sentence in the document is represented as multiple bags of words independently to the word order correlation between words in the sentence and the ones in concept names. According to their evaluation, they concluded that the multi-terminology approach outperforms the indexing relying on a single terminology in terms of recall for the concept extraction task. Similarly, authors in [9] presented a multi-terminology approach for indexing documents in the CISMeF portal but the concept extraction between free text and terminologies is based on the simple bag-of-words representation. The drawback of their extraction method, which may decrease the concept extraction accuracy, concerns the generation of all possible combinations of words in a given phrase that could be mapped to all possible bags-of-words of concepts in terminologies.

Our work presented in this paper aims at evaluating the impact of using multiple terminologies for biomedical IR. Our approach differs from previous works [8, 9] in two important ways: first, we use an approximate concept extraction method to identify concepts in each document using a mono terminology. Candidate concepts are weighted to measure their relevance to the document using a particular term weighting model (e.g., probabilistic model [18]). Second, we apply the concept extraction process on several terminologies and combine several concept lists using voting techniques. We see each concept identified from each document using multiple terminologies as an implicit vote for the document. Therefore, the multi-terminology based concept extraction can be modeled as a voting problem. The final concept list is considered to be revealing the document's subject matter(s) and could be used for document/query expansion.

3 A Voting Approach for a Multi-terminology Based IR

3.1 Multi-terminology Based Indexing and Retrieval Algorithms

Figure 1 depicts the two main stages of our biomedical IR framework.

Stage 1. Multi-terminology Indexing

```
Input: Collection C, Terminologies T
Output: Index I
for all document D in C do
    # Mono-terminology extraction
    for all terminology T_i in T do
        R(D,T_i) ← extract(D,T_i);
    end for
    # Concept fusion
    R(D,T) ← ∪_{i=1}^{n} R(D,T_i);
    # Document expansion
    D' ← expand(D, R(D,T));
    # Document indexing
    I ← addIndex(D');
end for
return I;
```

Stage 2. Document Retrieval

```
Input: Query Q, index I
Output: Result set S
# Query normalization:
# stemming, stopword removals
Q ← normalization(Q);
# First retrieval
S0 ← search(Q,I);
# Extract λ best terms from
# θ top-ranked documents
Γ ← extract(S0, λ, θ);
# Query expansion
Q^e ← expand(Q,Γ);
# Second retrieval
S ← search(Q^e, I);
return S;
```

Fig. 1. The multi-terminology based indexing and retrieval process

During the indexing stage, documents in the collection are indexed using terms in the documents that are expanded with relevant extracted concepts. Let $C(D)$ be the set of concepts extracted from document D and $C(T_i)$ be the set of concepts defined in terminology T_i. For each document D, the list of candidate concepts, denoted $R(D,T_i) = \{c_j | \forall c_j \in C(D) \wedge c_j \in C(T_i)\}$, is extracted using terminology T_i. We need to find the final set $R(D,T)$ containing the most relevant concepts for document D among the ones identified from several terminologies: $R(D,T) = \cup_{i=1}^{n} R(D,T_i)$, where $T = \{T_1, T_2, ..., T_n\}$, n is the number of terminologies used for indexing. During the retrieval stage, the top λ terms from the θ top-ranked documents retrieved from the first retrieval stage are used to expand the original user's query. We then detail our IR framework of two components: (1) *multi-terminology based indexing* and (2) *document retrieval.*

3.2 Multi-terminology Based Indexing as a Voting Problem

Our voting model for concept extraction is based on well known data fusion techniques (CombMAX, CombMIN, CombSUM, CombANZ ...) that have been used to combine data from different information sources [11]. They allow to produce optimal fused lists (terminological concepts in our current problem) using either the ranks of the retrieved documents (concepts), their scores or both of them. Our purpose here is to select the best multi-terminological concepts as a fusion of mono-terminological concepts by means of voting scores assigned to candidate concepts. For this purpose, we propose to combine rankings of the extracted concepts for each document using their matching scores and/or their ranks from the extraction stage. Intuitively speaking, the concept fusion can be seen as the voting problem described as follows. We compute the combined score of the candidate concept c_j voting for document D, given its score w_{ji}^D and rank r_{ji}^D when using terminology T_i, as the aggregation of votes of all identified concepts. We consider two sources of evidence when aggregating the votes to each candidate concept: (E1) Scores of the identified concept voting for each document; (E2) Ranks of the identified concept voting for each document.

We evaluate 8 voting techniques based on known data fusion methods [11], which aggregate the votes from several rankings of concepts into a single ranking of concepts, using both the ranks and/or scores of candidate concepts. The lists of extracted concepts from each document using several terminologies are merged together to obtain a final single concept list representing the document's subject matter(s). The optimal number of extracted concepts is retained for expanding the document content, namely document expansion (DE) [19], in an attempt to enhance the semantics of the document the document. Table 1 depicts all the voting techniques that we use and evaluate in this work. They are grouped into two categories according to the source of evidence used. The $\|.\|$ operator indicates the number of concepts having non-zero score in the described set; r_{ji}^D is the rank of concept c_j defined in terminology T_i and extracted from document D; and w_{ji}^D is the score of concept c_j, defined in T_i and extracted from document D, computed using the probabilistic BM25 scheme [18]. Formally:

$$w_{ji}^D = 1/\ell * \sum_{k=1}^{\ell} tf(w_k) * \frac{log\frac{N-n_k+0.5}{n_k+0.5}}{k_1 * ((1-b) + b\frac{dl}{avg\_dl}) + tf(w_k)} \quad (1)$$

where w_k is the constituent of concept c_j defined in terminology T_i; $tf(w_k)$ is the number of occurrences of word w_k in document D; N is the total number of documents in the collection; n_k is the number of documents containing word w_k; *dl* is the document length; *avg_dl* is the average document length; k_1, and b are parameters; ℓ is the number of words comprising concept c_j.

Table 1. Description of the voting techniques used for concept fusion

Category	Technique	score(c_j, D)	Description
Rank-based	CombRank	$\sum_{i=1}^{n}(\|R(D,T_i)\| - r_{ji}^D)$	Sum of concept ranks
	CombRCP	$\sum_{i=1}^{n} 1/r_{ji}^D$	Sum of inverse concept ranks
Score-based	CombSUM	$\sum_{i=1}^{n} w_{ji}^D$	Sum of concept scores
	CombMIN	$\min\{w_{ji}^D, \forall i = \overline{1..n}\}$	Minimum concept sores
	CombMAX	$\max\{w_{ji}^D, \forall i = \overline{1..n}\}$	Maximum concept scores
	CombMED	$median\{w_{ji}^D, \forall i = \overline{1..n}\}$	Median of concept scores
	CombANZ	$\sum_{i=1}^{n} w_{ji}^D \div \|\{c_j \in R(D,T)\}\|$	$CombSUM \div \|\{c_j \in R(D,T)\}\|$
	CombMNZ	$\sum_{i=1}^{n} w_{ji}^D \times \|\{c_j \in R(D,T)\}\|$	$CombSUM \times \|\{c_j \in R(D,T)\}\|$

3.3 Document Retrieval

The document retrieval aims at matching the user's query representation to the documents' one in order to retrieve a list of results that may satisfy the user information need. In our work, query terms are weighted using the well established BM25 model [18], where the score of document D for query Q is:

$$score(D,Q) = \sum_{t \in Q} \frac{(k_1+1) * tfn}{k+1+tfn} * \frac{(k_3+1) * qtf}{k_3+qtf} * w^{(1)} \tag{2}$$

where

- tfn is the normalized within-document term frequency given by:

$$tfn = \frac{tf}{(1+b) + b * \frac{dl}{avg\_dl}}, (0 \leq b \leq 1) \tag{3}$$

  where tf is the within-document term frequency, dl and avg_dl are respectively the document length and average document length in the collection
- k_1, k_3 and b are parameters (default values are $k_1 = 1.2, k_3 = 8.0, b = 0.75$),
- qtf is the within-query term frequency,
- $w^{(1)}$ is the *idf* (inverse document frequency) factor computed as follows:

$$w^{(1)} = log_2 \frac{N - N_t + 0.5}{N_t + 0.5} \tag{4}$$

  N is the total number of document in the collection; N_t is the number of documents containing term t,

As pointed out in our previous work [19], document expansion (DE) should come with query expansion (QE) for achieving a better IR effectiveness. The difference between DE and QE is basically the timing of the expansion step. In DE, terms are expanded during the indexing phase for each individual document while in QE only query terms are expanded at the retrieval stage. For QE, we used a pseudo or blind feedback technique to select the best terms from the top-ranked expanded documents. In our work, the term selection for QE is based on the Bose-Einstein statistics [20] for weighting terms in the expanded query Q^e derived from the original query Q.

4 Experimental Evaluation

4.1 Data Sets

We validate our multi-terminology based IR using two collections: TREC Genomics 2004 and 2005, which are the subset of about 4.6 millions MEDLINE citations from 1994 to 2003, under the Terrier IR platform[2]. However, human relevance judgments were merely made to a relative small pool, which were built from the top-precedence run from each of the participants. Our prototype IR system only indexes and searches all human relevance judged documents, i.e. the union of 50 single pools that contains total 48,753 citations in TREC 2004 and 41,018 ones in TREC 2005, without using manually assigned MeSH tags.

There are 50 queries in the TREC Genomics 2004 and 49 queries in TREC Genomics 2005. Table 2 depicts two examples of the TREC Genomics queries.

In our experiments described later, we used the latest version of four terminologies namely MeSH, SNOMED, ICD-10 and GO released in 2010.

Table 2. Examples of TREC Genomics queries

<ID>2</ID> <TITLE>Generating transgenic mice</TITLE> <NEED>Find protocols for generating transgenic mice.</NEED> <ID>15</ID> <TITLE>ATPase and apoptosis</TITLE> <NEED>Find information on role of ATPases in apoptosis</NEED>

4.2 Evaluation Protocol

This investigation aims at determining the utility of our multi-terminology IR approach within a conceptual IR framework. For this purpose, we designed two mono-terminology based indexing scenarios using state-of-the art concepts extractors namely MTI [13] and MaxMatcher [15]. The third scenario concerns our multi-terminology based concept extraction for biomedical IR. We detail in what follows the three indexing and retrieval scenarios leading to three series of experiments.

1. the first one concerns the mono-terminology indexing where MeSH concepts are extracted by the MTI tool, denoted MTI,
2. the second one concerns the mono-terminology indexing where MeSH concepts are extracted by MaxMatcher, denoted $MaxMatcher$,

[2] Terabyte Retriever (`http://terrier.org/`)

3. the third one concerns our multi-terminology IR approach where four terminologies MeSH, SNOMED, ICD-10 and GO are built into four dictionaries employed by MaxMatcher, which generates four concept lists for each document. We then applied the voting techniques for merging the final list of identified concepts as described in section 3.2.

According to our previous work [19], we extract the 20 most informative terms from 20 top returned documents, which are expanded with the top 5 identified concepts. The original query terms may appear in the 20 extracted terms.

For measuring the IR effectiveness, we used the MAP metrics representing the *Mean Average Precision* calculated over all the queries. The average precision of a query is computed by averaging the precision values computed for each relevant retrieved document of rank $x \in (1..N)$, where $N = 1000$ is the number of retrieved documents.

We compare the experimental results to the median official runs in each TREC year and then discuss each scenario.

4.3 IR Effectiveness Evaluation Results

Table 3 shows the IR performance of both the mono-terminology indexing task, i.e., the MTI tool [13], MaxMatcher [15] and the multi-terminology indexing task using 8 voting techniques on both the TREC Genomics 2004 and 2005. According to the results, we see that most of the voting techniques lead to a consistent improvement over the median runs. For instance, applying the $CombMNZ$ on the TREC Genomics 2004 collection results in an increase up to +118.37 % in terms of MAP over the median run. The improvement rate is even better than using a mono terminology (+94.12% for MTI and +112.73% for MaxMatcher). The $CombMNZ$ technique takes into account the score of the extracted concept as well as the number of terminologies where the concept is defined. Therefore, we think that highly weighted concepts that are defined in several terminologies tend to give the most important vote for the document and so to represent better the semantics of the document. For the TREC Genomics 2005 collection, the improvement rates of the voting techniques (ranging from +19.33 % to +23.56 %) are smaller but always result in a statistically significant increase in terms of MAP. The best MAP values are obtained using the $CombMIN, CombMAX$ or $CombMED$ techniques probably because the task of TREC Genomics 2005 focused more on finding gene and protein names that are mostly found in the Gene Ontology (GO) but not in the others.

As shown in Table 3, the paired-sample T-tests computed between MAP rankings of the median run in TREC Genomics 2004 and each of our run (e.g., $CombMNZ : M = 0.2455, t = 6.8517, df = 49, p = 0.001$) shows that our multi-terminology based IR approach is extremely statistically significant compared to the baseline. For the TREC Genomics 2005, our indexing approach yields smaller MAP improvements but that are always statistical significant compared to the baseline (e.g., $CombMIN : M = 0.0513, t = 2.1407, df = 48, p = 0.0374$). The obtained results are also superior to the best run in TREC Genomics 2004

(MAP=0.4075) and are found in the top four of automatic best runs in TREC Genomics 2005 (MAP of the fourth-best run is 0.2580) given that the MAP results of the top three best runs (0.2888, 0.2883, 0.2859) are very competitive.

Table 3. Retrieval effectiveness of MTI, MaxMatcher and the 8 voting techniques on the TREC Genomics 2004 and TREC Genomics 2005 collections

Run	**TREC Genomics 2004** MAP	Improvement (%)	**TREC Genomics 2005** MAP	Improvement (%)
Median	0.2074		0.2173	
	Mono-terminology indexing and retrieval			
MTI	0.4026†††	(+94.12)	0.2390	(+09.99)
MaxMatcher	0.4412†††	(+112.73)	0.2639	(+21.45)
	Multi-terminology indexing and retrieval			
CombANZ	0.4435†††	(+113.84)	0.2647	(+20.89)
CombMAX	0.4387†††	(+111.52)	0.2684†	(+23.52)
CombMED	0.4459†††	(+115.00)	0.2683†	(+23.47)
CombMIN	0.4440†††	(+114.08)	**0.2685**†	(+23.56)
CombMNZ	**0.4529**†††	(+118.37)	0.2593	(+19.33)
CombRank	0.4407†††	(+112.49)	0.2594	(+19.37)
CombRCP	0.4371†††	(+110.75)	0.2601	(+19.70)
CombSUM	0.4470†††	(+115.53)	0.2601	(+19.70)

Significant changes at $p \leq 0.05, 0.01$ and 0.001 are denoted †,†† and ††† respectively.

5 Conclusion

In this paper, we have proposed a novel multi-terminology approach to biomedical information retrieval. We argued that concept extraction using multiple terminologies can be regarded as a voting problem taking into account the rank and score of identified concepts. The extracted concepts are used for DE and QE in an attempt to close the semantic gap between the user's query and documents in the collection. The results demonstrate that our multi-terminology IR approach shows a significant improvement over the median runs participating in TREC Genomics 2004-2005 tracks. We conclude that conceptual IR in conjunction with an efficient way of identifying appropriate concepts in terminologies for DE/QE purposes would significantly improve the biomedical IR performance.

Our future work aims at incorporating our multi-terminology IR into a semantic model taking into account the concept centrality and specificity, which we believe to be able to overcome the limits of the bag-of-words based models. We also plan to combine several dictionary-based and statistical concept extraction methods by leveraging the advantages of each method. We believe that concepts extracted from several methods would enhance the concept extraction accuracy.

References

1. Zhou, X., Hu, X., Zhang, X.: Topic signature language models for ad hoc retrieval. IEEE Transactions on Knowledge and Data Engineering 19(9), 1276–1287 (2007)
2. Krauthammer, M., Nenadic, G.: Term identification in the biomedical literature. Journal of Biomedical Informatics 37, 512–528 (2004)
3. Keizer, N.F., et al.: Understanding terminological systems I: Terminology and Typology. Methods of Information in Medicine, 16–21 (2000)
4. Cornet, R., de Keizer, N.: Forty years of SNOMED: a literature review. BMC Medical Informaticas and Decision Making, pp. 268–272 (2008)
5. Nyström, M., et al.: Enriching a primary health care version of ICD-10 using SNOMED CT mapping. Journal of Biomedical Semantics, 7–28 (2010)
6. Taboada, M., et al.: An automated approach to mapping external terminologies to the UMLS. IEEE Transactions of Biomedical Engeenering, 605–618 (2009)
7. Avillach, P., Joubert, M., Fieschi, M.: A Model for Indexing Medical Documents Combining Statistical and Symbolic Knowledge. In: Proc. AMIA Symp., pp. 31–35 (2007)
8. Pereira, S., Neveol, A., et al.: Using multi-terminology indexing for the assignment of MeSH descriptors to health resources. In: Proc. AMIA Symp., pp. 586–590 (2008)
9. Darmoni, S.J., Pereira, S., Sakji, S., Merabti, T., Prieur, É., Joubert, M., Thirion, B.: Multiple terminologies in a health portal: Automatic indexing and information retrieval. In: Combi, C., Shahar, Y., Abu-Hanna, A. (eds.) AIME 2009. LNCS, vol. 5651, pp. 255–259. Springer, Heidelberg (2009)
10. Ingwersen, P.: Cognitive perspectives of information retrieval interaction-elements of cognitive theory. Journal of Documentation 52, 3–50 (1996)
11. Fox, E.A., Shaw, J.A.: Combination of Multiple Searches. In: TREC 1994, pp. 243–252 (1994)
12. Krauthammer, M., Rzhetsky, A., et al.: Using BLAST for identifying gene and protein names in journal articles. Gene, 245–252 (2000)
13. Aronson, A.R., Mork, J.G., Gay, C., Humphrey, S.M., Rogers, W.J.: The NLM Indexing Initiative's Medical Text Indexer. In: Medinfo 2004, pp. 268–272 (2004)
14. Ruch, P.: Automatic assignment of biomedical categories: toward a generic approach. Bioinformatics 22(6), 658–664 (2006)
15. Zhou, X., Zhang, X., Hu, X.: MaxMatcher: Biological Concept Extraction Using Approximate Dictionary Lookup. In: Yang, Q., Webb, G. (eds.) PRICAI 2006. LNCS (LNAI), vol. 4099, pp. 1145–1149. Springer, Heidelberg (2006)
16. Frantzi, K., Ananiadou, S., Mima, H.: Automatic recognition of multi-word terms: the C-value/NC-value method. Int. Journal on Digital Libraries 3, 115–130 (2000)
17. Hliaoutakis, A., et al.: The AMTEx approach in the medical document indexing and retrieval application. Data Knowledge Engineering, 380–392 (2009)
18. Robertson, S.E., Walker, S., Hancock-Beaulieu, M.: Okapi at TREC-7: Automatic Ad Hoc, Filtering, VLC and Interactive. In: TREC-7, pp. 199–210 (1998)
19. Dinh, D., Tamine, L.: Combining global and local semantic contexts for improving biomedical information retrieval. In: Clough, P., Foley, C., Gurrin, C., Jones, G.J.F., Kraaij, W., Lee, H., Mudoch, V. (eds.) ECIR 2011. LNCS, vol. 6611, pp. 375–386. Springer, Heidelberg (2011)
20. Amati, G.: Probabilistic models for Information Retrieval based on Divergence from Randomness. PhD thesis, University of Glasgow (2003)

Mapping Orphanet Terminology to UMLS

Maja Miličić Brandt[1,*], Ana Rath[2], Andrew Devereau[1], and Ségolène Aymé[2]

[1] NGRL Manchester
[2] Orphanet INSERM SC11, Paris

Abstract. We present a method for creating mappings between the Orphanet terminology of rare diseases and the Unified Medical Language System (UMLS), in particular the SNOMED CT, MeSH, and MedDRA terminologies. Our method is based on: (i) aggressive normalisation of terms specific to the Orphanet terminology on top of standard UMLS normalisation; (ii) semantic ranking of partial candidate mappings in order to group similar mappings and attribute higher ranking to the more informative ones. Our results show that, by using the aggressive normalisation function, we increase the number of exact candidate mappings by 7.1-9.5% compared to a mapping method based on MetaMap. A manual assessment of our results shows a high precision of 94.6%. Our results imply that Orphanet diseases are under-represented in the aforementioned terminologies: SNOMED CT, MeSH, and MedDRA are found to contain only 35%, 42%, and 15% of the Orphanet rare diseases, respectively.

1 Introduction

Creating mappings between different biomedical terminologies is essential for data integration and terminology curation. Mappings provide links between concepts of terminologies that are developed for different purpose, thus facilitating data integration and enabling better exploitation of knowledge encoded in different terminologies. Considering terminology curation, the mapping process itself and its evaluation may reveal inaccuracies in both the source and target terminologies, such as wrong synonyms, redundancies, or errors in concept hierarchies.

In this paper, we present our results on mapping the Orphanet Terminology of rare diseases to the Unified Medical Language System (UMLS).[1] The Orphanet portal[2] [2] and database of rare diseases contain comprehensive data on more than 7000 rare, mostly genetic, diseases. The data includes classification of rare diseases, the association of clinical signs and genes with diseases, their inheritance modes and epidemiological data. Orphanet data is becoming a standard for the classification of rare and genetic diseases and it is going to be incorporated into the next edition of ICD (International Classification of Diseases).[3]

* Supported by the EU project DG Sanco A/101112.

[1] `http://www.nlm.nih.gov/research/umls/`

[2] `http://www.orpha.net`

[3] `http://www.who.int/classifications/icd/en/`

M. Peleg, N. Lavrač, and C. Combi (Eds.): AIME 2011, LNAI 6747, pp. 194–203, 2011.

Our goal is to improve the representation and traceability of rare diseases in medical terminologies, health records and systems. By cross-referencing Orphanet with UMLS terminologies, we are providing the first step towards importing Orphanet data on rare diseases and their classification into established medical terminologies, such as SNOMED CT.[4]

Our task was to map 7558 Orphanet rare diseases to SNOMED CT, MeSH[5] and MedDRA[6] terminologies, all of which are integrated into UMLS. UMLS 2010AB incorporates around 100 medical terminologies in English and provides a rich source of synonyms. We are looking both for *exact* mappings (to equivalent UMLS concepts), and *partial* ones (to less specific UMLS concepts). Our mappings need to be re-computed when Orphanet and UMLS are updated as well as assessed manually before being used, which is extremely time consuming. In order to tackle this problem we invested effort to reduce the amount of manual work by developing a mapping method which: (i) has a high precision and recall; (ii) distinguishes clearly between exact and partial candidate mappings; (iii) smartly ranks partial candidate mappings in order to attribute higher ranking to the more informative ones. Fulfilment of conditions (ii) and (iii) significantly facilitates quality assessment in scenarios when only exact mappings are needed: in this case it suffices to check exact candidate mappings and the partial ones with the highest scores. Moreover, (iii) enables a better pre-selection of partial mappings for each Orphanet disease.

Comparison of different mapping approaches for biomedical terminologies[4] shows that since biomedical terminologies have strongly controlled vocabularies and share little structure, simple lexical methods perform best for these terminologies. Our mapping method is based on a more aggressive string normalisation on top of standard UMLS normalisation. Here exact mapping candidates correspond to strings with the same normal form, and partial ones to those whose normal forms are related by subset relation. By performing more aggressive normalisation we are able to detect candidate mappings that go unnoticed by methods based on standard UMLS normalisation or by MetaMap[1]. For example, since the words "autosomal" and "form" are removed in the aggressive normalisation step, the UMLS concept

Pseudohypoaldosteronism, type 1, recessive form [C0268438]

has the same normal form as the Orphanet concept

Autosomal recessive pseudohypoaldosteronism type 1 [ORPHA 171876]

and thus provides an exact candidate mapping for this concept.

Concerning score assignment to mappings, we find the standard ones based on string distance metrics such as Levenshtein distance, and even the sophisticated one by MetaMap, not suitable. For example, MetaMap assigns score 944 to the wrong mapping

[4] `http://www.ihtsdo.org/snomed-ct/`

[5] `http://www.nlm.nih.gov/mesh/`

[6] `http://www.meddramsso.com/`

Genetic disorder → Genital disorder,

while it assigns score 901 to the mapping

Congenital Hypothalamic Hamartoma → Hypothalamic Hamartoma .

which turns out to provide an exact match, since Hypothalamic Hamartoma is always congenital. Moreover, MetaMap assigns score 913 to the mapping

Congenital **Hypothalamic** Hamartoma → Congenital hamartoma,

thus failing to put the better match forward. Instead, we attempt to classify partial mappings and score more informative ones higher by qualifying the difference words between the string and its match. In the previous example, the difference "congenital" will imply a higher score than the difference "hypothalamic".

By using the aggressive normalisation in our method we obtain 9.5% more exact candidate mappings compared to MetaMap. The quality control of our mappings has shown a high precision of 94.6%. We have found that SNOMED CT, MeSH, and MedDRA contain 35%, 42%, and 15% of the Orphanet rare diseases, respectively. This implies that rare diseases are still under-represented in general medical terminologies. We hope that cross-referencing Orphanet with other medical terminologies and possibly its integration into UMLS will improve visibility of rare diseases in health records and systems.

In the remainder of the paper we describe the related work and then present our mapping method and obtained results in more detail. Finally, we discuss how computed mappings may help terminology curation.

2 Related Work

In [5] Merabti et al. present results on mapping French version of Orphanet to UMLS, in particular MeSH. It is shown that NLP methods in French perform significantly better that those based on manual mapping from Orphanet to ICD-10 and cross-referencing of ICD-10 and MeSH provided by UMLS.

In [7] Pasceri et al. investigate representation of Orphanet and ORDR[7] rare diseases in established medical terminologies, including SNOMED CT, MeSH, OMIM[8], and ICD-10. For this purpose, the authors automatically map rare diseases into these terminologies via UMLS and develop a sophisticated disambiguation algorithm for the cases where more than one exact mapping is found for the same rare disease. Mappings are used to perform a comprehensive analysis of the represenation of rare diseases in UMLS as well as to compare the structure of rare disease terminologies with the established ones. The authors come to a similar conclusion that rare diseases are insufficiently represented in medical terminologies.

[7] `http://rarediseases.info.nih.gov`

[8] `http://www.ncbi.nlm.nih.gov/omim/`

3 Mapping Orphanet

Since the target terminologies we are interested in – SNOMED CT, MeSH, and MedDRA – are a part of UMLS, we map Orphanet rare diseases to the concepts of these terminologies via UMLS. Concepts of different terminologies within UMLS are cross-referenced by means of sharing the same UMLS codes. Thus UMLS provides a rich source of synonyms, collected from around 100 English terminologies which it integrates. We restrict the search space within UMLS in two ways, by considering only UMLS codes:

(a) with corresponding sources in SNOMED CT, MeSH, or MedDRA;
(b) with one of the following 11 semantic types:
'Acquired Abnormality', 'Anatomical Abnormality', 'Cell or Molecular Dysfunction', 'Congenital Abnormality', 'Disease or Syndrome', 'Finding', 'Injury or Poisoning', 'Mental or Behavioral Dysfunction', 'Neoplastic Process', 'Pathologic Function', 'Sign or Symptom'.

UMLS allows for 135 different semantic types, and without restricting them, we get numerous wrong mappings, such as:

Ring Chromosome (Syndrome) → Ring Chromosomes (Cell Component)

We introduce a function rank on the selected semantic types, which ranks them in the order of preference. It assigns the highest rank to 'Disease or Syndrome' and the lowest to 'Finding'.

Our mapping algorithm is based on string normalisation. For every Orphanet disease, we compute its normal form by using standard UMLS normalisation, and then perform further, more aggressive, normalisation steps (denoted with **orpha-norm**).

The *UMLS normalisation* is producing a version of the original string in lower case, without punctuation, genitive markers, or stop words (prepositions and articles), diacritics, ligatures, with each word in its uninflected (citation) form, the words sorted in alphabetical order, and normalising non-ASCII Unicode characters to ASCII. We will refer to it as **umls-norm**. The UMLS normalisation procedure is available in the package of NLM lexical tools[9] and also distributed with UMLS. It is used to identify equivalent concepts within UMLS and assign them the same String Unique Identifier (SUI). UMLS distributions contain precomputed tables with normal forms of all its concepts.

The aggressive normalisation, **orpha-norm**, includes, among other steps:

(i) removing further stop words: type, form, onset, autosomal, origin, syndrome, disease, disorder, associate, isolated, unspecified.
(ii) converting Roman into Arabic numbers, e.g. iii → 3; ixa → 9a,
(iii) shortening the karyotype format, e.g. 46 xx → xx; 48 xxxy → xxxy
(iv) converting Latin adjectives into English noun form, e.g. renal → kidney ; palpebral → eyelid ; ocular → eye,

[9] `http://lexsrv3.nlm.nih.gov/LexSysGroup/Projects/lvg/current/web/`

(v) converting English adjectives into noun forms, e.g. arterial → artery, muscular → muscle, sexual → sex,
(vi) sorting words alphabetically in the end.

We developed **orpha-norm** empirically, by inspecting mapping candidates produced by MetaMap[1]. MetaMap is a sophisticated NLM tool for mapping biomedical texts and terms to UMLS. It generates phrase variants by consulting UMLS Specialist Lexicon and thus computes mappings that simple UMLS normalisation cannot detect.

Let $\mathbf{norm}^+$ denote the composition of **umls-norm** and **orpha-norm**, i.e. $\mathbf{norm}^+(s) = \mathbf{orpha\text{-}norm}(\mathbf{umls\text{-}norm}(s))$[10]. Let s be a string (Orphanet disease) that we want to map to UMLS, and let m be a UMLS concept. We call (s, m) an *exact candidate mapping* iff $\mathsf{norm}^+(s) = \mathsf{norm}^+(m)$, and we call it a *partial candidate mapping* iff $\mathsf{norm}^+(m) \subset \mathsf{norm}^+(s)$. Intuitively, an exact candidate mapping is expected to provide a link to an equivalent concept, while a partial one is expected to provide a link to a less specific concept.

3.1 Exact Mappings

For every Orphanet disease, we compute the list of exact candidate mappings for its preferred name and its synonyms, by comparing their normal forms with normal forms of UMLS concepts (computed w.r.t. $\mathbf{norm}^+$). We assign scores to the produced mappings such that those computed for Orphanet preferred terms score higher than those computed for synonyms. Moreover, we score higher mappings computed for "standard" synonyms over those computed for acronyms. Mappings computed for acronyms where the UMLS match is not exactly the same (case sensitive) are not taken into account. If two mappings (s, m_1) and (s, m_2) have the same score we compare the ranks of semantic types of m_1 and m_2, and pick the one with the higher ranked semantic type. Going back to our example from the introduction, we obtain that:

$$\begin{aligned} &\mathbf{norm}^+(\text{Autosomal recessive pseudohypoaldosteronism type 1}) \\ &= \text{“1 recessive pseudohypoaldosteronism”} \\ &= \mathbf{norm}^+(\text{Pseudohypoaldosteronism, type 1, recessive form}) \end{aligned}$$

thus providing an exact candidate mapping:

Autosomal recessive pseudohypoaldosteronism type 1 [ORPHA 171876]
→ Pseudohypoaldosteronism, type 1, recessive form [C0268438]

Similarly, we obtain the following exact candidate mapping:

Brachydactyly type B [ORPHA 93383]
→ Brachydactyly syndrome type B[C1300267]

since these two concepts share the normal form "b brachydactyly".

[10] For simplicity, we are abstracting away the fact that **umls-norm**(s) may have more than one result. Moreover, we may treat a result of normalisation as a set of words rather than a string.

Although we attempt at choosing one "best" candidate mapping for an Orphanet disease in order to simplify the quality assessment, this is not always possible. Multiple exact candidate mappings are particularly important pointers to errors in both the source and target terminology and thus invaluable in terminology curation process. For this reason, we list all exact mappings for assessment. We will discuss multiple exact mappings in more detail in the next sections. Moreover, since we are looking for exact mappings to three different terminologies within UMLS, it might happen that exact matches to different terminologies computed for the same Orphanet disease are found via different UMLS concepts. Two possible reasons for this unexpected outcome are missed synonymy or code duplication within UMLS.

3.2 Partial Mappings

If no exact candidate mappings is found, we try to find a partial one. Let (s, m) be a partial candidate mapping. If $s_n = \mathsf{norm}^+(s)$ and $m_n = \mathsf{norm}^+(m)$, then $s_n \subset m_n$. We define *difference* between s and m as $d_{s,m} := s_n \setminus m_n$ and introduce around 20 groups that classify possible differences and corresponding mappings. Our score is then assigned to a partial mapping (s, m) based on the group the difference $d_{s,m}$ belongs to. Below we list some of the groups in the descending order of their assigned scores:
(i) Group describing a missing qualifier "classical" or "classic". For example:

Classic Pfeiffer syndrome → Pfeiffer Syndrome

We expect that these mappings will provide a reliable informative partial match, and in some cases, even exact matches.
(ii) Missing qualifier "familial", "congenital", "hereditary", "genetic". For example:

Congenital Hypothalamic Hamartoma → Hypothalamic Hamartoma (1)

Familial Scheuermann disease → Scheuermann disease (2)

Congenital prekallikrein deficiency → prekallikrein deficiency (3)

Expert assessment of the listed mappings has revealed that some of them correspond to exact matches. This holds for mappings (1) and (3) since Hypothalamic Hamartoma and prekallikrein deficiency are always congenital. This shows that the qualifier "congenital" is redundant in the names of these diseases and may be removed.
(iii) Missing qualifier "rare". Around 90 mappings are associated with this group, including:

Rare respiratory disease → Respiratory disease

Rare otorhinolaryngologic disease → Disease, Otorhinolaryngologic

We believe that such mappings provide the best possible, though never exact, matches for these diseases (or rather disease groups), as the disease qualifier "rare" is specific to Orphanet and seldom found in other terminologies.
(iv) Missing disease subtype:

Spinocerebellar ataxia **type 10** → Ataxia, Spinocerebellar
Spondyloepiphyseal dysplasia, **Kimberley type** → Spondyloepiphyseal Dysplasia
Craniometadiaphyseal dysplasia,**wormian bone type** → Craniometadiaphyseal dysplasia

(v) Missing inheritance mode:

Autosomal recessive palmoplantar keratoderma → Keratoderma, Palmoplantar
X-linked severe congenital neutropenia → Spondyloepiphyseal Dysplasia

(vi) Missing disease onset:

Juvenile sialidosis type 2 → Sialidosis, type 2
Late-onset retinal degeneration → Retinal Degeneration

(vii) Missing other common disease qualifiers, such as "acquired", "non-acquired", "syndromic", "non-syndromic", etc:

Acquired peripheral neuropathy → Peripheral Neuropathy
Syndromic Palpebral Coloboma → Palpebral coloboma

We assign lower scores to mappings whose difference cannot be classified by any of the created groups, and these scores get lower with increasing number of words in the mapping difference. Returning to our example from the introduction,

Congenital Hypothalamic Hamartoma → Hypothalamic Hamartoma

would be assigned the score 935, based on the difference "congenital", while

Congenital **Hypothalamic** Hamartoma → Congenital hamartoma,

would be assigned the lower score 850, since the difference is one, unclassified, word "hypothalamic".

The lowest scores are assigned to particularly uninformative UMLS matches, such as Malformation, Anomaly, Rare Disease, Genetic Disease, in order to give preference to other mappings found for a particular Orphanet disease, if any exist. As in the case of exact candidate mappings, here we also consult the semantic types of UMLS matches in order to rank mappings, if necessary. Where it is impossible to pick "the best" mapping with high certainty, we list the alternative mappings we computed as well. We believe, however, that our ranking of partial mapping is putting more informative mappings forward, facilitating the manual assessment and providing more structure to the set of computed mappings.

4 Results and Evaluation

We computed candidate mappings for 7558 Orphanet diseases to the subset of UMLS (version 2010AB) corresponding to SNOMED CT, MeSH, and MedDRA terminologies. We found candidate mappings for 7410 diseases, where exact candidate mappings are found for 3801 diseases (50.3%), and partial ones for a further 3609 diseases (47.7%) For 730 Orphanet diseases, we found more than one exact candidate mapping. The number of all exact candidate mappings (counting the multiple ones for the same Orphanet disease) is 4578.

Concerning distribution of mappings over single terminologies, we found 2634 (35%), 3186 (42%) and 1475 (15%) of the Orphanet rare diseases to have equivalent counterparts in SNOMED CT, MeSH (2011) and MedDRA, respectively. This implies that rare diseases are still under-represented in general medical terminologies. We have noticed a positive trend, though, as the previous version of MeSH (2010) was found to contain only 19.5% of Orphanet rare diseases, compared to 42% in the 2011 version. This is due to the fact that the work of merging rare diseases by the Office of Rare Diseases Research into MeSH vocabulary is ongoing.

In the table below we summarize our results and compare them to those obtained by MetaMap. MetaMap is used with options "–ignore_word_order –term_processing" and other appropriate options to set the UMLS version and restrict source terminologies and semantic types. Since MetaMap does not define the notion of an exact candidate mapping (and considering only those with MetaMap scores of 1000 would be too restrictive), in order to perform a comparison we counted all candidate mappings produced by MetaMap that are exact by our definition. The comparison shows, that, by performing more aggressive normalisation, we were able to find exact mappings for 252 diseases more, which is an improvement of 7.1% w.r.t. MetaMap results. If we compare the numbers of all exact candidate mappings, counting multiple ones for the same Orphanet disease (shown in column UMLS (all)), we obtain an even more significant increase of 9.5%. In the last three columns of the table, we compare the numbers of Orphanet diseases with exact candidate mappings in SNOMED CT, MeSH, and MedDRA, respectively.

	UMLS	UMLS (all)	SNOMED CT	MeSH	MedDRA
MetaMap	3549	4083	2464	3001	1426
UMLS+Orpha Norm	3801	4578	2634	3186	1475
improvement	252(7.1%)	391 (9.5%)	170(6.8%)	185(6.1%)	49(3.4%)

To date, clinical experts have evaluated 2476 exact candidate mappings for different Orphanet diseases. Out of these, 2343 (94.6%) were marked as correct, 42 as wrong and 91 as partial. A closer inspection has shown that a significant number of wrong or partial mappings were created due to wrong synonyms coming from OMIM (33 cases) or ambiguous acronyms (8 cases) within UMLS. For 29 of those marked as partial or wrong, exact matches are found among alternative mappings provided for corresponding Orphanet diseases. Thus, out of the selected 2476 diseases, 2362 (95.3%) are found to have an exact match.

5 Curating Terminologies

Ambiguous (multiple) exact mappings are particularly valuable for detecting errors in the source and target terminologies, and thus they facilitate terminology curation process. We suggest several reasons that explain ambiguous mappings:

(a) Missed synonymy within UMLS. For example, for ORPHA 585 Disease, the preferred term Mucosulfatidosis and its synonym Sulfatidosis juvenile, Auston type are mapped to two different UMLS concepts, however these correspond to synonyms both within SNOMED CT and MeSH. Note that in MeSH, a disease and its subcategories often share the same code, however neither of Mucosulfatidosis and Sulfatidosis juvenile, Auston type is a subcategory of each other.

(b) Existence of redundant codes within UMLS due to imprecise integration of single terminologies. Aggressive normalisation in our mapping method helps reveal such cases, e.g.

48,XXYY Syndrome [C2936741] (MeSH)
XXYY syndrome [C0856043](SNOMED, MedDRA)

Crigler Najjar syndrome, type 2 [C2931132] (MeSH)
Crigler-Najjar syndrome, type II (disorder) [C0268311](SNOMED, MedDRA)

Pseudohypoparathyroidism Type 2 [C2932717](MeSH)
Pseudohypoparathyroidism type II [C0271870] (SNOMED)

Ichthyosis hystrix, Curth Macklin type [C1840296](MeSH)
Ichthyosis hystrix of Curth-Macklin [C0432307] (SNOMED)

(c) Different granularity of terminologies. We found several cases where synonyms from Orphanet are mapped to parent and a child in SNOMED CT hierarchy. For example, for ORPHA 1201, the preferred term Artresia of small intestine is mapped to Congenital artresia of small intestine (SCT 84296002), while its Orphanet synonym Jejunal Artresia is mapped to Congenital artresia of jejunum (SCT 360491009) the child of the former SNOMED CT concept. Since jejunum is a part of small intestine, this indicates that Jejunal Artresia should be a child of Artresia of small intestine within Orphanet as well, rather than its synonym.

(d) wrong or ambiguous synonyms in UMLS or Orphanet.

The above examples show that, by detecting reasons for the existence of ambiguous mappings, we pinpoint errors and inaccuracies in terminologies and help their revision.

6 Conclusion and Future Work

We found that only over a half of Orphanet rare diseases have an equivalent counterpart in SNOMED CT, MeSH or MedDRA. Our results show that rare diseases are still not well represented in general medical terminologies. We hope that the mappings we produced can be used to integrate Orphanet into UMLS and thus raise the profile and visibility of rare diseases in medical systems.

In order to increase the mapping coverage, we plan to use Orphanet disease hierarchy and produce further mappings by going one or two steps higher in the hierarchy. Moreover, we will use manually produced mappings from Orphanet to OMIM to find further mappings. We also plan to compare our mappings with those produced for the French version of Orphanet[5,6] and integrate them.

Our future work will include utilising computed mappings from Orphanet to SNOMED CT to revise and update SNOMED data on rare diseases. In order to revise SNOMED's hierarchy of rare disease, we will use exact mappings to import it into Orphanet's hierarchy. Orphanet data include constraints on diseases that are used for checking the consistency of Orphanet disease hierarchy (by constructing its OWL[3] model). By performing a consistency check on the merged hierarchies, we will be able to detect possible errors in SNOMED/Orphanet classification of rare diseases. Once the SNOMED CT and Orphanet classifications of rare diseases are revised and synchronised, mappings can be used to import missing Orphanet rare diseases as well their hierarchy into SNOMED CT.

Acknowledgements. Many thanks to Alan Rector, Jeremy Rogers, Stéfan Darmoni and Tayeb Merabti for their support and advice. The authors would also like to thank Olivier Bodenreider, Bastien Rance and Erika Pasceri for discussions and their valuable advice on UMLS normalisation. Finally, the authors would like to thank Kathryn Leask, Siddharth Banka and Catherine Mercer for performing quality control of computed mappings.

References

1. Aronson, A.: Effective Mapping of Biomedical Text to the UMLS Metathesaurus: The MetaMap Program. In: AMIA 2001 Symposium Proc. (2001)
2. Ayme, S., Urbero, B., Oziel, D., Lecouturier, E., Biscarat, A.: Information on rare diseases: the Orphanet project. Rev. Med. Interne. 19 Suppl 3, 376–377 (1998)
3. Bechhofer, S., van Hamerlen, F., Hendler, J., Horrocks, I., McGuinness, D.L., Patel-Schneider, P., Stein, L.: OWL Web Ontology Language reference. W3C Recommendation (2004), `http://www.w3.org/TR/owl-ref/`
4. Ghazvinian, A., Noy, N., Musen, M.: Creating Mappings For Ontologies in Biomedicine: Simple Methods Work. In: AMIA 2009 Symposium Proc. (2009)
5. Merabti, T., Joubert, M., Lecroq, T., Rath, A., Darmoni, S.: Mapping biomedical terminologies using natural language processing tools and UMLS: Mapping the Orphanet thesaurus to the MeSH. IRBM 31(4), 221–225 (2010)
6. Merabti, T.: Methods to map health terminologies: contribution to the semantic interoperability between health terminologies. PhD thesis, University of Rouen (2010)
7. Pasceri, E., Rance, B., Rath, A., Lewis, J., Snyder, M., Bodenreider, O.: Representation of Rare Diseases in Biomedical Terminologies (submitted)

The FMA in OWL 2

C. Golbreich[1], J. Grosjean[2], and S.J. Darmoni[2]

[1] LIRMM CNRS 5506, Montpellier & University Versailles Saint-Quentin, France
[2] CISMeF & TIBS, LITIS EA 4108, Rouen University Hospital, Rouen, France
cgolbrei@gmail.com, Julien.Grosjean@chu-rouen.fr,
Stefan.Darmoni@chu-rouen.fr

Abstract. Representing the Foundational Model of Anatomy (FMA) in OWL 2 is essential for semantic interoperability. The paper describes the method and tool used to formalize the FMA in OWL 2. One main strength of the approach is to leverage OWL 2 expressiveness and the naming conventions of the native FMA to make explicit some implicit semantics, meanwhile improving its ontological model and fixing some errors. A second originality is the flexible tool developed. It enables to easily generate a new version for each Protégé FMA update. While it provides one 'standard' FMA-OWL version by default, many options allow for producing other variants customized to users applications. To the best of our knowledge, no complete representation of the entire FMA in OWL DL or OWL 2 existed so far.

Keywords: Ontology, OWL, Life Sciences, Health, Anatomy.

1 Introduction

The Foundational Model of Anatomy (FMA) is "a reference ontology about human anatomy" [1-2]. The FMA is intended to model *canonical* human anatomy that is, "the ideal or prototypical anatomy to which each individual and its parts should conform" [1]. It contains more than 85,000 classes, 140 relationships connecting the classes and over 120,000 terms. Most entities are anatomical structures composed of many parts interconnected in complex ways, described in terms of their regions, constituents, innervations, blood vessels, boundaries etc. For example, a Heart has two regions – its *left and right side* -, several constitutional parts – *Wall of Heart, Interatrial, Interventricular*, and *Atrioventricular septum, Mitral Valve*, etc. -, is innervated by the *Deep cardiac plexus, Right and Left coronary nerve plexus*, etc. Thus the FMA is a very large and perhaps one of the most complex ontology in the biomedical sciences.

OWL 2 is the W3C standard for ontologies on the Semantic Web [8]. OWL 2 provides several advantages for Life Sciences ontologies: interoperability, semantics, reasoning services. (1) *Interoperability* is important for shared use across different domains. Once converted to OWL 2, ontologies become more easily connected or combined with other ontologies. (2) *Semantics* (meaning) of terms is formally specified thanks to the underlying description logics. (3) Another practical benefit is that it allows the exploitation of the multitude of existing OWL tools, in particular

M. Peleg, N. Lavrač, and C. Combi (Eds.): AIME 2011, LNAI 6747, pp. 204–214, 2011.

powerful *reasoners*. Furthermore OWL 2's higher *expressiveness*, in particular its new metamodeling abilities, is of major interest as shown next.

The objective of the work is to represent the FMA in OWL 2, in order to make it interoperable with the increasing number of OWL ontologies available. Formalizing the FMA in OWL 2 provides a precise and rigorous meaning to the anatomical entities, crucial for example to share annotated resources. Making an OWL 2 version available is also an indispensable step for being able in the future to assist the FMA maintenance and to assure its quality thanks to OWL reasoning services and tools. The aim of the work is not to simply convert the FMA (for example by a script) from a format to another one, but to leverage OWL underlying description logic for enriching the FMA entities with formal definitions and axioms having a sound anatomical meaning.

A first strength of the approach consists in exploiting naming conventions and lexical patterns of the native FMA to make explicit the implicit semantics (meanwhile improving its ontological model and fixing some errors). A second originality is that the tool developed makes it possible to generate a new version each time the Protégé FMA is updated by its authors. As they are not very familiar with OWL and may prefer to continue to use existing Protégé frame editor, this friendly and easy to use converter is very useful for them to automatically create the OWL conversion. Additionally, while it is possible to provide one 'standard' FMA-OWL version, many options allow for producing by a simple click other variants customized to applications, if needed. The next sections describe the method and tool achieved for representing the FMA in OWL 2 and presents the results obtained so far.

2 Method

The FMA ontology is implemented in Protégé frames[1] and stored in a MySQL database backend. Transforming it into OWL 2 is not a simple translation. It requires to specify the meaning of its terms in logic and to express by logical statements (axioms) some knowledge about the anatomical entities, which is not explicit in the native FMA. This raises several issues. The first one is that different types of information are embedded in Protégé FMA. Indeed, apart from the domain knowledge concerning the anatomical entities, the FMA also includes meta-level knowledge. The problem is that interpreting both knowledge in the same model might lead to undesired consequences because of their interactions. Two solutions are proposed thereafter: an OWL 1 DL ontology *without* metaclasses and an OWL 2 ontology *with* metaclasses (§2.1). The second challenge is to guarantee that the formal definitions and axioms created are semantically correct from an *anatomical* viewpoint. The idea for it is to use lexical patterns (§0). The third issue is that, given the large size of the FMA, it is essential to *automatically* generate the OWL axioms. A friendly tool (§3) has been achieved for that. An interesting feature of this tool is that it enables to create (by default) a 'standard' ontology from the native FMA frames and also other customized variants useful for specific applications, if wanted.

[1] The frame-based system developed by Stanford Center for Biomedical Informatics Research.

2.1 Metamodeling

In FMA Protégé frames each anatomical entity is modeled both as a class and a metaclass[2]. At the domain level, classes describe the anatomical entities. At the meta-level, metaclasses serve several purposes. They associate metadata to the anatomical entities, for example they attach to the class *Heart* its author 'JOSE MEJINO, MD', preferred-terms 'Heart' in English, 'Cor' in Latin, Non-English equivalent 'coeur' in French, its definition, synonyms, FMAID, etc. Metaclasses are also used to define 'templates' specifying some given types of entities. For example, the metaclass *Organ With Cavitated Organ Parts*, is intended to specify the common template of all the organ types (species) that have cavitated organ parts. Metaclasses are organized into a subclass hierarchy. The metaclass *Heart*, is a subclass of *Organ with cavitated organ parts*, itself subclass of *Organ*, of which it inherits the slots, facets, e.g.; *bounded by* with range *Surface of organ*, or *arterial supply* with range *Artery, Arteriole, Arterial plexus* etc. At the class level, the own slots, e.g.; *part of, bounded by, arterial supply*, are assigned particular values. Thus, an anatomical entity, e.g.; a canonical *Heart,* can be specified as being an *Organ With Cavitated Organ Part* with a particular structure fulfilled by its individuals: any heart is composed of a *Right atrium, Left atrium, Right ventricle, Left ventricule*, is *bounded by* a *Surface of heart,* has a *Right coronary artery* and *Left coronary artery*, etc., as *arterial supply*.

To avoid undesired effects caused by interpreting both knowledge in the same model, it is offered to have either *(a)* an OWL 1 (2) DL ontology *without* metaclasses but capturing their knowledge otherwise, or *(b)* an OWL 2 ontology *with* metaclasses:

(a) An OWL 1 DL Ontology *Without Metaclasses* was initially proposed earlier [3] before OWL 2. OWL DL requires the deletion of the FMA higher order structure. The solution adopted to remain at first order while still capturing the information embedded at metaclasses, is to replace the metaclass instantiations by subclass axioms and to transform metaclasses into ordinary OWL classes. This did not introduce significant change, because "*all concepts in the Anatomy Taxonomy are subclass of a superclass and also an instance of a metaclass*". As metaclasses specify a given "template" of classes while classes specify the structure of their instances, property restrictions at metaclasses are approximated by universal restrictions dedicated to limit the allowed types, while restrictions at classes are translated into existential restriction (for details see [3]). *(b)* Now, thanks to the OWL 2 metamodeling new features, punning and enhanced annotations [9], it is possible to have an OWL 2 Ontology *With Metaclasses,* which (partly) better reflects the FMA authors original design. Indeed, while OWL 1 DL required a strict separation between the names of classes and individuals. OWL 2 relaxes this separation [9]. Now punning makes it possible to use the same term to refer to a class and an individual, while retaining decidability. Thus, it is possible to use metaclasses that reflect more accurately the FMA templates: the name `Heart` can be used both for the metaclass `Heart` and for the class `Heart` instance of `Organ with cavitated organ parts`. On the other hand, OWL 2 enhanced annotations are used for representing the metadata attached to the FMA entities. While OWL 1 allowed extralogical annotations, such as

[2] In FMA frames, each anatomical entity is modeled both as a metaclass and as a class. "*... for enabling the selective inheritance of attributes*" [1 2].

a label or a comment, OWL 2 additionally allows for annotations of axioms and of annotations themselves. In FMA frames, properties such as preferred name, synonyms, non-English equivalents, etc. are modeled as slots, whose values are not strings but individuals of the Concept name class. As they do not concern data of the domain of anatomy but metadata, using OWL 2 annotations of annotation is more appropriate than FMA metaclasses. Thus, the domain and meta-level data are no more confused and do not interact. Besides, doing so, a huge number of individuals are removed. For example, the class `Heart` (Fig.1 1) is annotated by the label `"Coeur"@fr` (Fig.1 4), the labeling itself being annotated by its creator JOSE MEJINO MD (Fig.1 2), date (Fig.1 3), its FMAID "217079" (Fig.1 4), publisher, etc.

```
(1) Declaration(Class(:Heart))
(2) AnnotationAssertion(Annotation(dc:creator "JOSE MEJINO MD"^^xsd:string)
(3) Annotation(dc:date "Thu May 12 142434 GMT-0800 2005"^^xsd:date)
(4) Annotation(:FMAID "217079"^^xsd:string).. rdfs:label :Heart "Coeur"@fr)
```

Fig. 1. OWL 2 annotations

2.2 Formal Semantics

The second main challenge is to enrich the FMA with formal definitions and axioms that have a sound anatomical meaning. The formalization is achieved in two steps. The first step focuses on the transformation of the FMA frames syntax and the second step on the FMA anatomical entities semantics. While the first transformation closely mirrors the FMA native model, the latter pushes the logical formalization further: new definitions and axioms are added that express some knowledge, which was not explicitly stated in frames, but was implicit. Partly for historical reasons (OWL 2 did not exist before), the first step transforms the FMA ontology from frames to OWL 1 DL (*FMA-OWL v1*), the second step brings it to OWL 2 (*FMA-OWL 2*).

The transformation of the frames syntax in OWL reuses the 2005 rules defined in [3]. In short, Protégé classes and slots are converted into OWL classes and properties, with the specified domain and range. Slot characteristics (inverse, symmetric, functional) are translated using corresponding OWL constructs. Values of own slots of classes are converted either into OWL values of annotation properties or into existential property restrictions. As said above, property restrictions defined at metaclasses or classes are respectively transformed into universal or existential property restrictions. Metaclass instantiation is replaced by a subclass relation.

At the second step the logical formalization is pushed forwards and the FMA ontology is enriched in several ways: (a) classes definitions are automatically generated from lexical patterns; (b) numerous related axioms are automatically created or moved; (c) new properties characteristics are added - for details see the next paragraphs (a) (b) (c); (d) OWL annotations of annotation are used for metadata (cf. §2) (e) OWL 2 metaclasses are created, but they can be omitted on demand.

(a) Class definitions. An important shortcoming of the 2005 ontology was its class definitions. Class expressions were built from one uniform property, e.g. *constitutional part*. However, all anatomical entities cannot be uniformly defined

from the same properties [3]. Now new formalization rules are defined for creating the definitions. The key idea is to exploit *lexical* patterns of the FMA vocabulary and implicit properties omitted in such names (joined to the inference power of OWL). For example, it is very likely that the pattern `Left_A` (e.g., `Left_Hand`) denotes all A (`Hands`) that have left *laterality*, that `Left_superior_cervical_ganglion` means all the left and superior cervical_ganglion, `Region_of_cytoplasm` all the regional parts of cytoplasm etc. The new rules create different forms of definition depending on each pattern. The patterns are basically unambiguous and moreover, their meaning was checked with FMA authors[3], all class definitions and axioms introduced in this manner are fully reliable. At the moment, two types of patterns are supported: (i) Pattern `P_A` denoting symmetrical siblings with an opposite anatomical_coordinate, e.g., `Left_A/Right_A`, `Anterior_A/Posterior_A`, `Inferior_A/Superior_A` etc., or an opposite gender, e.g.; `MaleA/FemaleA` and (ii) Pattern `A_of_B` denoting parts of entity, e.g., `Lobe_of_Lung`. Classes are incrementally defined as follows.

• Pattern P_A. At first, the `Anatomical_coordinate` subclasses are defined. `Primary_Anatomical_coordinate` are specified via property value restrictions, for example, axiom Fig. 2. (1) states that *`Left`* denotes all objects with left laterality. `Binary_Anatomical_coordinate` are defined as an intersection of `Primary_Anatomical_coordinate` classes. For example axiom Fig. 2 (2) states that `Left_superior` refers to all objects having a left and superior anatomical_coordinate. Entities of pattern `P_A`, where `P` is a `Primary_Anatomical_coordinate` subclass, are then provided definitions. For example, axiom Fig. 2 (3) states that `Left_Hand` (resp. `Right_Hand`) denotes all hands having left laterality.

```
(1) EquivalentClasses(:Left ObjectHasValue(:laterality:individual_Left))
(2) EquivalentClasses(:Left_superior ObjectIntersectionOf(:Superior :Left))
(3) EquivalentClasses(:Left_Hand ObjectIntersectionOf(:Hand :Left))
(4) EquivalentClasses(:Lobe_of_Lung
        ObjectIntersectionOf(:Anatomical_Lobe
        ObjectSomeValuesFrom(:regional_part_of :Lung)))
(5) EquivalentClasses(:Region_of_cytoplasm
        ObjectIntersectionOf(:Region_of_cell_component
        ObjectSomeValuesFrom(:regional_part_of :Cytoplasm)))
(6) SubClassOf(:Hand ObjectExactCardinality(1 :laterality
        ObjectOneOf(:individual_right :individual_left)))
```

Fig. 2. OWL 2 axioms

• Pattern A_of_B. In most cases a name A_of_B is a contraction formed from A and B that omits some property `p` relating the two entities A and B. The idea for providing

[3] In a very few cases, ambiguity was solved via discussions with FMA's authors.

semantics to entities A_of_B is to build a class expression from that implicit relation. The missing property p is recovered from scanning the list of property restrictions attached to the class. For example, it is *regional_part_of* for Lobe_of_Lung. Axiom Fig. 2 (4) states that Lobe_of_Lung means all the *anatomical lobe* that are a *regional_part_of* some *lung*. A particular process is defined for A_of_B where A is Region, Zone, Segment, Subdivision. From FMA authors, all 'region' classes denote *regional parts,* further distinguished on the types of boundary used to define the region, for example *Organ segment* is a region with one or more anchored fiat boundaries, *Organ zone* is a region with one or more floating fiat boundaries. At the moment, the p handled are only the part_of properties and subproperties (e.g.; regional_part_of) but this will next be extended to other relationships.

(b) Axioms. The lexical patterns are not only used for class definitions, but also for handling - creating/removing/moving - axioms:

Disjointness and subclass axioms. While the sibling symetrization process provides semantics to classes of pattern P_A, it achieves other tasks at the same time: 1° it adds relevant subclass axioms. 2° it detects and repairs errors or omission in the native FMA (for details see Algorithm 1). For example, while the meaning of Left_Hand is defined by the equivalent class axiom Fig. 2 (3), meanwhile several axioms are created: axiom Fig. 2 (6) asserts that each hand necessary has exactly one left or right laterality while DisjointClasses(*Left Right*) states that nothing can be both left and right. Hence, all Left_A and Right_A, e.g.; left and right hands are inferred to be exclusive. For each modality, only one single disjointness axiom is created stating that nothing can have two opposite modalities. Thus much less axioms are used. The algorithms implemented for each pattern are quickly sketched below.

Algorithm 1. The process for symmetrical siblings first parses all names of classes to get the terms matching a specific prefix P_ where P is a subclass of Primary_Anatomical_coordinate (e.g. Left). For each class P_A, (e.g. Left_A/Right_A), if A exists and A (or Anatomical_A) is a direct superclass of P_A, then several axioms are created respectively for P_A, its sibling and its father, according to the following rules: (1.1) each time A has a child P_A, A should have the pair as children, unless exceptions; (1.2) each time A has two symmetrical children, e.g.; Left_A and Right_A, and A has an existential restriction on a *part* property or subproperty, the two siblings should have symmetrical restrictions (modulo symmetry); (1.3) if a (symmetrical) restriction is present in two symmetrical siblings but not in their direct superclass, the relevant abstracted restriction is added to it. For example, as Left_Hand and Right_Hand have restrictions ObjectSomeValuesFrom(:*constitutional_part: Investing+fascia+of+left+hand*) (resp. *Investing+fascia+of+right+hand*), the missing axiom subclassOf(*Hand* ObjectSomeValuesFrom(:*constitutional_part*:*Investing+fascia+of+ +hand*)) is created; (1.4) as explained above, for each P_A, two axioms are created: a class axiom EquivalentClasses(:*P_A* ObjectIntersectionOf(:P :A)) and a subclassOf axiom like (6) for example, which asserts that each A necessary has exactly one left or right laterality SubClassOf*(:A* ObjectExactCardinality*(1 :laterality* ObjectOneOf*(:individual_Left :individual_Right)))*.

Algorithm 2. Similarly, the process first parses all names of classes to get the terms that match the pattern A_of_B. The EquivalentClasses(:*A_of_B* ObjectIntersectionOf(:*A* ObjectSomeValuesFrom(*:p_of :B*))) axiom is created in any of the following cases: (2.1) if the direct superclass of A_of_B is A or Anatomical_A and A has a restriction on a *part_of* property or subproperty p_of: SubClassOf(:A ObjectSomeValuesFrom(*:p_of :B'*)) with B' direct superclass of B (e.g. Ganglion_of_cranial_nerve). (2.1b) if B' is not a direct superclass of B (it may be a distant ancestor) but A or Anatomical_A exists and B' has a restriction for the *inverse* p of p_of: SubClassOf(:B' ObjectSomeValuesFrom(*:p : A_of_B'*)); (2.2) if the direct superclass of A_of_B is A or Anatomical_A and A_of_B has a restriction SubClassOf(:*A_of_B* ObjectSomeValuesFrom(*:p_of : B*)) (e.g. Tendon_of_biceps_femoris). For example, as the direct superclass of Lobe_of_Lung is Anatomical_Lobe and Lobe_of_Lung is a subclass of regional_part_of some Anatomical_Lobe the axiom EquivalentClasses(*:Lobe_of_Lung* ObjectIntersectionOf(*:Anatomical_Lobe* ObjectSomeValuesFrom(*:regional_part_of: Lung*))) is created. (2.3) A specific process handles classes A_of_B where A is *Region_of, Zone_of, Segment_of, Subdivision_of* (1273 classes). It defines A_of_B as regional_part of B, like axiom (5) for Region_of_cytoplasm.

• **Completing or compacting axioms.** In canonical anatomy, if an entity A has some part B, then reversely B should also be a part of some A (which is not logically equivalent). 669 missing subclassOf axioms expressing such 'symmetrical' restrictions are created. On the other hand, based on inference power, several axioms are removed: if all the subclasses of A have the same existential restriction, it is removed from the subclasses and moved up to A instead.

(c) Properties characteristics. OWL 2 offers new properties characteristics. According to FMA authors, *part, regional_part, constitutional_part, systemic_part, member* and their inverse are asserted to be transitive, irreflexive, asymmetric, *continuous_with* and *connected_to* are symmetric, and *continuous_with* is reflexive.

3 The FMA-OWLizer Tool

The third issue was to achieve a formalization tool that can deal with the sheer size and the frequent incremental updates of the FMA. FMA-OWLizer is a friendly and easy to use tool that automatically generates on a simple click a 'standard' FMA ontology in OWL[4]. It can process *all* existing public FMA versions, FMA 2005 version, FMA3.0 (2008), April 2010 FMA 3.1 update. It is highly flexible, allowing providing also a customized ontology adapted to the users' needs and their application. The main parameters are selected via a friendly *graphical user interface* (http://www.lirmm.fr/tatoo/IMG/pdf/FMA-OWLizer.pdf), while the other ones are

[4] Which one should be the 'standard', the ontology with or without metaclass, depends on the native FMA, mainly of the future improvements of its templates.

configured in configuration files. For example, the file 'classes_to_delete.txt' states the classes to be removed. FMA-OWLizer includes many options. It is possible to select the chosen source file as input, to have metaclasses or not, to choose the properties to be included, to customize the class and property axioms in various ways: to supply particular class definitions by designating the properties, e.g.; *constitutional_part, bounded_by* etc. for the equivalent classes axioms, to include/remove all the subclass axioms (e.g. for performance tests), to configure properties characteristics. For example, to get an OWL 2 DL ontology that reasoners can process, it is recommended to select 'ignore irreflexive and asymetric'. Otherwise, as the properties *part* and their inverse are transitive, asymmetric and irreflexive, the ontology would violate the OWL 2 restriction, which requires that only simple roles can be used in asymetric and irreflexive object property axioms. It is also possible to choose which concrete syntax is used to store the ontology (RDF/XML, OWL/XML, Functional Syntax), to select French or English for the GUI. FMA-OWLizer is a local Java program designed and developed specifically for the FMA. All processes are performed via the OWL API 3.0, benefiting of its functionalities. The GUI is achieved with the Swing/AWT Java graphics libraries and is multilingual support (bundle files) thanks to the CISMeF Utils platform.

4 Results

Complete representations of the entire FMA are now available in OWL 2. An OWL 2 ontology[5] without metaclasses (*FMA-OWL2*_noMTC Table 1 #3) has been generated from FMA 3.0. It includes all FMA classes and properties (except *homonym_of* and *homonym_for,* discarded in agreement with FMA's authors). The new class definitions and axioms retain transitivity but voluntarily ignore irreflexivity and asymetry. This ontology offers 15,084 new definitions of classes, 16,113 disjointness axioms; 85,467 axioms are removed and replaced by one single axiom next inherited, 15 subproperties axioms and 228,263 annotations. 7664 class definitions are obtained from the pattern `A_of_B`, while 7333 from the pattern `Left_A/Right_A`. Another OWL 2 ontology *with* metaclasses[6] is also available (*FMA-OWL2*_noMTC

Table 1. Metrics of FMA-OWL ontologies

File		Size (MB)	Classes	**Class axioms**	Expressivity
		FMA-OWL 1 from FMA frames - 2005			
#1	without N&S	41,6	41648	236208	$\mathcal{ALCOIF}(\mathcal{D})$
#2	with N&S	40,8	41648	230690	$\mathcal{ALCOIF}(\mathcal{D})$
		FMA-OWL 2 from FMA 3.0 frames - 2008			
#3	without MTC	256	85005	263389	$\mathcal{SROIQ}(\mathcal{D})$
#4	with MTC	314	85005	261331	$\mathcal{SROIQ}(\mathcal{D})$

[5] http://gforge-lirmm.lirmm.fr/gf/download/docmanfileversion/214/747/FMA_3.0_noMTC_100702.owl.zip

[6] http://gforge-lirmm.lirmm.fr/gf/download/docmanfileversion/215/748/FMA_3.0_MTC_100701.owl.zip

Table 1 #4). The FMA-OWLizer tool (§3) can generate both a standard FMA-OWL ontology and other ontologies of various size and complexity that better fit specific applications needs. For example, *FMA-OWL v1* are OWL 1 partial (smaller) ontologies (41 MB) issued from the FMA 2005, of which left/right leaves are cut, without or with class definitions (Table 1 #1 or #2) built from the *constitutional_part* property. Ontologies obtained from the FMA 3.1 update have also been generated.

5 Discussion

There has been several efforts since 2005 for translating the FMA in OWL [3] [4] [5]. But earlier conversions to OWL were no fully satisfying. A main limitation of [4] [5] is the metaclasses representation. The difficulty is that translating FMA metaclasses into OWL 1 leads to OWL Full. [4] offers two components: an OWL DL and an OWL Full component. The former is obtained in omitting the metaclasses to remain in OWL DL, thus is incomplete. The latter is a complete representation that imports the OWL DL module, but is an OWL Full component. In contrast, the FMA ontology [3] is OWL DL, while including the metaclass knowledge. However, it had different limitations: the left/right leaves were cut for memory and tools limitation reasons, thus it was incomplete; the class definitions were not "semantically" satisfying for all classes: all anatomical entities cannot be uniformly defined solely in terms of their constitutional parts. The present approach offers more satisfying solutions: the FMA-OWL (DL) ontology without metaclasses captures the metaclass knowledge like [3] but is now complete; the FMA-OWL 2 (DL) ontology with metaclasses keep the metaclass structure thanks to OWL 2 new metamodeling features. Second, the formalization is pushed much forwards, eliciting further the FMA underlying semantics. Presently, as they are based on lexical patterns, the class definitions and axioms created are semantically correct and reliable from an *anatomical* viewpoint. Besides, while the earlier conversion program [3] did not scale up and was not robust, the new mapping of the syntax now handles the *entire* FMA and can overcome the changes of FMA successive updates. Regarding the pattern approach, a few patterns are shared with [11] but the goal of Abstracting and Generalizing is clearly different, it is to reduce the FMA size or abstract it. Automatically generating axioms is partly shared with [6], but our approach is more general.

However, the ontologies are still unstable and exhibit errors (present in the original FMA). Though it was not the objective of this work, we made an attempt to check the FMA-OWL ontologies with a reasoner. But reasoning with FMA-OWL proved to be a real challenge. The FMA-OWL ontologies are perhaps the largest and most complex OWL ontologies available. Firstly no reasoner could classify them. Recently, the special 'core blocking' strategy of HermiT [7] that was developed for FMA like ontologies with lots of unsatisfiable classes, succeeded to process them in a reasonable time. *FMA-OWL* 2 (Table 1 #3 - 2010-03-11) has 65,753 unsatisfiable classes out of 85,005. The time for classification, including loading and preprocessing was 58m 12s 929ms (by Birte Glimm*)*. *FMA-OWL* v1 with constitutional-part for N&S (#1) had 33,433 unsatisfiable classes out of 41,648, and the time for classification was 33m 46s 55ms. At the time of this work, no explanation tool compatible with OWL 2 and the OWL API 3.0 was available. Due to the large size of the FMA-OWL, it was difficult to go further in debugging it. This is obviously an interesting perspective, as soon as friendly reasoning and explanation tools will be available for large ontologies. Modules may also be extrcted to trace the errors down.

6 Conclusion

We have presented a method to represent the FMA in OWL 2 and a friendly and flexible tool. Complete representations of the entire FMA in OWL 1 or OWL 2 DL are now available and over 15,500 FMA classes have a reliable logical definition. It was a real challenge to design automatic procedures that correctly encode the semantics and that DL reasoners can process. Although many classes are unsatisfiable, this work is an important step forwards. This is a major achievement for making the FMA more coherent in the future. The tool allows for automatically producing new FMA-OWL updates and customized variants on demand. Future perspectives are to push the formalization in OWL 2 or its extension [12] further, to exploit OWL reasoners and explanation tool to improve the FMA. The 'pattern' approach is general and it might be worth to apply it to other ontologies as well.

Acknowledgments. We are grateful to C. Rosse and O. Mejino for their advice and support and to Oxford team for their specialized classification algorithm, special thanks to B. Glimm.

References

1. Rosse, C., Mejino Jr, J.L.: The Foundational Model of Anatomy Ontology. In: Burger, A., et al. (eds.) Anatomy Ontologies for Bioinformatics: Principles and Practice, pp. 59–118. Springer, New York (2008) ISBN 978-1-84628-884-5
2. Rosse, C., Mejino Jr, J.L.: A reference ontology for biomedical informatics: the Foundational Model of Anatomy. J. Biomed. Inform. 36(6), 478–500 (2003)
3. Golbreich, C., Zhang, S., Bodenreider, O.: The Foundational Model of Anatomy in OWL: experience and perspectives. Journal of Web Semantics, Web Semantics: Science, Services and Agents on the World Wide Web 4(3), 181–195 (2006)
4. Dameron, O., Rubin, D.L., Musen, M.A.: Challenges in converting frame based ontology into OWL: the Foundational Model of Anatomy case-study. In: AMIA Annual Symposium, Washington DC, pp. 181–185 (2005)
5. Natalya, F., Noy, D.L.: Rubin, Translating the Foundational Model of Anatomy into OWL. Journal of Web Semantics, Web Semantics: Science, Services and Agents on the World Wide Web 6, 133–136 (2008)
6. Dameron, O., Chabalier, J.: Automatic generation of consistency constraints for an OWL representation of the FMA. In: 10th International Protégé Conference (2007)
7. Glimm, B., Horrocks, I., Motik, B.: Optimized Description Logic Reasoning via Core Blocking. In: Giesl, J., Hähnle, R. (eds.) IJCAR 2010. LNCS, vol. 6173, pp. 457–471. Springer, Heidelberg (2010)
8. W3C, O.W.L., Working Group, O.W.L.: 2 Web Ontology Language Document Overview W3C Recommendation October 27 (2009), `http://www.w3.org/TR/owl2-overview/`

9. Golbreich, C., Wallace, E.K.: OWL 2 Web Ontology Language New Features and Rationale W3C Recommendation October 27 (2009), http://www.w3.org/TR/owl2-new-features/
10. Darmoni, S.J., Pereira, S., Névéol, A., Massari, P., Dahamna, B., Letord, C., Kedelhué, G., Piot, J., Derville, A., Thirion, B.: French Infobutton: an academic and business perspective. In: AMIA Symp., p. 920. IOS Press, Amsterdam (2008)
11. Mikroyannidi, E., Rector, A., Stevens, R.: Abstracting and Generalizing the Foundationql Model of Anatomy ontology. In: Bio-ontologies 2009 (2009)
12. Motik, B., et al.: Representing Ontologies Using Description Logics, Description Graphs, and Rules. Artificial Intelligence 173(14), 1275–1309 (2009)

Improving Information Retrieval by Meta-modelling Medical Terminologies

Lina F. Soualmia[1,2], Nicolas Griffon[2], Julien Grosjean[2], and Stéfan J. Darmoni[2]

[1] LIM&Bio, University of Paris 13, Sorbonne Paris Cité, 93017 Bobigny, France
Lina.Soualmia@gmail.com
[2] TIBS, LITIS & CISMeF, Rouen University, 76031 Rouen, France
{Nicolas.Griffon,Julien.Grosjean,Stefan.Darmoni}@chu-rouen.fr

Abstract. This work aims at improving information retrieval in a health gateway by meta-modelling multiple terminologies related to medicine. The meta-model is based on meta-terms that gather several terms semantically related. Meta-terms, initially modelled for the MeSH thesaurus, are extended for other terminologies such as IC10 or SNOMED Int. The usefulness of this model and the relevance of information retrieval is evaluated and compared in the case of one and multiple terminologies. The results show that exploiting multiple terminologies contributes to increase recall but lowers precision.

Keywords: Meta-modelling, controlled vocabularies, information retrieval.

1 Introduction

In the context of the increasing preeminence of the Internet as a source of health information, several health gateways have been developed to help users to find the information they are looking for. They rely on thesauri which are a proven key technology for effective access to information since they provide a controlled vocabulary for indexing. The main thesaurus used for health documents is the Medical Subject Headings thesaurus (MeSH) [1]. The MeSH in French is exploited in the CISMeF (Catalogue and Index of Online Health Resources in French), a gateway which indexes the most important sources of institutional health information in French. Several improvements have been introduced to adapt this scientific publication-oriented indexing vocabulary to internet resources [2]. One enhancement is to gather all MeSH terms that are related to a given specialty, since they can be dispersed among the 16 MeSH branches. The use of multiple terminologies is recommended [3] to increase the number of the lexical and graphical forms of a biomedical term recognised by a search tool. Since 2007, CISMeF resources are indexed using the vocabulary of 23 other terminologies [4]. This work aims at evaluating information retrieval by meta-modelling the MeSH thesaurus and the 23 other terminologies, by evaluating the relevance on using multiple terminologies *versus* only the MeSH. The remainder of the paper is organized as follow: in the section 2 we start by describing the meta-model of the MeSH and the multiple terminologies. The results of information retrieval evaluation and relevance are in the section 3. Finally, we give some related work and conclusions in the section 4.

M. Peleg, N. Lavrač, and C. Combi (Eds.): AIME 2011, LNAI 6747, pp. 215–219, 2011.

2 Meta-modelling Terminologies and Controlled Vocabularies

The MeSH thesaurus is partitioned at its upper level into 16 branches (e.g. diseases). The core of MeSH is a hierarchical structure that consists of sets of descriptors. At the top level we find general headings (e.g. diseases), and at deeper levels we find more specific headings (e.g. asthma). A MeSH heading is placed in multiple hierarchies. Together with a main heading, a subheading (e.g. diagnosis, complications) allows us to specify which particular aspect of the main heading is addressed in a document. For example, the pair [hepatitis/diagnosis] specifies the diagnosis aspect of hepatitis.

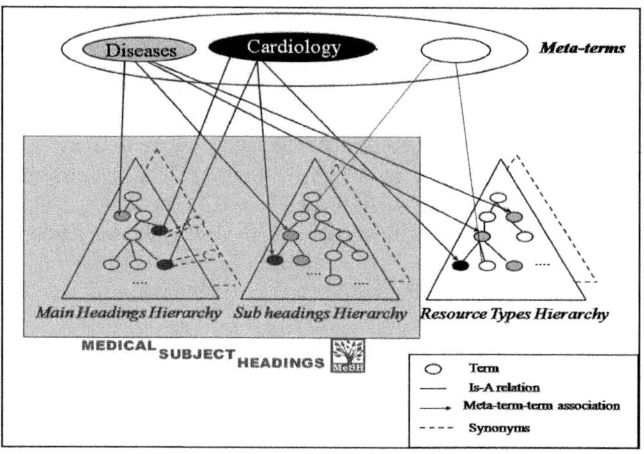

Fig. 1. Gathering MeSH *main headings* and *subheadings* under *meta-terms*

MeSH main headings and subheadings hierarchies do not allow a complete view concerning a specialty. They are gathered in CISMeF under *meta-terms* (e.g. cardiology) as described in Fig. 1. Meta-terms (n=73) concern medical specialties and it is possible by browsing to know sets of MeSH main headings and subheadings which are semantically related to the same specialty but dispersed in several trees. Meta-terms have been created to optimize information retrieval in CISMeF. Introducing "cardiology" as meta-term is an efficient strategy to obtain more results because instead of exploding one single MeSH tree, the use of meta-terms results in an automatic hierarchical expansion of the queries by exploding other related MeSH trees besides the current tree [2]. A comparison of the results of MeSH term-based queries and meta-terms-based queries showed an increased recall with no decrease in precision [5].

To increase the number of the lexical and graphical forms of a biomedical term recognised, CISMeF evolved from a single terminology approach to a multiple terminologies using, in addition to the MeSH thesaurus, vocabularies and classifications that deal with various aspects of health. Among them, SNOMED, French CCAM for procedures, Orphanet for rare diseases and classifications from the World Health Organization : ICD 10 for diseases, ATC for drugs, ICF for handicap, ICPS for patient safety, MedDRA for drug adverse effects. New terminologies have been linked to meta-terms manually by experts. For instance, the meta-term "cardiology" was initially linked to MeSH main headings such as "cardiology", "stents", and their descendants. With the integration of new terminologies, additional links completed the definition of the meta-term “cardiology”: links to "cardiovascular system", "Antithrombotic agents" and others from ATC, links to "Cardio-myopathy", "Heart" and their descendants from ICD10 and so on.

3 Information Retrieval

Our aim is to compare the precision and recall of multiple terminologies meta-terms (mt-mt) to MeSH meta-terms (M-mt) in CISMeF. Since mt-mt are based on M-mt plus semantic links to some terms in other terminologies, the query results for M-mt are all included in the query results for mt-mt, which is thus the gold standard for recall. On one hand, we have to evaluate the precision of the query retrieving resources indexed by a term linked to M-mt and on the other hand by a term linked to mt-mt and not to M-mt (i.e. Δ query). For this purpose, Boolean queries were built using the meta-terms. For example, for the "surgery" meta-term, the M-mt query is "`surgery[M-mt]`". The Δ query is "`surgery[mt-mt] NOT surgery[M-mt]`". For each query an automatic expansion is performed. The resources returned by automatic query expansion were assessed for relevance according to a three modality scale used in other standard information retrieval test sets : irrelevant (+0), partly relevant (+1) or fully relevant (+2). Relevance scores are assigned manually to the top 20 resources returned for each meta-term query. The results of the evaluation are given in the Table 2. (95% of the end-users do not go beyond the top 20 results when using a search engine [6]). For the purpose of assessing meta-terms for information retrieval, we have developed a test collection comprising relevance judgments for the top 20 resources returned for a selection of 20 meta-terms queries. 788 of the 126,587 documents retrieved by the 20 meta-terms queries, were assessed for relevance(0.6%).

Weighted precisions for MeSH meta-terms queries and for Δ queries were computed given the level of relevance considered and compared using χ^2 test. Indexing methods and meta-terms were compared too. Relative recall for MeSH meta-terms queries were computed given the level of relevance considered. The mean weighted precision of Δ queries was 0.33 and 0.76 for full and partial relevance, respectively. The mean precision of MeSH meta-terms queries was 0.66 and 0.80 for full and partial relevance respectively. The difference between MeSH meta-terms and multiple terminologies meta-terms was significant for full relevance (0.66 vs 0.61; $p<10^{-4}$, χ^2) but not for partial relevance (both 0.80; p=0.3, χ^2). The mean recall of MeSH meta-terms queries was 0.92 and 0.86 for full and partial relevance. Whatever the relevance considered was, results varied significantly according to the indexing method: manual (precision of 0.50 and 0.81 for full and partial relevance) perform better than automatic (precision of 0.38 and 0.48 for full and partial relevance), and to the studied meta-term. For full relevant resources, the precision decreases with the shift from MeSH meta-terms to multiple terminologies meta-terms (from 0.66 to 0.61) for an 8% improvement in recall. For partial relevance, the increase of recall with multiple terminologies is even higher (14%) at no cost in terms of precision (0.80). Overall, the multiple terminologies paradigm for meta-terms definition increases the recall but lowers the relevance of retrieved resources.

Table 1. Number of documents retrieved by 20 meta-terms queries, MeSH and Δ and their relevance

Meta-Term Query	Total of documents	query type	Number of documents	Relevance of the top 20 documents		
				Not	Partially	Totally
Diagnosis	13,482	MeSH Δ	13,132 350	0 14	2 1	15 5
Toxicology	12,462	MeSH Δ	11,980 482	0 16	0 1	20 3
Neurology	11,493	MeSH Δ	9,325 2,168	8 11	4 5	8 4
Infectious Diseases	9,130	MeSH Δ	6,557 2,573	0 3	0 16	20 1
Paediatrics	7,811	MeSH Δ	7,560 251	4 2	4 4	12 13
Cardiology	7,676	MeSH Δ	5,288 2,388	1 4	0 10	18 6
Oncology	6,689	MeSH Δ	5,626 1,063	0 2	1 14	18 4
Surgery	5,824	MeSH Δ	5,504 320	1 5	0 0	3 15
Rheumatology	5,264	MeSH Δ	4,408 856	3 11	8 5	9 4
Gastroenterology	5,175	MeSH Δ	4,069 1,106	0 8	0 11	20 1
Allergies and Immunology	5,171	MeSH Δ	4,598 573	1 2	17 17	2 1
Metabolism	4,646	MeSH Δ	3,797 849	14 0	2 2	4 18
Dermatology	4,623	MeSH Δ	3,196 1,427	7 0	0 4	13 16
Nutrition	4,482	MeSH Δ	3,455 1,027	0 0	1 9	19 11
Pneumology	4,050	MeSH Δ	3,466 584	0 0	7 14	12 6
Gynaecology	4,036	MeSH Δ	3,186 850	6 0	1 1	12 19
Haematology	3,981	MeSH Δ	2,906 1,075	13 7	2 10	5 3
Endocrinology	3,834	MeSH Δ	3,168 666	15 0	1 9	4 11
Obstetrics	3,379	MeSH Δ	3,063 316	5 20	1 0	12 0
Virology	3,379	MeSH Δ	3,122 257	1 0	11 20	6 0
Total	**126,58 7**	**MeSH Δ**	**107,406 19,181**	**95 105**	**62 153**	**232 141**

4 Discussion

There exist as many different terminologies, controlled vocabularies, thesauri and classification systems as fields of application. A joint semantic repository is necessary to render these terminologies "interoperable" with effective interaction and a minimum loss of meaning. It requires a shared model representing the terms, whatever the original terminology is. The richest source of biomedical terminologies is the UMLS Metathesaurus [7]. It does not allow interoperability between terminologies since it integrates the various terminologies as they stand, without making any connection between the terms other than by linking equivalent terms to a single concept. In CISMeF, a terminology meta-model into which every terminology model can be integrated was developed. The meta-model in OWL, the process and the method to align multiple terminologies are detailed in [8]. In contradistinction to terminology, a formal ontology gives precise information and describes a domain independently of human language. The OBO platform is an online library of biomedical ontologies (n=60). It is a community initiative to create interoperable biomedical ontologies adhering to good ontology design principles [9]. Several upper-level ontologies such as BFO [10] or Bio-Top [11] has been devised. Our meta-model for terminologies is quite similar to these upper-level ontologies. But, as well-described in [12], terminologies and ontologies do not have the same objectives. Terminologies are well-adapted to a wide range of applications and users, in particular to resources indexing and retrieval. Nonetheless, actually some efforts are developed to include lexicons of ontologies for completing the already existing terminologies in CISMeF. Among these, SNOMED CT, LOINC and FMA.

References

1. Nelson, S.J., et al.: Relationships in Medical Subject Heading. Relationships in the Organization of Knowledge, 171–184 (2001)
2. Soualmia, L.F., Darmoni, S.J.: Combining Different Standards and Different Approaches for Health IR in a Quality-controlled Gateway. Int. J. Med. Inf. 74(2-4), 141–150 (2005)
3. Wagner, M.: An Automatic Indexing Method for Medical Documents. In: Symp. on Computer Application in Medical Care, pp. 1011–1017 (1991)
4. Darmoni, S.J., Pereira, S., Sakji, S., Merabti, T., Prieur, É., Joubert, M., Thirion, B.: Multiple Terminologies in a Health Portal: Automatic Indexing and Information Retrieval. In: Combi, C., Shahar, Y., Abu-Hanna, A. (eds.) AIME 2009. LNCS, vol. 5651, pp. 255–259. Springer, Heidelberg (2009)
5. Gehanno, J., et al.: Evaluation of Meta-Concepts for Information Retrieval in a Quality-Controlled Health Gateway. In: AMIA, pp. 269–273 (2007)
6. Spink, A., Jansen, B.J.: Web Search: Public Searching on the Web. Kluwer Ac. Pub., Dordrecht (2004)
7. Nelson, S.J., et al.: The Unified Medical Language System (UMLS) of the National Library of Medicine. J. Am. Med. Ass. 61, 40–42 (2006)
8. Joubert, M., et al.: Modelling and Integrating Terminologies into a French Multi-terminology Server. In: Medinfo (2010)
9. Smith, B., et al.: The OBO Foundary: coordinated Evolution of Ontologies to Support Biomedical Data Integration. Nature Biotechnology (11), 1251–1255 (2007)
10. Smith, B., et al.: Relations in Biomedical Ontologies. Genome Biology 6(5) (2005)
11. Stenzhorn, H., et al.: Towards a Top-Domain Ontology for Linking Biomedical Ontologies. In: Medinfo, pp. 1225–1229 (2007)
12. Freitas, F., Schulz, S.: Survey of Current Terminologies and Ontologies in Biology and Medicine. Journal of Comm. Information and Innovation in Health 1(3), 7–18 (2009)

Improving the Mapping between MedDRA and SNOMED CT

Fleur Mougin[1], Marie Dupuch[2], and Natalia Grabar[3]

[1] LESIM, INSERM U897, ISPED, University Bordeaux Segalen, France
fleur.mougin@isped.u-bordeaux2.fr
[2] Centre de Recherche des Cordeliers, Université Pierre et Marie Curie - Paris6; INSERM U872, Paris, F-75006 France
marie.dupuch@crc.jussieu.fr
[3] STL, CNRS UMR 8163, Université Lille 3, France
natalia.grabar@univ-lille3.fr

Abstract. MedDRA is exploited for the indexing of pharmacovigilance spontaneous reports. But since spontaneous reports cover only a small proportion of the existing adverse drug reactions, the exploration of clinical reports is seriously considered. Through the UMLS, the current mapping between MedDRA and SNOMED CT, this last being used for indexing clinical data in many countries, is only 42%. In this work, we propose to improve this mapping through an automatic lexical-based approach. We obtained 308 direct mappings of a MedDRA term to a SNOMED CT concept. After segmenting MedDRA terms, we identified 535 full mappings associating a MedDRA term with one or more SNOMED CT concepts. The direct approach resulted in 199 (64.6%) correct mappings while through segmentation this number raises to 423 (79.1%). On the whole, our method provided interesting and useful results.

Keywords: mapping of terminologies, MedDRA, SNOMED CT, UMLS.

1 Introduction

The spontaneous reporting of adverse drug reactions completely depends on healthcare professionals for identifying and sending the reports to the national pharmacovigilance (PV) center or to the manufacturer [1]. Once spontaneous reports are submitted, they are coded with MedDRA [2] or WHO-ART [3] terms and then sent to the surveillance processes. But since spontaneous reports cover only a small proportion of the existing adverse drug reactions, the exploration of clinical reports is seriously considered because they may contain explicit information on causes of diseases and symptoms. The detection of such data depends on the capacity to extract them and also on the capacity to link clinical reports with PV facts. This last need especially relies on the alignment of the dedicated terminologies, i.e., MedDRA (exploited in PV databases) and SNOMED CT [4] (exploited for encoding the clinical documents). Through the UMLS® [5], the current mapping between these two terminologies is only 42%, which seriously impedes the situation. In this work, we propose an automatic lexical-based approach to improve this mapping.

M. Peleg, N. Lavrač, and C. Combi (Eds.): AIME 2011, LNAI 6747, pp. 220–224, 2011.

2 Background

MedDRA. The Medical Dictionary for Regulatory Activities (MDR) [2] has been designed for the encoding of adverse drug reactions chemically induced by drugs. It contains a large set of terms (signs and symptoms, diagnostics, therapeutic indications, complementary investigations, medical and surgical procedures, medical, surgical, family and social history), which are structured into five hierarchical levels: 26 System Organ Classes, 332 High Level Group Terms, 1,688 High Level Terms, 18,209 Preferred Terms, and 66,587 Low Level Terms.

SNOMED CT. The Systematized Nomenclature of Medicine – Clinical Terms (SNCT) is a biomedical terminology, which is maintained by the International Health Terminology Standards Development Organisation [4]. It contains 291,205 current concepts and 750,880 synonyms. The concepts are related through hierarchical relations and defining relations. Thanks to its logic-based organization, the SNCT concepts are compositional and follow the post-coordination approach: the simple concepts are recorded while the complex concepts are either recorded and linked to simple concepts or not recorded but possibly composed with these simple concepts.

UMLS. The Unified Medical Language System® (UMLS) [5] includes two sources of semantic information: the Metathesaurus® and the Semantic Network. The UMLS Metathesaurus integrates over 150 source vocabularies, including MDR and SNCT. The 2010AA version contains more than two million concepts which correspond to clusters of terms coming from the different vocabularies. Nearly 46 million relations exist among these concepts. The Semantic Network is a much smaller network of 133 semantic types organized in a tree structure. The semantic types have been aggregated into fifteen coarser semantic groups [6], which represent subdomains of biomedicine (*e.g.*, **Anatomy**, **Disorders**). Each Metathesaurus concept has a unique identifier (CUI) and is assigned at least one semantic type.

Related works. The mapping between terminologies and ontologies is an active research area, as indicated by the existence of the UMLS and its intensive international exploitation. Nevertheless, very few works have addressed the mapping between MDR and SNCT explicitly. Three experiments aimed at improving the current alignment rate. The exploitation of hierarchical relations has been performed: (1) when mapping MDR to SNCT, instead of considering an unmapped MDR term, they considered its mapped ancestor [7], which showed a 71% success rate; and (2) when mapping SNCT to MDR, hierarchical relations from SNCT, which are far more fine-grained than those from MDR, were exploited [8] and allowed on the whole over 100,000 new mappings. However, these two studies attempted to find mappings of the MDR terms as such, without trying to decompose and then map them to more than one SNCT term. Finally, a specific browser was designed in order to align the frequent MDR terms with the SNCT terms [9]. It was enriched with simple synonyms from the UMLS and it also considered a decomposition of the MDR terms. The approach allowed to propose 599 new mappings to one or more SNCT terms.

3 Methods

Selecting MedDRA and SNOMED CT terms. We first identified the UMLS concepts, which contained at least one term from MDR and no term originating from

SNCT. Then, we selected all MDR terms, which belong to these corresponding concepts. This provided us with a set of MDR terms that are not mapped to any SNCT term in the exploited version of the UMLS. From now on, we call *SNCT concepts* those UMLS concepts that contain at least one SNCT term.

Preparing and mapping the terms. We designed a lexical approach for the mapping of terms. First, terms were segmented into words and then normalized according to: variation of word order *{Accident household; Household accident}*, punctuation *{Precipitate labour, with delivery; Precipitate labor - delivered}*, stopwords *{Injury to diaphragm without mention of open wound into cavity; Injury diaphragm without open wound cavity}*, inflectional *{Ichthyoses; Ichthyosis}* and derived *{Acetabular dysplasia; Dysplasia of acetabulum}* forms, and also synonyms *{Dilated veins; Distended vein}*. With this approach, we exploited several resources: a list of stopwords (n=181), a morphological lexicon (85,628 pairs), and synonyms (101,225 pairs). The MDR terms were mapped either directly or through their decomposed elements. The decomposition was performed through several approaches, exemplified through *Ear and labyrinth disorders*: (1) a decomposition on stopwords called *segmented set* gave *ear* and *labyrinth disorders*; (2) a decomposition on stopwords with a special processing of the coordination called *coo-segmented set* gave *ear disorders* and *labyrinth disorders*; (3) a decomposition was performed through the Part-of-Speech tagging, the syntactic analysis and the exploitation of various syntactic phrases (*e.g.*, NP, VP, ADJP). This set was called *syntax-segmented set* and gave: *ear*, *and*, *labyrinth* and *disorders*. The decomposition provided us with three sets of MDR components.

Filtering mappings according to their semantic groups. The UMLS semantic groups (SGs) are expected to realize a partition of the UMLS concepts. We exploited this information for filtering out the wrong mappings among those generated by the previous step. This was possible only for 1-1 mappings, *i.e.*, when a MDR term was associated with a SNCT concept. In this case, we searched for the UMLS concept the MDR term belongs to and we recovered its corresponding SG. If the latter was not the same as the SG the SNCT concept belongs to, we considered the proposed mapping as wrong and eliminated it from the list of candidate mappings.

Evaluating the mappings. We performed a quantitative and a qualitative evaluations of the remaining mappings. For each processed set, we counted the number of 1-1 mappings and the number of MDR terms which components could all be mapped to one or more SNCT concepts, called "full mappings". We also compared the full mappings obtained by the three segmentation sets. Finally, we manually examined the 1-1 and full mappings and assessed their quality as "correct", "incorrect", or "hierarchically-related". The latter category corresponded to cases where the proposed mapping was not judged incorrect because it denoted a hierarchical relation between the MDR term and the SNCT concept(s), which is not set in the UMLS.

4 Results

Mapping results. 30,023 MDR terms were extracted from the 23,102 UMLS concepts containing no SNCT term. Table 1 presents the number of MDR components generated by each segmentation approach and the number of full and 1-1 mappings which were obtained within each processed set. An example of full mapping is the one found between the MDR term hematuria aggravated (C0856126) and the SNCT concepts Haematuria (C0018965) and Aggravated (C0436331).

Table 1. Mapping results obtained for each processed set

	Direct	Segmented	Coo-segmented	Syntax-segmented
# of MDR components		28,227	30,116	21,056
# of full mappings		52	234	361
# of 1-1 mappings	308	10	211	137

Comparing the segmentation approaches. Surprisingly, we found a low overlap between full mappings obtained within the three segmentation sets (Fig. 1). One of the 13 mappings common to the three approaches is the mapping of Suicide of sibling (C0860090) to the two SNCT concepts Suicide (C0038661) and Sibling (C0037047). The mapping of Chronic osteomyelitis involving hand (C0158384) to Chronic osteomyelitis (C0008707) and Hand (C0018563) is among the nine which were found only through the segmented and coo-segmented approaches. This mapping was not obtained through the syntax approach because the latter kept the word *involving*. Finally, one of the 135 mappings found only by the coo-segmented approach is Somatoform and factitious disorders (C0851579) which was efficiently mapped to Somatoform disorder (C0037650) and Factitious disorder (C0015480).

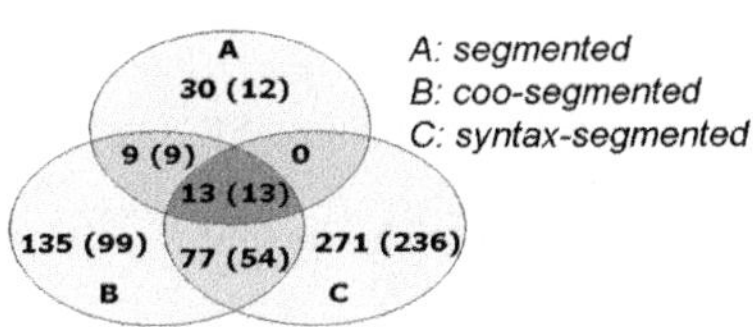

Fig. 1. Overlap of full mappings obtained within the three segmentation approaches. The number of mappings, which are deemed "correct", are displayed in brackets.

Evaluation. The 1-1 mappings generated by the direct approach corresponded to 199 correct mappings (64.6%), 45 incorrect (14.6%), and 64 hierarchically-related (20.8%). For example, Acute myringitis without mention of otitis media (C0155459) was correctly mapped to Acute myringitis without otitis media (C0395846). In contrast, the mapping of Eighth rib fracture (C0920007) to Fracture of eight OR more ribs (C0272566) is incorrect ("eight" and "eighth" were both normalized to *eight*).

Most of the full mappings obtained by the segmentation approaches were deemed "correct" (see numbers in brackets Fig. 1). For example, Drain of cerebral subdural space (C0948933) was correctly mapped to Drain (C0180499) and Subdural space of brain (C1284568). Only 68 mappings were hierarchically-related, which however provided useful propositions. For example, we found such a mapping between Polyradiculoneuritis (C0936254) and Polyneuritis (C0032541), while no relation currently exists between these concepts in the UMLS. Finally, some MDR terms containing a negation resulted in incorrect mappings, such as Vertigo (excluding dizziness) (C0852858) mapped to Vertigo (C0042571) and Dizziness (C0852858).

5 Discussion

On the whole, the proposed method provided several new and correct mappings, which resulted in a more complete alignment between MDR and SNCT. The assumption on the compositionality of the MDR terms has proved to be correct. However, our method displayed errors. The use of NLP tools may cause wrong segmentations and then result in incorrect mappings. For example, *ankle* was considered as an article (in the MDR term Ankle stiffness) instead of a noun. But because we did not consider this POS tag during the segmentation, *ankle* was lost and the mapping of Ankle stiffness could not be full. Other errors were induced through our semantic resources, where synonymous pairs may provide a correct link in some but not in all the contexts.

In our study, the exploitation of the SGs was useful to eliminate wrong mappings (approximately 1/4 of the initially proposed mappings). For example, an incorrect mapping was first proposed between Pleocytosis measurement (C1509130 / semantic type: *Laboratory Procedure*) and Pleocytosis (C0151857 / semantic type: *Finding*). We eliminated this mapping automatically because the concepts belong to distinct SGs (**Procedures** and **Disorders**, resp.). Conversely, we identified inconsistencies in the UMLS, which is a well-known problem in this system [10]. As an illustration, a synonymy relation between Photophobia aggravated (C0853637) and Photophobia (C0085636) is set in the UMLS while a hierarchical relation would be more accurate . In contrast, our segmentation-based approach was more precise and allowed to map Photophobia aggravated to both Photophobia and Aggravated (C0436331).

References

1. Lindquist, M.: VigiBase, the WHO Global ICSR Database System: Basic Facts. Drug Information Journal 42, 409–419 (2008)
2. Brown, E.G., Wood, L., Wood, S.: The medical dictionary for regulatory activities (MedDRA). Drug Saf. 20, 109–117 (1999)
3. The WHO Adverse Reaction Terminology – WHO-ART, `http://www.umc-products.com/graphics/3149.pdf`
4. SNOMED CT. IHTSDO, Copenhagen (2007), `http://www.ihtsdo.org/`
5. Bodenreider, O.: The Unified Medical Language System (UMLS): integrating biomedical terminology. Nucleic Acids Res. 32, D267–D270 (2004)
6. Bodenreider, O., McCray, A.T.: Exploring semantic groups through visual approaches. J. Biomed. Inform. 36, 414–432 (2003)
7. Alecu, I., Bousquet, C., Mougin, F., Jaulent, M.C.: Mapping of the WHO-ART terminology on Snomed CT to improve grouping of related adverse drug reactions. Stud. Health Technol. Inform. 124, 833–838 (2006)
8. Bodenreider, O.: Using SNOMED CT in combination with MedDRA for reporting signal detection and adverse drug reactions reporting. In: AMIA Annu. Symp. Proc. 2009, pp. 45–49 (2009)
9. Nadkarni, P.M., Darer, J.D.: Determining correspondences between high-frequency MedDRA concepts and SNOMED: a case study. BMC Med. Inform. Decis. Mak. 10, 66 (2010)
10. Zhu, X., Fan, J., Baorto, D.M., Weng, C., Cimino, J.J.: A review of auditing methods applied to the content of controlled biomedical terminologies. J. Biomed. Inform. 42, 413–425 (2009)

COPE: Childhood Obesity Prevention [Knowledge] Enterprise

Arash Shaban-Nejad[1], David L. Buckeridge[1], and Laurette Dubé[2]

[1] McGill Clinical & Health Informatics, Department of Epidemiology and Biostatistics, Faculty of Medicine, McGill University, 1140 Pine Ave. W., Montreal, Canada, H3A 1A3
{arash.shaban-nejad,david.buckeridge}@mcgill.ca
[2] Desautels Faculty of Management, McGill University, 1001 Sherbrooke St. West, Montreal, Canada H3A 1G5
laurette.dube@mcgill.ca

Abstract. This paper presents our work-in-progress on designing and implementing an integrated ontology for widespread knowledge dissemination in the domain of obesity with emphasis on childhood obesity. The COPE ontology aims to support a knowledge-based infrastructure to promote healthy eating habits and lifestyles, analyze children's behaviors and habits associated with obesity and to prevent or reduce the prevalence of childhood obesity and overweight. By formally integrating and harmonizing multiple knowledge sources across disciplinary boundaries, we will facilitate cross-sectional analysis of the domain of obesity and generate both generic and customized preventive recommendations, which take into consideration several factors, including existing conditions in individuals and communities.

Keywords: Biomedical ontologies, Childhood obesity prevention, Knowledge modeling, Behavioral analysis.

1 Introduction

Obesity is well known [1] as one of the major risk factors for several diseases, including: hypertension or high blood pressure; coronary heart disease; type 2 diabetes; stroke; gallbladder disease; osteoarthritis; sleep apnea and other breathing problems; some cancers, such as breast, colon, and endometrial cancer; and mental health problems, such as low self-esteem and depression. Addressing childhood obesity prevention as one of today's most complex health and socioeconomic challenges is tied to the need for better alignment between different sources of data on human behavior, the health system, nutrition and nutrition-related health problems (e.g., child and maternal nutrition, food safety), media, and markets at local, national, and global levels. It does not seem feasible to deal with such complexity without a clear understanding of the active components and parameters, their interactions at different levels, and how they shape individual, organizational, and collective choice, at any point in time and under varying conditions. While obesity traditionally has been described as "an excess amount of body fat" in general population, no consensus exists on the description and classification of obesity in children [2]. A prerequisite for decision making

M. Peleg, N. Lavrač, and C. Combi (Eds.): AIME 2011, LNAI 6747, pp. 225–229, 2011.

and policy analysis in a domain is capturing the domain's knowledge and standardization of terminologies. One way to achieve this in modern knowledge-based systems is through ontologies, which are used as a formal medium for sharing common vocabularies, providing semantic annotation and integration, indexing and reasoning support [3], and capturing behavioral knowledge. In order to facilitate collaborative medical-social research in the domain of healthy eating and child obesity prevention, the Childhood Obesity Prevention [Knowledge] Enterprise (COPE) project aims to employ state of the art techniques, tools and skills and generate a consistent multidisciplinary semantic platform to capture the social, environmental, economical and behavioral knowledge in this domain.

2 The COPE Ontology Design

Our approach employs the emerging technologies in Knowledge Representation (KR) and Semantic Web, including OWL 2.0 [4], advanced logical reasoning services, and social networking to develop an integrated knowledge base for the obesity domain. We classify the domain into five major categories that describe the areas of a healthy lifestyle in terms of food and nutrition, associated diseases (i.e., obesity and related chronic diseases), social- environmental factors, behavioral parameters and media (Figure 1). Defining appropriate rules and axioms along with different associated relationships between the individuals of those categories enables us to derive non-trivial inferencing from our ontology to support decision making in this area. As an example, the concepts such as "overweight person" should be defined based on several parameters, such as the person's height, age, body mass, and gender. The ontology defines the semantic relationship between different dependent components and regulates their interactions through a set of rules.

As the formal representation language we use OWL 2.0 along with Description Logics (DLs). OWL 2.0 is the extension of OWL to support more expressive knowledge modeling by adding features such as the possibility of defining property chains, richer data types, data ranges, and qualified cardinality restrictions. Using OWL 2.0 as one of the World Wide Web Consortium (W3C) recommendations enables us to model classes, properties, and individuals, and define the new datatypes through more expressive semantics (in comparison to classic OWL) for developing ontologies that are exchanged as RDF (Resource Description Framework) graphs. For the reasoning we have used logical reasoners such as RACER [5], and Pellet [6]. The iterative, collaborative nature of an ontology development life cycle requires that ontologies go through one or more processes, such as matching, mapping, merging, alignment, integration, debugging, and versioning. To develop an integrated ontology that can be reused, in whole or in part, by different tools and algorithms, we study different relationships (explicit or implicit) and potential matching between components of different knowledge sources. When integrating existing controlled vocabularies and ontologies from different domains, we also needed to deal with several mismatches at the language (syntax), and conceptual (semantics) levels.

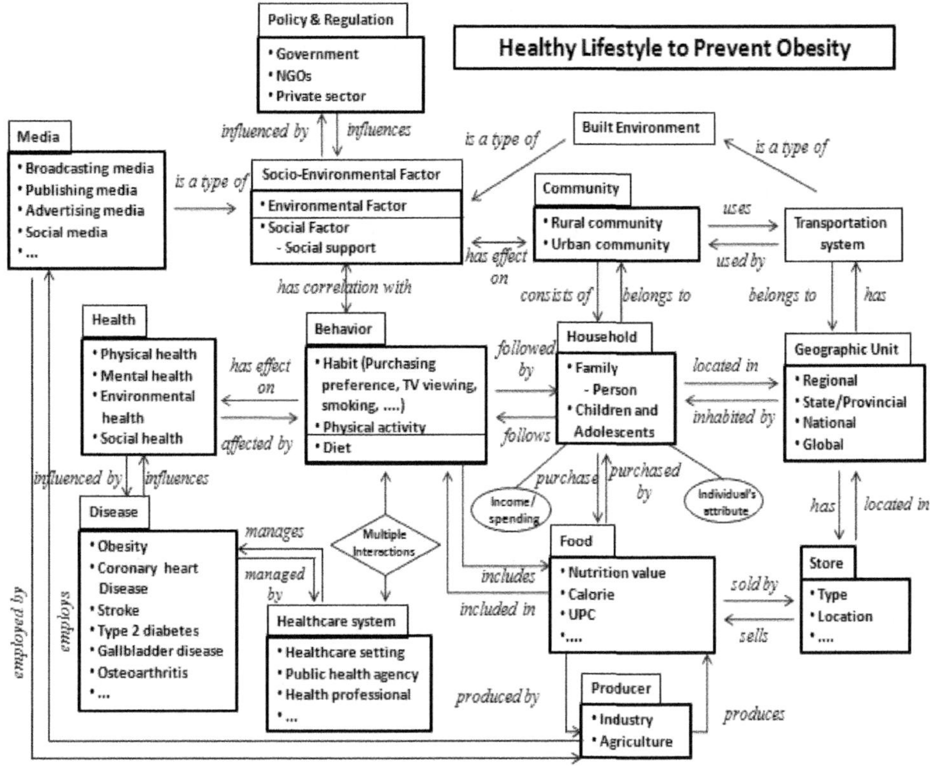

Fig. 1. An abstract representation of the major components and their interactions in the COPE ontology

2.1 Target Data Sources

Due to the interdisciplinary nature of the domain, the COPE ontology as an integrated knowledge base, is implemented on the basis of several textual resources, existing controlled vocabularies and thesauruses, blogs and databases, including RAMQ[1] (physician services and pharmaceutical prescriptions), Canadian Community Health Survey (CCHS[2]) (population health database that represents information on health status, health care utilization, and health determinants for Canadians), CARTaGENE[3], AGROVOC[4] (FAO agricultural thesaurus), and more. CARTaGENE provides information on medical history, genealogical data (to study family medical history), lifestyles, laboratory blood tests, biological samples, and physical measurements. Other important resources to analyze and determine consumer behavior outcomes are

[1] Régie de l'assurance maladie du Québec: `http://www.ramq.gouv.qc.ca/index_en.shtml`

[2] Canadian Community Health Survey (CCHS): `http://www.statcan.gc.ca/concepts/health-sante/index-eng.htm`

[3] `http://www.cartagene.qc.ca/index.php?lang=english`

[4] AGROVOC : `http://aims.fao.org/agrovoc/`

Statistics Canada[5] and Statistics Quebec (ISQ)[6], consisting of the Survey of Household Spending (SHS)[7], the National Population Health Survey (NPHS)[8] (provides socio-demographic information about health of Canadians through different time-stamps and related parameters) and private sectors. Also, several other surveys, such as those on regional transportation, living standards, and physical activities for different communities, will be used for cross-community comparison at different levels of granularity. Moreover we obtain the data on how people get information, consume media and buy goods and services through our collaboration with our partner in private sector. These datasets (e.g. data on retail measurement, demographics and store locations, and media/advertising measurement) can be linked together using demographic "hooks" or geographic coordinates and fused to third party data sets such as the BMI Survey. We will also collect our own primary data through multi-purpose individual-level questionnaires whenever we face a gap in the available resources.

3 Discussion

The availability of an integrated consensus knowledge on different (biological, nutritional, geographical, environmental, behavioral and social) factors relating to childhood obesity should be regarded as a vital component of any national/global surveillance system that continuously "tracks progress toward meeting the overall health objective of reducing and/or eliminating health problems across populations" [7]. COPE as an integrated data model consisting of nutrition, obesity and chronic diseases, behaviors, media, and marketing can be used as a basis for data integration and knowledge discovery for multidisciplinary researches. The COPE ontology can be used in various knowledge-based systems at both individual and community levels. It can provide a semantic backbone for a healthy diet recommender system to promote healthy eating habits. The dietary recommendations can be performed not only based on the existing food guides, which mainly focuses on the amount and types of foods, but also on other important factors personalized to the individuals' information (e.g. income, dietary restrictions, behaviors) and environmental parameters (e.g., family- and parent-associated interventions). As an application scenario, from the behavioral point of view, we are currently studying the impact of the new advances in social media on the general dietary behavior of children. In our scenario we emphasize on the dietary patterns associated with selection/consumption of low/high added-sugar food choices. Several types of behaviors (i.e. regulatory, social, habitual, and etc.) involve in a typical food selection/consumption process. The excessive use of social media may give rise to the abnormal behaviors in children (i.e. social media addiction) that affect their ingestive behavior and cause several childhood psychiatric disorders. Many of these mental disorders are also known as the major risk factors for obesity. An individual can regulate her behaviors (i.e. eating behavior) through her choices (e.g. selection of food, life style, etc.) in response to the environment [8]. For example increasing the level of physical activity [9] is recommended as a conscious

[5] http://www.statcan.gc.ca/start-debut-eng.html

[6] http://www.stat.gouv.qc.ca/default_an.htm

[7] http://www.statcan.gc.ca/imdb-bmdi/3508-eng.htm

[8] http://www.statcan.gc.ca/concepts/nphs-ensp/index-eng.htm

regulatory behavior to adjust the energy balance and improve behavioral outcome. Our future work will be focused on two aspects: i) enriching the COPE ontological structure with adding more components and more complex axioms to study multifaceted interactions between different components in the domain; ii) incorporating advanced social networking, social marketing and policy development techniques along with Web 2.0 methodologies to support decision making not only at the individual level but also at the community and society level.

Acknowledgments. COPE is a part of the Brain-to-Society (BtS) [8] research agenda within the McGill World Platform for Health and Economic Convergence (MWP) [10] initiative.

References

1. OBESITY, Health Canada Catalogue # H13-7/20-2006E-PDF (2006) ISBN # 0-662-44192-3
2. HCF Health Report on obesity and weight loss, No 9 (2003), `http://www.hcf.com.au/pdf/obesity.pdf`
3. Smith, B., Ashburner, M., et al.: The OBO Foundry: Coordinated Evolution of Ontologies to Support Biomedical Data Integration. Nature Biotechnol. 25(11), 1251–1255 (2007)
4. OWL 2.0 Overview, `http://www.w3.org/TR/owl2-overview/`
5. Haarslev, V., Möller, R.: RACER System Description. In: Goré, R.P., Leitsch, A., Nipkow, T. (eds.) IJCAR 2001. LNCS (LNAI), vol. 2083, pp. 701–706. Springer, Heidelberg (2001)
6. Pellet: OWL 2 Reasoner for Java, `http://clarkparsia.com/pellet/`
7. Singh, G.K., Kogan, M.D., van Dyck, P.C.: Changes in state-specific childhood obesity and overweight prevalence in the United States from 2003 to 2007. Arch. Pediatr. Adolesc. Med. 164(7), 598–607 (2010)
8. Dubé, L., Bechara, A., Böckenholt, U., Ansari, A., Dagher, A., et al.: Towards a brain-to-society systems model of individual choice. Market Lett 19, 323–336 (2008)
9. Ng, C., Marshall, D., Willows, N.D.: Obesity, adiposity, physical fitness and activity levels in Cree children. Int. J. Circumpolar Health 65(4), 322–330 (2006)
10. McGill World Platform for Health and Economic Convergence, `http://www.mcgill.ca/mwp/`

Repeated Prognosis in the Intensive Care: How Well Do Physicians and Temporal Models Perform?

Lilian Minne[1], Evert de Jonge[2], and Ameen Abu-Hanna[1]

[1] Academic Medical Center, Department of Medical Informatics, P.O. Box 22660, 1100 DD Amsterdam, The Netherlands
[2] Leiden University Medical Center, Department of Intensive Care, P.O. Box 9600, 2300 RC Leiden, The Netherlands
{L.Minne,A.Abu-Hanna}@amc.uva.nl, E.de_Jonge@lumc.nl

Abstract. Recently, we devised a method to develop prognostic models incorporating patterns of sequential organ failure to predict the eventual hospital mortality at each day of intensive care stay. In this study, we aimed to understand, using a real world setting, how these models perform compared to physicians, who are exposed to additional information than the models. We found a slightly better discriminative ability for physicians (AUC range over days: 0.73-0.83 vs. 0.70-0.80) and a slightly better accuracy for the models (Brier score range: 0.14-0.19 vs. 0.16-0.19). However when we combined both sources of predictions we arrived at a significantly superior discrimination as well as accuracy (AUC range: 0.81-0.88; Brier score range: 0.11-0.15). Our results show that the models and the physicians draw on complementary information that can be best harnessed by combining both prediction sources. Extensive external validation and impact studies are imperative to further investigate the ability of the combined model.

Keywords: Prognostic models, calibration, discrimination, human intuition, temporal patterns.

1 Introduction

In the Intensive Care Unit (ICU), physicians are daily challenged with the complex task of *prognosis*. Prognosis can be defined as the prediction of (the probability of) an event, such as death, before its possible occurrence [1,2]. Patient preferences to undergo intensive life sustaining treatments highly depend on their prognosis. In fact, they often prefer palliative care aiming at comfort and relief of pain if their chances of survival are very low [3,4] and clinicians' perceptions of survival chances strongly influence provision of life support [5]. Survival in the ICU is usually defined as *hospital survival*, which is the probability that a particular patient will be discharged alive from the hospital. This means that a patient that was discharged alive from the ICU to a hospital ward but died in the ward will be considered as a non-survivor.

Predictions of survival can be obtained either subjectively (e.g. expert opinion) or objectively (e.g. mathematical models). The main advantage of an *objective* approach

M. Peleg, N. Lavrač, and C. Combi (Eds.): AIME 2011, LNAI 6747, pp. 230–239, 2011.

is that mathematical models are extremely consistent and able to optimally combine information into a global judgment [6]. Commonly used mathematical models in the ICU are the Acute Physiology and Chronic Health Evaluation (APACHE) I-IV [7], the Simplified Acute Physiology Assessment (SAPS) I-III [8] and the Mortality Prediction Model (MPM) I-II [9]. These models are mostly used to adjust for severity of illness when comparing hospital performance based on their mortality rates. In comparison to objective predictions, *subjective* predictions may be inexact or even inconsistent [10,11]. There can be substantial disagreement between different clinicians, even if they are both very experienced [12], and prognosis is the part of medical practice they feel most insecure about [13]. On the other hand, clinicians are able to incorporate important implicit knowledge outside the scope of mathematical models and react quickly to changing situations [6].

Several of these mathematical models have been compared to clinicians (i.e. expert opinion). In general, clinicians seem to have good discriminative ability [12,14-24], which is superior compared to objective models [25]. Objective models tend however to be better calibrated [16,17]. Capitalizing on the individual strengths of both subjective and objective predictions by using a *combined* approach seems to yield superior discrimination and calibration over either one alone [16,18,22,23,26,27]. However, the problem of comparing repeated predictions for the same patient over time between the two approaches has not been studied before, and in fact there is paucity of work on repeated predictions in either approach (subjective or objective).

Repeated predictions are important to better individualize the prognosis for a patient as more information obtained over time can be used. For example, the chance of surviving until hospital discharge will decrease in patients who suffer major complications during their ICU stay. The present ICU models are less suitable for individual prognosis because they are based on only physiologic data from the first 24 hours after ICU admission. We recently suggested a method for developing *"temporal"* prognostic models for providing hospital survival predictions at each day of ICU stay [28]. Specifically, we showed that the use of specific patterns of sequential data (e.g. the transition from normal renal function to renal failure) lead to models that can better discriminate between survivors and non-survivors and more accurate than the present *"static"* models [29,30].

The aim of this study is to investigate and compare daily prognostication in adult ICU patients based on subjective and objective prognostic information. In particular we address the following sources of predictions: 1) Expert opinion (daily survival estimates by physicians) and 2) Three types of temporal models including different levels of objective and subjective information.

2 Methods

2.1 Data Collection

We designed a prospective comparative study in which we included all consecutive patients admitted between October 2007 and April 2008 to a 28-bed multidisciplinary mixed adult ICU of a 1002-bed university hospital in Amsterdam. We extracted demographics, patient outcomes and all data necessary to calculate the severity of illness score in the first 24 hours (SAPS-II, which ranges between 0 and 163) and the daily organ failure scores (SOFA scores, ranging between 0 and 24) from the Dutch National Intensive Care Evaluation (NICE) registry [31]. Each 24 hours, physicians' estimates of the likelihood of survival up to ICU discharge were elicited and recorded in a software module that we developed and integrated into the Patient Data Management System (PDMS; a computerized system that automatically collects and stores vital parameters from the patient monitor and provides digital patient charts [32]). After completion of routine data collection, a question regarding the patient's chance of survival popped up automatically in which physicians could choose between 10 probability categories (0-10%, 10-20%, 20-30%, 30-40%, 40-50%, 50-60%, 60-70%, 70-80%, 80-90% and 90-100%) or state that they did not have any clue. Categories were indicated by red (low survival probabilities) and green (high survival probabilities) color-scales. The predictions were transformed to predictions of mortality for comparison to the mathematical models. The scoring moment was typically between 9 and 12 am, but estimates could be changed until 12 pm.

2.2 Physicians

At the time we started this study, our ICU employed 10 critical care attendings, 8 fellows and approximately 14 residents, all of which participated in the study. Critical care attendings are specialists (e.g. neurologists or cardiologists) who have completed an additional intensive care specialization of two years. Fellows and residents have completed at least two years of post-MD training. Fellows are in training for the intensive care specialization and residents are in training for anaesthesiologist. Physicians were blinded for the predictions of the objective models and were unaware of their colleagues' assessments. They were not trained to estimate survival probabilities and did not receive feedback. Physicians were notified of this study by email and by an announcement during their staff meeting.

2.3 Development of Mathematical Models

A model was developed for each day of ICU stay from day 2 to day 7 by the procedure described in [29]. This procedure involves two steps: 1) data-driven discovery of temporal patterns of sequential organ failure scores, and 2) embedding them in the familiar logistic regression model. As in the original work in [29], SOFA scores were categorized as low (*L*) if SOFA ɑ {0, …, 6}, medium (*M*) if SOFA Œ {7, 8} or high (*H*) if SOFA Œ {9, …, 24} and patterns were aligned to the day of prediction. For example, the pattern *M,H* on day 4 (the day of prediction) means a high SOFA score on day 4 preceded by a medium score on day 3. In our systematic review on SOFA-based models [33], we found two strategies leading to good performing models (not necessarily for repeated predictions): our approach based on temporal patterns (described above) and combining SOFA abstractions with admission scores (e.g. SAPS-II). Commonly used abstractions of SOFA are its mean, maximum (from admission to day of prediction *d*), and delta (difference in scores between day *d* and day of admission). In this study, we developed logistic regression models containing three levels of information: Type A) SAPS-II score and SOFA patterns, Type B) SAPS-II score, SOFA patterns and mean, max and delta SOFA scores, and Type C) SAPS-II score, SOFA patterns, mean, max and delta SOFA scores and mean, max and delta in expert opinion (i.e. the physician's prediction of mortality). The Akaike Information Criterion (AIC) [34] was used to select the optimal subset of covariates yielding the best model (i.e. the one with the lowest possible AIC). The AIC is defined as $-2ln(L) + 2k$ where L is the maximized likelihood of the model and k is the number of free parameters in the model. The AIC trades off predictive performance for parsimony by penalizing for the number of variables included in the model in order to avoid overfitting [29]. The variable selection procedure starts by including all variables and incrementally eliminating the least predictive covariate in each round (i.e. the one associated with the highest AIC) until the AIC cannot be decreased any further.

2.4 Statistical Analysis

Discrimination (i.e. the ability of the model to distinguish between survivors from non-survivors) was measured by the Area Under the Receiver Operating Characteristic Curve (AUC). An AUC ranges between 0 to 1 with higher values indicating better discriminative ability. Although the AUC is dependent on the prevalence of the event in the sample, it is common to consider an AUC between 0.6 and 0.7 as poor, between 0.7 and 0.8 as fair, between 0.8 and 0.9 as good and above 0.9 as excellent. The Brier score is a measure of accuracy, which has both aspects of discrimination and calibration (i.e. the degree of correspondence between predicted risks and patients' actual risks of death). The formula of the Brier score is:

$$BS = \frac{1}{N}\sum_{i=1}^{N}(p_i - o_i)^2$$

where N is the number of observations, p the forecasted probability and o the observed outcome. Outcome measures and confidence intervals were obtained by calculating the bootstrap sampling distributions of the respective statistics based on 1,000 bootstrap samples. Missing values of SAPS-II were excluded from the dataset, while missing physicians' predictions were imputed by taking the value of the previous day or, when not available, the mean of all predictions available for the patient involved. Analyses were conducted in the R statistical environment.

3 Results

The baseline characteristics of the 397 patients admitted during the study period are shown in Table 1. For 397 admissions, 1966 physicians-estimations were registered, and 349 values (15%) were missing. Physicians recorded that they had no idea regarding a patient's chance of survival in 55 cases (2.4%). There were no missing values in SOFA scores and only two missing values in SAPS-II scores (0.5%). Hospital mortality was 21.4%.

Table 1. Patient characteristics. LOS = Length of Stay, SAPS = Simplified Acute Physiology Score, SOFA = Sequential Organ Failure Assessment, SD = Standard deviation.

	Survivors *n=312*	Non-survivors *n=85*	Total population
Admission type (%)			
Medical	35.9	71.8	43.6
Urgent	13.5	18.8	14.6
Planned	50.6	9.4	41.8
Mean age +/- SD (years)	61.7 +/- 14.6	66.3 +/- 13.7	62.7 +/- 14.5
Male/female (%)	61.2/38.8	51.8/48.2	59.2/40.8
Mean SAPS-II +/- SD	50 +/- 16.7	67.8 +/- 19.8	53.8 +/- 18.9
Mean SOFA +/- SD	6.6 +/- 3.5	9.6 +/- 4.3	7.4 +/- 4.0
Mean estimate +/- SD (%)	33.6 +/- 27	55.9 +/- 29.7	39.8 +/- 29.5

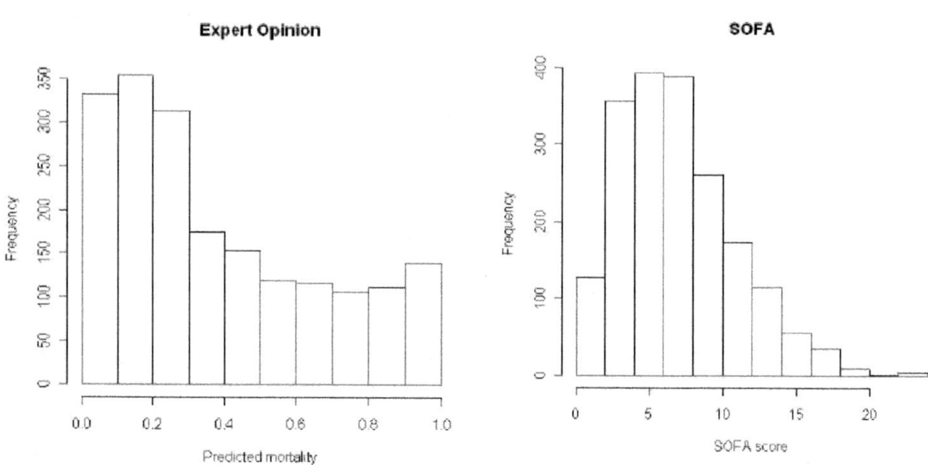

Fig. 1. Distribution of Expert Opinion and SOFA scores

Figure 1 shows histograms of expert opinion (i.e. the physician's predictions of mortality) and SOFA scores. Mean predicted mortality by physicians was 39.8% (1.86 times the actual mortality). To assess whether expert opinion could reliably identify high-risk patients, all patients with predicted mortality above 90% were obtained yielding 55 patients. Of these only 69.1% actually died (this is the positive predictive value at 0.9). Mean standard deviation per patient was 1.68 for expert opinion and 2.27 for the SOFA score model.

Table 2. Description of the developed logistic regression models. SAPSII = Simplified Acute Physiology Score-II, L = Low (score of 0-7), M = Medium (score of 8-11), H = High (score of 12-24), expert = expert opinion, i.e. the physician's predictions of mortality.

Day	Model type	Model description
2	Type A model	-3.10 + 0.04 SAPSII - 0.09 M,M - 1.48 L,L
	Type B model	-3.35 + 0.05 SAPSII + 0.42 mean SOFA 0.34 max SOFA - 1.30 M,M - 1.48 L,L
	Type C model	-3.74 + 0.03 SAPSII - 0.51 mean SOFA + 4.22 mean expert - 0.51 max SOFA + 3.44 delta expert - 1.25 M,M - 2.24 L,L
3	Type A model	-2.53 + 0.04 SAPSII - 1.57 L - 0.83 M,M
	Type B model	-5.29 + 0.04 SAPSII + 0.22 mean SOFA + 0.91 M - 0.88 M,M
	Type C model	-5.97 + 0.03 SAPSII + 0.12 mean SOFA + 5.21 mean expert + 2.36 delta expert - 1.28 L,L,L
4	Type A model	-2.21 + 0.04 SAPSII + 1.46 L - 1.05 M
	Type C model	-4.72 + 0.02 SAPSII + 5.20 mean expert + 1.57 delta expert - 1.89 L,L,L,L
5	Type A model	-3.03 + 0.04 SAPSII - 1.26 L,L,L,L
	Type B model	-4.34 + 0.04 SAPSII + 0.15 mean SOFA
	Type C model	-4.64 + 0.03 SAPSII + 4.64 mean expert - 1.63 L,L,L,L
6	Type A model	-2.78 + 0.04 SAPSII - 1.63 L + 1.58 L,L,L - 1.50 L,L,L,L,L
	Type C model	-5.44 + 0.03 SAPSII + 5.84 mean expert + 1.88 delta expert - 2.15 L,L,L,L,L
7	Type A model	-1.43 + 0.03 SAPSII - 1.89 L - 1.04 M + 1.31 L,L,L,L -2.00 L,L,L,L,L,L
	Type B model	-4.40 + 0.02 SAPSII + 0.18 max SOFA + 1.13 L,L,L,L - 1.56 L,L,L,L,L,L
	Type C model	-4.09 + 7.81 mean expert - 3.27 L,L,L,L,L,L

The logits (log odds) of the best temporal models for days 2-6 are summarized in Table 2. For example the best temporal model of type A on day 2 is described by the following logistic regression model:

$$\frac{e^{-3.10+0.04SAPS-II-0.09M,M-1.48L,L}}{1+e^{-3.10+0.04SAPS-II-0.09M,M-1.48L,L}}$$

where *M,M* means medium SOFA score on day 1 and on day 2 (the day of prediction), and *L,L* means low SOFA score on day 1 and 2. Predictive performance of the temporal models and expert opinion is summarized in Figure 2.

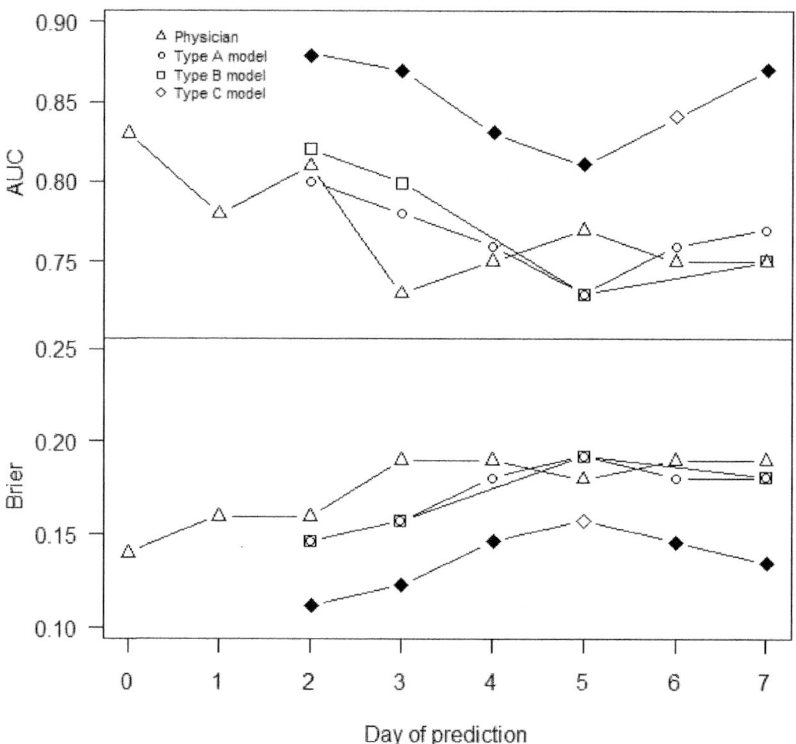

Fig. 2. Predictive performance of physicians and temporal models. SAPS = Simplified Acute Physiology Score, AUC = Area Under the Receiver Operating Curve. Filled icons in model C indicate statistically significant differences with results of model B for that particular day. No statistically significant differences were found between models of type B and type A or between models of type A and physicians.

The AUC of expert opinion ranged from 0.73 on day 3 to 0.83 on the day of admission, while the Brier score ranged from 0.14 on the day of admission to 0.19 on days 3, 4, 6 and 7. Models of type C had significantly higher (better) AUCs than physicians on day 2 to day 7 and significantly lower (better) Brier scores for days 2, 3 and day 4 to 7. These were also better than all other temporal models (which were more or less comparable to physicians), and significantly so for all says except for the AUC on day 6.

4 Discussion

In this study, we compared the performance of physicians and mathematical models in predicting mortality in the ICU. Physicians had fair to good discriminative ability

(AUC range: 0.73-0.83), which was comparable (only slightly higher but without statistical significance) to the mathematical models (AUC range: 0.70-0.80). The accuracy of physicians (Brier score range: 0.16-0.19) was comparable to the accuracy of the mathematical models without subjective information (Brier score range: 0.14-0.19). Nevertheless, physicians seem to markedly overestimate mortality. The mean predicted mortality by physicians (39.8%) was much higher than the observed mortality (21.4%) and patients estimated as high risk patients (> 0.9 probability of death) still had a realistic chance to survive (30.9%). Mathematical models were significantly improved by adding subjective information (AUC range 0.81-0.88 and Brier score range: 0.11-0.15) which made them superior to physicians.

To our knowledge the present pilot study is unique, and the first in comparing models with daily predictions of physicians. The idea of models with repeated predictions is relatively new, and these models have not been combined with subjective information before, at least not in the ICU. Another strength of this study is the use of bootstrapping techniques to correct for optimistic estimates of predictive performance because of similarities in train and test data. Weaknesses of this study include the use of a relatively small dataset and the fact that different physicians provided estimates for the same patients.

Other studies scrutinizing expert opinion on a daily basis either validated the most recent prediction only [26] or did not provide direct measures of predictive performance, such as the AUC or error rates [5,35]. In general, other studies validating predictive ability of physicians also found fair to good discrimination [12,14-24] and superior predictive performance of a combined approach of subjective and objective information [16,18,22,23,26,27]. In our study, the difference in discriminative ability between physicians and objective models without subjective information was not significant, however.

We found that the mathematical models can be significantly improved by the inclusion of subjective information. These models have the potential to provide some patient groups with reliable information about survival probabilities, and in the future may be useful to support individual decision-making in these patient groups with very high risk of dying. Although some of these patients may prefer palliative care and will decide to stop treatment, the models might also help physicians not to withdraw therapy. As physicians tend to overestimate mortality, the models might be able to prevent unjust decisions leading to withdrawal of treatment in patients who would otherwise survive. An advantage of including expert opinion in the final prognosis is that it may lead to higher acceptance of the models by physicians and patients or their families. Before they can make their way into clinical practice, however, extensive external validation and studies on their impact on clinical decisions and patient outcomes are imperative [36].

Future research needs to focus on questions about how to optimize these temporal models, the potential value of including nurses' predictions of mortality, their external validity, their acceptability by clinicians and their potential impact on clinical decisions and patient outcomes. Note also that in our study the AUC and Brier scores were generally better on the first days of admission, but that the patients in later days form subsets of those in earlier days because on each day some patients leave the ICU (they are either discharged alive or die). Investigating the behavior of the AUC and Brier scores over time for the same patient group merits future research.

References

1. Lucas, P.J., Abu-Hanna, A.: Prognostic methods in medicine. Artif. Intell. Med. 15, 105–119 (1999)
2. Abu-Hanna, A., Lucas, P.J.: Prognostic models in medicine. AI and statistical approaches. Methods Inf. Med. 40, 1–5 (2001)
3. Fried, T.R., Bradley, E.H., Towle, V.R., Allore, H.: Understanding the treatment preferences of seriously ill patients. N. Engl. J. Med. 346, 1061–1066 (2002)
4. Murphy, D.J., Burrows, D., Santilli, S., Kemp, A.W., Tenner, S., Kreling, B., et al.: The influence of the probability of survival on patients' preferences regarding cardiopulmonary resuscitation. N. Engl. J. Med. 330, 545–549 (1994)
5. Rocker, G., Cook, D., Sjokvist, P., Weaver, B., Finfer, S., McDonald, E., et al.: Clinician predictions of intensive care unit mortality. Crit. Care Med. 32, 1149–1154 (2004)
6. Whitecotton, S.M., Sanders, D.E., Norris, K.B.: Improving Predictive Accuracy with a Combination of Human Intuition and Mechanical Decision Aids. Organ Behav. Hum. Decis. Process 76, 325–348 (1998)
7. Knaus, W.A., Draper, E.A., Wagner, D.P., Zimmerman, J.E.: APACHE II: a severity of disease classification system. Crit. Care Med. 13, 818–829 (1985)
8. Le Gall, J.R., Lemeshow, S., Saulnier, F.: A new Simplified Acute Physiology Score (SAPS II) based on a European/North American multicenter study. JAMA 270, 2957–2963 (1993)
9. Lemeshow, S., Teres, D., Klar, J., Avrunin, J.S., Gehlbach, S.H., Rapoport, J.: Mortality Probability Models (MPM II) based on an international cohort of intensive care unit patients. JAMA 270, 2478–2486 (1993)
10. Christakis, N.A., Lamont, E.B.: Extent and determinants of error in doctors' prognoses in terminally ill patients: prospective cohort study. BMJ 320, 469–472 (2000)
11. McClish, D.K., Powell, S.H.: How well can physicians estimate mortality in a medical intensive care unit? Med. Decis. Making 9, 125–132 (1989)
12. Poses, R.M., Bekes, C., Copare, F.J., Scott, W.E.: The answer to "What are my chances, doctor?" depends on whom is asked: prognostic disagreement and inaccuracy for critically ill patients. Crit. Care Med. 17, 827–833 (1989)
13. Christakis, N.A., Iwashyna, T.J.: Attitude and self-reported practice regarding prognostication in a national sample of internists. Arch. Intern. Med. 158, 2389–2395 (1998)
14. Scholz, N., Basler, K., Saur, P., Burchardi, H., Felder, S.: Outcome prediction in critical care: physicians' prognoses vs. scoring systems. Eur. J. Anaesthesiol. 21, 606–611 (2004)
15. Garrouste-Orgeas, M., Montuclard, L., Timsit, J.F., Misset, B., Christias, M., Carlet, J.: Triaging patients to the ICU: a pilot study of factors influencing admission decisions and patient outcomes. Intensive Care Med. 29, 774–781 (2003)
16. Knaus, W.A., Harrell Jr., F.E., Lynn, J., Goldman, L., Phillips, R.S., Connors Jr., A.F., et al.: he SUPPORT prognostic model. Objective estimates of survival for seriously ill hospitalized adults. Study to understand prognoses and preferences for outcomes and risks of treatments. Ann. Intern. Med. 122, 191–203 (1995)
17. Christensen, C., Cottrell, J.J., Murakami, J., Mackesy, M.E., Fetzer, A.S., Elstein, A.S.: Forecasting survival in the medical intensive care unit: a comparison of clinical prognoses with formal estimates. Methods Inf. Med. 32, 302–308 (1993)
18. Marks, R.J., Simons, R.S., Blizzard, R.A., Browne, D.R.: Predicting outcome in intensive therapy units–a comparison of Apache II with subjective assessments. Intensive Care Med. 17, 159–163 (1991)

19. Poses, R.M., Bekes, C., Copare, F.J., Scott, W.E.: What difference do two days make? The inertia of physicians' sequential prognostic judgments for critically ill patients. Med. Decis. Making 10, 6–14 (1990)
20. Poses, R.M., Bekes, C., Winkler, R.L., Scott, W.E., Copare, F.J.: Are two (inexperienced) heads better than one (experienced) head? Averaging house officers' prognostic judgments for critically ill patients. Arch. Intern. Med. 150, 1874–1878 (1990)
21. Poses, R.M., McClish, D.K., Bekes, C., Scott, W.E., Morley, J.N.: Ego bias, reverse ego bias, and physicians' prognostic. Crit. Care Med. 19, 1533–1539 (1991)
22. McClish, D.K., Powell, S.H.: How well can physicians estimate mortality in a medical intensive care unit? Med. Decis. Making 9, 125–132 (1989)
23. Brannen, A.L., Godfrey, L.J., Goetter, W.E.: Prediction of outcome from critical illness. A comparison of clinical judgment with a prediction rule. Arch. Intern. Med. 149, 1083–1086 (1989)
24. Kruse, J.A., Thill-Baharozian, M.C., Carlson, R.W.: Comparison of clinical assessment with APACHE II for predicting mortality risk in patients admitted to a medical intensive care unit. JAMA 260, 1739–1742 (1988)
25. Sinuff, T., Adhikari, N.K., Cook, D.J., Schunemann, H.J., Griffith, L.E., Rocker, G., et al.: Mortality predictions in the intensive care unit: comparing physicians with scoring systems. Crit. Care Med. 34, 878–885 (2006)
26. Chang, R.W., Lee, B., Jacobs, S., Lee, B.: Accuracy of decisions to withdraw therapy in critically ill patients: clinical judgment versus a computer model. Crit. Care Med. 17, 1091–1097 (1989)
27. Meyer, A.A., Messick, W.J., Young, P., Baker, C.C., Fakhry, S., Muakkassa, F., et al.: Prospective comparison of clinical judgment and APACHE II score in predicting the outcome in critically ill surgical patients. J. Trauma 32, 747–753 (1992)
28. Toma, T., Bosman, R.J., Siebes, A., Peek, N., Abu-Hanna, A.: Learning predictive models that use pattern discovery–a bootstrap evaluative approach applied in organ functioning sequences. J. Biomed. Inform. 43, 578–586 (2010)
29. Toma, T., Abu-Hanna, A., Bosman, R.J.: Discovery and inclusion of SOFA score episodes in mortality prediction. J. Biomed. Inform. 40, 649–660 (2007)
30. Toma, T., Abu-Hanna, A., Bosman, R.J.: Discovery and integration of univariate patterns from daily individual organ-failure scores for intensive care mortality prediction. Artif. Intell. Med. 43, 47–60 (2008)
31. de Jonge, E., Bosman, R.J., van der Voort, P.H., Korsten, H.H., Scheffer, G.J., de Keizer, N.F.: [Intensive care medicine in the Netherlands, 1997-2001. I. Patient population and treatment outcome]. Ned Tijdschr Geneeskd 147, 1013–1017 (2003)
32. Fretschner, R., Bleicher, W., Heininger, A., Unertl, K.: Patient data management systems in critical care. J. Am. Soc. Nephrol. 12 suppl 17, S83–S86 (2001)
33. Minne, L., Abu-Hanna, A., de Jonge, E.: Evaluation of SOFA-based models for predicting mortality in the ICU: A systematic review. Crit. Care 12, R161 (2008)
34. Burnham, K.P., Anderson, D.R.: Model selection and multimodel inference: a practical-theoretic approach. Springer, Heidelberg (2002)
35. Frick, S., Uehlinger, D.E., Zuercher Zenklusen, R.M.: Medical futility: predicting outcome of intensive care unit patients by nurses and doctors–a prospective comparative study. Crit. Care Med. 31, 456–461 (2003)
36. Moons, K.G., Royston, P., Vergouwe, Y., Grobbee, D.E., Altman, D.G.: Prognosis and prognostic research: what, why, and how? BMJ 338, b375 (2009)

Automating the Calibration of a Neonatal Condition Monitoring System

Christopher K.I. Williams and Ioan Stanculescu

School of Informatics, University of Edinburgh,
10 Crichton Street, Edinburgh EH8 9AB, UK
c.k.i.williams@ed.ac.uk, i.a.stanculescu@sms.ed.ac.uk
http://www.inf.ed.ac.uk

Abstract. Condition monitoring of premature babies in intensive care can be carried out using a Factorial Switching Linear Dynamical System (FSLDS) [15]. A crucial part of training the FSLDS is the manual *calibration* stage, where an interval of normality must be identified for each baby that is monitored. In this paper we replace this manual step by using a classifier to predict whether an interval is normal or not. We show that the monitoring results obtained using automated calibration are almost as good as those using manual calibration.

Keywords: Condition monitoring, switching linear dynamical system, intensive care, logistic regression, decision tree, Naïve Bayes.

1 Introduction

Condition monitoring often involves the analysis of systems with hidden factors that "switch" between different modes of operation and collectively determine the observed data. Given the monitoring data, we are interested in recovering the state of the factors that gave rise to it. In our work condition monitoring is performed on premature babies receiving intensive care, with the data coming from second-by-second measurements of their vital signs. The factors correspond to physiological events (such as bradycardia, a spontaneous slowing of the heart) or artifactual events (such as taking a blood sample).

The Factorial Switching Linear Dynamical System (FSLDS) [15] has the ability to model a system which switches between multiple modes of operation conditioned on a set of factors. More precisely, given a sequence of observations, the FSLDS outputs the filtering distribution of the switch setting at each time step. The model has proved to be highly successful in inferring the hidden factors that govern the observations collected by cotside computers [10,12].

As a crucial part of training the FSLDS, a manual *calibration* stage is needed [12]. This requires finding an interval of normality for each examined baby. By normality, we generally understand a period in which the baby is in a stable physiological condition and there is no artifact corrupting the measurements [10]. The primary goal of this paper is *automating* the calibration stage. More precisely, we will build a binary classifier that predicts whether an interval of

M. Peleg, N. Lavrač, and C. Combi (Eds.): AIME 2011, LNAI 6747, pp. 240–249, 2011.

monitoring data is normal or not. The main reason for the feasibility of such a classification is that while the normal dynamics can be different for each baby, artifact is stereotypical.

The structure of the rest of the paper is as follows: An introduction to physiological monitoring in a neonatal intensive care unit is given in Section 2. Section 3 is dedicated to the Factorial Switching Linear Dynamical System (FSLDS) discussing the model, the application-specific setup, learning and inference. Section 4 details our approach for automating the calibration stage needed by the model. The results obtained by employing the classifiers built in the previous part are given in Section 5. A discussion of our main findings together with recommendations for future work concludes the paper in Section 6.

2 Neonatal Condition Monitoring Data

The physiological system can be thought of in terms of three partly independent sub-systems: the respiratory system, the cardiovascular system and the thermoregulatory system [10, §2.1.1]. Each of these systems has its associated set of measurement channels. The respiratory system is monitored by measuring the O_2 saturation in arterial blood (SO) and the partial pressures of O_2 ($TcPO_2$) and CO_2 ($TcPCO_2$). The flow of blood through the body is controlled by the cardiovascular system. This is traditionally monitored by obtaining heart rate (HR) measurements from an electrocardiogram. In addition, a transducer records the evolution of the blood pressure on two channels, systolic (BS) and diastolic (BD). The thermoregulatory system keeps the body at an adequate temperature. This is monitored by two channels: core temperature (TC) and peripheral temperature (TP). Along with this set of physiological measurements, clinicians also need the environment inside the incubator to function in normal parameters. Therefore, they record incubator temperature (IT) and incubator humidity (IH).

We now enumerate the physiological and artifactual events we plan to uncover by doing inference in the auto-calibrated FSLDS. *Bradycardia* (see Figure 2.b) is a physiological event characterized by a temporary drop in the heart rate measurements. *Probe disconnection* is a frequent artifactual event related to operating the monitoring equipment. Generally, when a probe is disconnected the measurements fall to zero. However, the current paper analyses *core temperature probe detachment*, when the disconnection is characterized by a decay of measurements towards incubator values. Periodically taking a *blood sample* is another artifactual event (see Figure 2.b). The procedure causes an artifactual ramp in the blood pressure measurements. Moreover, if the heart rate is also computed from the pressure sensor, readings will cease for the duration of the blood sampling event [10, §2.3.2]. A common artifactual event is *opening the incubator's* doors. This is caused by various medical procedures that need to be performed on the patient. During this operation, we usually see an increased variance in the physiological measurement channels. At the same time the incubator's temperature and humidity slowly adjust to room values. A great number of other factors can influence a patient's condition and precisely determining all of these is practically impossible. A solution is to introduce the *X-factor* [10], a factor responsible for all events that are neither normal nor correspond to a known factor.

3 The Factorial Switching Linear Dynamical System

Switching [3,8,13] and factorization [4] are two well-known ideas for relaxing the assumptions made by state-space models on the probability distribution of the data. The FSLDS [10,12,15] combines both with the advantages of autoregressive (AR) processes to model baby monitoring. In a traditional Switching Linear Dynamical System (SLDS) (see e.g. [13]), discrete hidden states, s_t, evolve according to Markovian transition probabilities, $p(s_t \mid s_{t-1})$, and determine which set of parameters is used by the dynamics and observation equations at the current time step:

$$\mathbf{x}_t \sim N(\mathbf{A}(s_t)\mathbf{x}_{t-1}, \mathbf{Q}(s_t)), \qquad \mathbf{y}_t \sim N(\mathbf{C}(s_t)\mathbf{x}_t, \mathbf{R}(s_t)), \tag{1}$$

where $\mathbf{x}_t$ is the continuous hidden state and $\mathbf{y}_t$ is the observed variable. The joint distribution of such a model is:

$$p(s_{1:T}, \mathbf{x}_{1:T}, \mathbf{y}_{1:T}) = p(s_1)p(\mathbf{x}_1)p(\mathbf{y}_1 \mid \mathbf{x}_1, s_1) \prod_{t=2}^{T} p(s_t \mid s_{t-1})p(\mathbf{x}_t \mid \mathbf{x}_{t-1}, s_t)p(\mathbf{y}_t \mid \mathbf{x}_t, s_t). \tag{2}$$

However, in problems such as physiological monitoring there are a large number

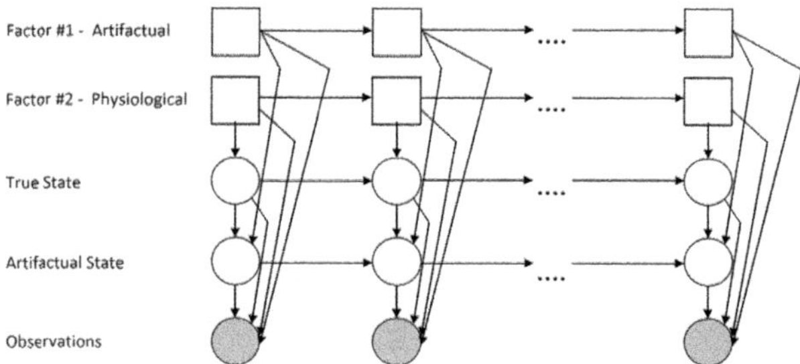

Fig. 1. The DAG of a FSLDS with 2 factors (one physiological and one artifactual). Each column represents a discrete time step. The state is divided into dimensions that approximate the "true" physiology and dimensions that approximate the artifactual patterns. Shaded variables are observed; circles represent continuous variables and squares represent discrete ones.

of factors influencing the dynamics of the system. The solution in [12] was to represent the switch variable as the cross product of M discrete factors, $s_t = f_t^{(1)} \otimes f_t^{(2)} \otimes ... \otimes f_t^{(M)}$. If the factors are assumed to be all a priori independent, the transition probabilities can be written as: $p(s_t \mid s_{t-1}) = \prod_{m=1}^{M} p(f_t^{(m)} \mid f_{t-1}^{(m)})$.

The FSLDS's structure (see Figure 1) allows valuable application-specific representational choices. For each of the measurement channels, there is precisely one visible dimension in the observation vector $\mathbf{y}_t$ at time t, and there are one or more hidden continuous dimensions in the state vector $\mathbf{x}_t$ at time t. The purpose is to increase the capability of the system to track the "true" physiological signals. Consequently, continuous hidden state dimensions can be associated either with true physiology or with artifact [12]. A similar rationale is applied to the discrete factors. However, artifactual factors can affect only artifactual states, while physiological factors can influence any state. In addition, the dynamics matrices, $\mathbf{A}(s_t)$, and dynamics noise matrices, $\mathbf{Q}(s_t)$, are chosen to have a "block diagonal" structure [12]. This is a great advantage, since the set of available observation channels usually varies from baby to baby based on the medical staff's prior beliefs about its physical condition.

Learning in the FSLDS model [10, §5] is facilitated by the fact that part of the regimes in the data are annotated by clinical experts. This means that when the hidden switch state is known, we can condition on it, making learning equivalent to training a simple Linear Dynamical System (LDS). Fortunately, there is no need to consider all possible switch settings because some factors overwrite the others [10,12]. We can also estimate the factor transition probabilities by simple data counting.

We now discuss learning the dynamics under the normal regime, which corresponds to the LDS obtained when all the other factors are off. This stage is called *calibration* and needs to be performed separately for each baby. It requires manually selecting a period of normal measurements on all channels. The parameters are obtained by independently fitting AR processes to each of these channels [12].

Exact inference is proved to be computationally intractable in many generalizations of the state-space model [6]. Among the approximate inference methods tested so far for the FSLDS, the Gaussian sum approximation [1,5,8] delivered the best performance and will be exclusively used below. The basic idea is to avoid the exponential growth in the number of terms needed at each time step by applying a moment matching approximation.

Clearly the FSLDS is one of many approaches to solving the problems of condition monitoring and artifact detection. A review of this related work is beyond the scope of the present paper, but can be found in [10, §3].

4 Automating Calibration

In order to automate the calibration stage, we rely on the following clinical considerations. The physiological patterns corresponding to normality are specific to each patient. On the other hand, physiological and artifactual factors like the ones introduced in Section 2 are stereotypical. This means that each occurrence of those events can be associated with a certain known pattern. In the following we describe our data, give a full problem formulation and then explain feature and classifier choices.

Exploratory Data Analysis: Our dataset consists of 24 hour recordings taken from each of fifteen premature born babies at Edinburgh Royal Infirmary. The babies were around 24 to 29 weeks gestation and aged 1 to 16 days post-partum. The data has been sampled at 1Hz and the set of measurement channels varies from baby to baby. Expert annotations are available for five known factors (Bradycardia, Blood Sample, Incubator Open, Core Temperature Probe Detachment and Transcutaneous Probe Recalibration) and for the X-factor. In addition, one period of Normal data is highlighted for each baby. These carefully chosen intervals have been used up to now to "manually" calibrate the FSLDS. As in [10,12], due to the scarcity of examples in the dataset we will not use the Transcutaneous Probe Recalibration factor in any of the following experiments.

Counting the number of incidences of each factor, we notice that factors such as opening the incubator and the X-factor are far more frequent than taking a blood sample or a detachment of the temperature probe. We also note that the mean durations of the various events are quite different as well. Although artifactual events always respect the same patterns, there is a great deal of variability in their duration (see [14]). The consequence is that the feature extraction task becomes more challenging.

We also know that a period for which there are no annotations is automatically considered a period of normality. Thus we can compute the total duration of normality in our data, which is 283 hours (79% of the total 360 hours). Note that this computation cannot be performed by summing up the total durations of the factors, since there is a significant overlap between factors.

Problem formulation: Since the objective is to extract some periods of normality from continuously recorded data, we begin by finding an appropriate length for these intervals. Based on the duration of annotated normality periods, we choose our intervals to have a length of 15 minutes (i.e. 900 seconds). For simplicity, no overlapping is permitted. A disadvantage of fixed length intervals is that we sometimes split a single event between intervals.

Examining our annotations, we have concluded that we can use at most four known factors (Bradycardia, Blood Sample, Incubator Open and Core Temperature Probe Detachment) to assess the performance of the FSLDS. Using the clinical information summarized in Section 2, we consider the union of all the channels that are influenced by the four factors of interest: HR, BS, BD, SO, TC, IH and IT. This set is the necessary and sufficient set of channels that need to be observed in order to set up a FSLDS capable to infer the discussed factors. Our original problem of finding an interval of normality by looking at all the available channels for a baby has just reduced to looking at all the channels enumerated above. Note that this does not imply that all the channels in the set above are present for all the babies. One may also notice that introducing an observation channel not influenced by any factor in the FSLDS will have no effect on inferences because of the block diagonal structure of $\mathbf{A}(s_t)$ and $\mathbf{Q}(s_t)$.

With all this in place, we explain the "channel-based" procedure we have chosen to use for classification. We break our classification problem into seven smaller classification problems, predicting normality/non-normality for each measurement channel. For these tasks, a new labelling of the data is required: If at least one of the factors has a non-empty intersection with the interval, it is labelled as being Non-Normal; otherwise it is labelled as Normal. Also note that when active, the Incubator Open and X-factor may not affect the whole set of factors they can influence, but only a subset of them. Thus, we decided to look at all available channels before making predictions for each channel.

Our reason for pursuing the "channel-based" approach is that it efficiently uses the limited amount of data on hand. An alternative "interval-based" approach making a single prediction regarding all the measurement channels would have been a poorer choice. The reason is that it is often the case that during a fifteen minute period, only a factor affecting a small subset of channels is active. This means that all the other channels are evolving normally during this period. In the "interval-based" approach this interval would have been labelled as Non-Normal, and we might have lost possibly valuable information about normality on the unaffected channels.

Feature extraction: Extracting good features is an essential requirement for success. This task is made difficult by the fact that periods of non-normailty can appear anywhere within a 15 minute interval, and that there is a significant amount of variability in the patterns of the known factors.

Normal heart rate (HR) measurements usually display a low amplitude, high frequency fluctuation around a slowly changing baseline. An event affecting this channel will generally result in a higher variance, so we chose the standard deviation as a feature. The baseline level of the heart rate signal is captured by the median feature. In order to detect bradycardia, we have chosen to record the difference between the minimum and average values of the observations. The most common event influencing blood pressure measurements (BS and BD) is taking a blood sample. The difference between the maximum and median values of these channels has been experimentally found to capture such variations. The oxygen saturation (SO) channel's dynamics can be recorded by computing the median and the difference between the median and the mean of the observations. Moving to the core temperature (TC) measurements, we are interested for these values to stay within some acceptable lower and upper limits. Thus we pick the minimum and maximum values of the channel as features. The standard deviation also offers valuable information about the baby's condition. When the incubator's doors are opened we usually see a drop in the humidity measurements (IH). Consequently, we keep track of the standard deviation of the channel and of the difference between the median and minimum values of the channel. A similar rationale is applied for the incubator temperature channel (IT).

Classifier setup: We now clarify the setting in which we have performed our experiments.

The classifiers employed for the task were logistic regression, Naïve Bayes and decision trees. These choices are mainly motivated by the simplicity, the easier interpretation of results and the reduced number of parameters associated with these classifiers. The optimization procedure used to get the maximum likelihood parameters for logistic regression is the Iterative Reweighted Least Squares Algorithm (IRLS) [2, §4.3.3]. Our Naïve Bayes implementation models each attribute's distribution as a Gaussian. The tree building algorithm we have employed is C4.5, which relies on the information gain criterion [9].

Considering the manner in which we have chosen our (baseline) set of features, dropout measurements may raise serious problems. However, as previously stated, they can be trivially detected. Since we clearly don't want to calibrate the FSLDS using an interval that contains dropouts, we will remove periods containing such artifact from the very beginning.

Moreover, there are babies for whom we do not have all seven channels on hand. Our solution was to always input as much information as possible into our classifiers. Theoretically, we make a Missing at Random (MAR) [7] assumption about the absent measurement channels. This means we had to train separate classifiers that work on feature sets with different dimensionalities (see [14]).

5 Results

Evaluation of the auto-calibration procedure is done in two phases. First, we assess the quality of the predictions produced by the classifiers. Second, we use these predictions in order to train the FSLDS, and then run inference in the model. The latter analysis is much more interesting since it allows a direct comparison between the manual and auto-calibrated systems.

In order to avoid over-fitting, all the experiments are performed in a 3-fold cross-validation setting. For each of the three tests, ten babies are used for training and the remaining five are left for testing.

The quality of our predictions is measured by two criteria. First, we draw Receiver Operating Characteristics (ROC) curves and compute the Area Under the ROC curve (AUC), noting that the larger the better. However, our primary objective is to extract some intervals of normality from the data. This means that we do not necessarily look for the most accurate classification between Normal and Non-Normal intervals; it is sufficient for the employed classifiers to deliver some intervals that we can confidently consider to be typical for the Normal dynamics of a baby and then utilize them to calibrate the FSLDS. This consideration motivates our second criterion. We will compare the classifiers based on how well they answer the following question: *"On a per baby basis, for how many positive instances (i.e. Normal intervals) does the classifier output a posterior probability of belonging to class Normal, $P(C = Normal \mid x)$, higher than the largest posterior of a negative instance (i.e. Non-Normal interval)?"*. We will call this criterion the Interval Ranking Criterion (IRC).

Using the baseline feature set described in the previous section, we now compare the performance of the three classifiers: logistic regression, Naïve Bayes and a decision tree. Since the features we are using display intrinsically different ranges and variances, we will standardize the input (i.e. zero mean, unit variance).

The results for the seven channel classification tasks are similar [14]. The general conclusion is that logistic regression always outperforms the other two methods on both criteria. A distinguishing observation about logistic regression is that it has always found, for each baby, at least one positive interval with higher posterior probability of being normal than any negative instance.

In other experiments, we have studied the Bayesian approach to logistic regression, and the introduction of other features like post-natal age, gestation or even LDS parameters trained on the 15 minute intervals [14]. None of those attempts managed to outperform the classifier consisting of the baseline feature set and maximum likelihood logistic regression. We emphasize that we do not need to fix a threshold in order to use any of the classifiers above in practice. Since we just need some Normal intervals for each observed channel, we simply sort the probabilities for all the intervals corresponding to a baby and pick the top k predictions.

As previously explained, we set up a FSLDS able to infer the posterior probability distribution for four hidden factors: Incubator Open, Bradycardia, Core Temperature Probe Detachment and Blood Sample. The quality of the inferences

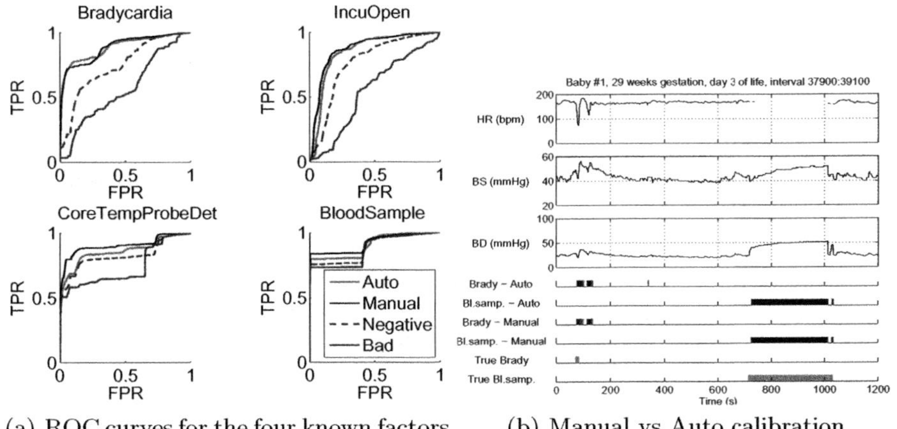

(a) ROC curves for the four known factors (b) Manual vs Auto calibration

Fig. 2. a) Classification results aggregated over the fifteen babies. b) Inferred distributions for Blood Sample and Bradycardia. For both methods, inference is correct. However, an inferred bradycardia instance around time $t = 125$ is in disagreement with the annotator's opinion.

will be assessed by the same two criteria as in [10,12]. The first one is the AUC already introduced in the previous section and the second one is the equal error rate (EER)[1]. Since the EER is an error, the smaller the value the better. For evaluation, we use the same setting as the one described in [12] and all the 360 hours of physiological monitoring data on hand[2]. The experiment is again done

[1] The EER is the error rate computed for the threshold value at which the false positive rate (FPR) is equal to the false negative rate (FNR).

[2] The experiments made use of John Quinn's code for the FSLDS [11].

with three-fold cross-validation: ten babies are used for training and the remaining five for testing. The auto-calibration system selects only the top prediction outputted by the classifier (i.e. $k = 1$). In Figure 2.a, we plot ROC curves aggergated over the fifteen babies corresponding to the four inferred factors for four methods of doing calibration: Auto, Manual[3] Negative and Bad. The last two are control conditions; in 'Negative' we randomly select a Non-Normal interval for calibration. In 'Bad' the we select a heavily corrupted interval for calibration. Table 1 shows that the quality of the inferences produced by the auto-calibrated

Table 1. Summary statistics for the two methods of calibration

Calibration	Statistic	Bradycardia	Incu Open	Core Temp Probe Det	Blood Sample
Auto	AUC	0.89	0.85	0.86	0.91
	EER	0.21	0.18	0.18	0.20
Manual	AUC	0.89	0.87	0.90	0.92
	EER	0.24	0.17	0.13	0.16
Negative	AUC	0.75	0.76	0.82	0.88
	EER	0.33	0.27	0.22	0.24
Bad	AUC	0.57	0.55	0.72	0.88
	EER	0.48	0.43	0.32	0.25

FSLDS is very close to the one of those produced by the manually calibrated version for three of the factors: Incubator Open, Core Temperature Probe Detachment and Blood Sample. For the remaining factor, Bradycardia, the AUC values are identical in both cases. Moreover, for this factor the auto-calibrated FSLDS manages to outperform the manual version in terms of EER. The performance deteriorates for the control conditions.

We also illustrate some comparative examples of inferences done with the manually- and auto-calibrated FSLDSs for physiological condition monitoring in Figure 2.b. The horizontal bars in the lower part of the figures indicate the posterior distributions of factors. Levels of grey from white to black indicate values from zero to one respectively. We observe that the two systems perform equally well at inferring Bradycardia and Blood Sample.

6 Discussion

In this paper we have introduced a classification-based approach to determining the normality/non-normality of intervals of monitoring data. Using carefully chosen features and a logistic regression classifier, we have demonstrated that the manual calibration stage used by the FSLDS for neonatal condition monitoring can be replaced by an automated procedure, with very little loss of performance. This reduction in the need for manual input (and consequent error) should be of great benefit in the clinical context.

[3] The results obtained with the manually-calibrated FSLDS are not identical to the ones in [12] due to using an updated version of both code and data annotations.

The work on auto-calibration can be extended in a number of directions. We can consider alternatives to the fixed-length no-overlapping constraint imposed on the intervals used for prediction. In terms of evaluation, we can use an event-based detection analysis, as opposed to the current second-by-second inference.

Acknowledgments. We thank John Quinn and the staff of the Simpson Centre for Reproductive Health, Royal Infirmary of Edinburgh for their assistance with this work. This work is supported in part by the IST Programme of the European Community, under the PASCAL2 Network of Excellence, IST-2007-216886. This publication only reflects the authors' views.

References

1. Alspach, D.L., Sorenson, H.W.: Nonlinear Bayesian Estimation Using Gaussian Sum Approximations. IEEE Transactions on Automatic Control 17(4), 439–448 (1972)
2. Bishop, C.M.: Pattern Recognition and Machine Learning. Springer, Heidelberg (2007)
3. Ghahramani, Z., Hinton, G.E.: Variational Learning for Switching State-Space Models. Neural Computation 12(4), 831–864 (2000)
4. Ghahramani, Z., Jordan, M.I.: Factorial Hidden Markov Models. Machine Learning 29, 245–273 (1997)
5. Kim, C.-J.: Dynamic Linear Models with Markov-Switching. J. Econometrics 60, 1–22 (1994)
6. Lerner, U., Parr, R.: Inference in hybrid networks: Theoretical limits and practical algorithms. In: UAI, pp. 310–318 (2001)
7. Little, R.J.A., Rubin, D.B.: Statistical analysis with missing data. Wiley, New York (1987)
8. Murphy, K.P.: Switching Kalman Filters. Technical report, U.C. Berkeley (1998)
9. Quinlan, J.R.: C4.5: Programs for Machine Learning. Morgan Kaufmann, San Mateo (1993)
10. Quinn, J.: Bayesian Condition Monitoring in Neonatal Intensive Care. PhD thesis, University of Edinburgh (2007), `http://hdl.handle.net/1842/2144`
11. Quinn, J.: Neonatal condition monitoring demonstration code (2008), `http://omnipresence.org/jq/software.html`
12. Quinn, J.A., Williams, C.K.I., McIntosh, N.: Factorial Switching Linear Dynamical Systems Applied to Physiological Condition Monitoring. IEEE Trans. Pattern Anal. Mach. Intell. 31(9), 1537–1551 (2009)
13. Shumway, R., Stoffer, D.: Dynamic linear models with switching. J. of the American Statistical Association 86, 763–769 (1991)
14. Stanculescu, I.: Auto-Calibration for Neonatal Condition Monitoring. Master's thesis, University of Edinburgh, School of Informatics (2010)
15. Williams, C.K.I., Quinn, J.A., McIntosh, N.: Factorial Switching Kalman Filters for Condition Monitoring in Neonatal Intensive Care. In: Weiss, Y., Schölkopf, B., Platt, J. (eds.) Advances in Neural Information Processing Systems, vol. 18. MIT Press, Cambridge (2006)

Mining Temporal Constraint Networks by Seed Knowledge Extension

M.R. Álvarez, P. Félix, and P. Cariñena

Centro de Investigación en Tecnoloxías da Información (CITIUS),
Universidade de Santiago de Compostela,
15782 Santiago de Compostela, Spain
miguel.rodriguez@usc.es

Abstract. This paper proposes an algorithm for discovering temporal patterns, represented in the Simple Temporal Problem (STP) formalism, that frequently occur in a set of temporal sequences. To focus the search, some initial knowledge can be provided as a seed pattern by a domain expert: the mining process will find those frequent temporal patterns consistent with the seed. The algorithm has been tested on a database of temporal events obtained from polysomnography tests in patients with Sleep Apnea-Hypopnea Syndrome (SAHS).

1 Introduction

Temporal data mining aims to discover interesting patterns in large collections of temporal data. The *Apriori* algorithm for sequence mining [1], based on the premise that if a sequence is frequent, all of its subsequences are also frequent, aims at finding frequent partial orderings of sets of events. Episodes providing information about event types frequently found together in the same temporal window, and episodes establishing a temporal order between events are obtained in [6,7]. Recent proposals try to enhance the representation of the temporal information by means of temporal patterns under the STP formalism[3]: a metric temporal constraint network between a set of events, where every constraint is an interval limiting the range of possible durations between two events; in [4] a unique STP is obtained among each set of events, even if they present different temporal arrangements corresponding to different patterns and interpretations. In [2] an algorithm that discriminates between patterns among the same set of events is proposed.

Some proposals consider using previous domain knowledge in the mining process: e.g. regular expressions to specify constraints [5]. The STP formalism seems a good choice for representing temporal knowledge, as it includes both qualitative and quantitative information. In this paper we present an algorithm for discovering frequent patterns from a set of data sequences, that are consistent with some initial knowledge expressed as STP patterns, which are extended and/or refined.

M. Peleg, N. Lavrač, and C. Combi (Eds.): AIME 2011, LNAI 6747, pp. 250–254, 2011.

2 Definitions

An **event type** E is a tuple $(o, a{=}v, T)$, being o an observable, a an attribute with value v, and T a temporal instant; $\mathcal{E}{=}\{E_1, ..., E_p\}$ is the set of event types provided by observation in a particular domain. An **event occurrence** $e_i{=}(o_i, v_i, t_i)$ of an event type $E_i{=}(o_i, v_i, T_i)$ is the result of observing v_i for o_i in $T_i{=}t_i$. For example, *(apnea,central,02:03:46)* represents the identification of the beginning of an *apnea*, being *(apnea,central,T)* its event type. Let $<$ be an order relation between event occurrences e_i and e_j such that $(e_i{<}e_j) \Leftrightarrow (t_i{<}t_j) \vee ((t_i{=}t_j) \wedge (o_i{<}o_j))$, assuming a lexicographical order between observable names; an **event sequence** is an ordered set $S{=}\{e_1, ..., e_m\}$, $e_i{<}e_j, \forall i{=}1, ..., m{-}1, i{<}j$. A **temporal window** of size ω in a sequence S is every subsequence $W{=}\{e_i, ..., e_k\}$ of S such that t_k-$t_i \leq \omega$, and $\forall t_j \in [t_i, t_k] \wedge\ e_j \in S \Rightarrow e_j \in W$.

A **temporal association** is an ordered set of event types $A{=}\{E_1, ..., E_n\}$ with event occurrences in the same window. Figure 1 shows two examples of the temporal association with event types A, B, C. Different temporal arrange-

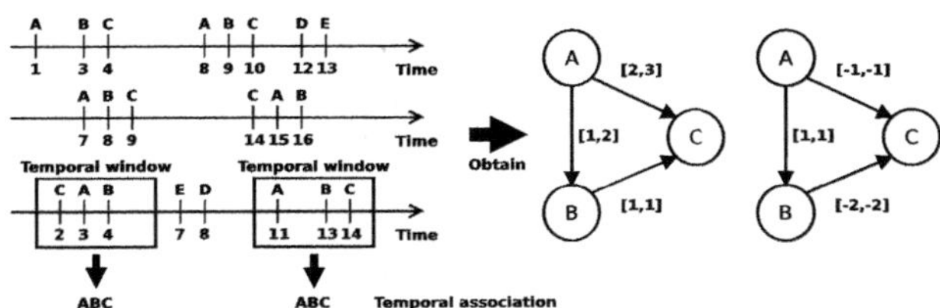

Fig. 1. Different occurrences of the same temporal association produce two frequent temporal patterns represented as STP

ments within temporal associations lead to different temporal patterns. A **temporal pattern** in STP formalism [3] is a directed graph $P{=}{<}D, \mathcal{L}{>}$ with $D{=}\{E_1, ..., E_n\} \subset \mathcal{E}$, $E_i{\neq}E_j, \forall i{\neq}j$, and $\mathcal{L}{=}\{L_{ij}; 1{\leq}i, j{\leq}n\}$ a set of temporal constraints between pairs of event types in D: $L_{ij}{=}[a_{ij}, b_{ij}]$, so that $a_{ij}{\leq}T_j$-$T_i{\leq}b_{ij}$, being $E_i{=}(o_i, v_i, T_i)$ and $E_j{=}(o_j, v_j, T_j)$. A **pattern occurrence** of pattern $P{=}{<}D, \mathcal{L}{>}$ is a subsequence $X{=}\{e_1, ..., e_n\}$ of $\mathcal{S}$ such that, $\forall i{=}1, ..., n$, e_i is an occurrence $E_i{\in}D$ satisfying all constraints in $\mathcal{L}$. Given two patterns $P{=}{<}D, \mathcal{L}{>}$ and $P'{=}{<}D', \mathcal{L}'{>}$, we say that P' is an **extension** of P, $P \preceq P'$, if $D{\subseteq}D'$ and $L'_{ij}{\subseteq}L_{ij}, \forall L_{ij}{\in}\mathcal{L}, L'_{ij}{\in}\mathcal{L}'$. A **seed-pattern** $F \preceq P$ is a STP pattern used as a starting point in the search procedure for pattern P: the user may indicate what event types are interesting and which initial constraints must apply between them. Given two temporal patterns $P{=}{<}D_p, \mathcal{L}_p{>}$ and $Q{=}{<}D_q, \mathcal{L}_q{>}$, their **combination**, $P \bowtie Q$, is a new pattern $R{=}{<}D_r, \mathcal{L}_r{>}$, where $D_r{=}D_p \cup D_q$ and constraints $\mathcal{L}_r = \{L^r_{ij} = L^p_{ij} \cap L^q_{ij} | L^p_{ij} \in \mathcal{L}_p, L^q_{ij} \in \mathcal{L}_q\}$. The **frequency** of a temporal pattern P in $\mathcal{S}$, $f(P)$, is defined as the number of occurrences of P in $\mathcal{S}$. The domain usually establishes the minimum frequency $f_{\min}$ that makes a pattern relevant: P is frequent if $f(P) \geq f_{\min}$. Figure 1 shows two frequent temporal patterns obtained with $f_{\min}{=}2$.

3 Algorithms

The PATTERN_SEARCH algorithm (Fig. 2(a)) extends the proposal in [2] allowing seed knowledge to be specified. The algorithm iteratively searches in collection of event sequences $\mathcal{S}$ for frequent STP patterns P, with frequency threshold $f_{\min}$, that extend a seed pattern F, and where events are, at most, ω time units apart.

The procedure INITIALIZATION (Fig. 2(b)) obtains all frequent patterns of size 2 consistent with F. Frequent event types in $\mathcal{S}$ are stored in P^1, and all temporal windows in $\mathcal{S}$ are checked for occurrences of F. For every pair j of event

```
procedure PATTERN_SEARCH(𝒮,ℰ,F,ω,f_min)
begin
  P² ← INITIALIZATION(𝒮,E,F,ω,f_min)
  i ← 3
  while (P^(i-1) ≠ ∅ ) do begin
    C^i ← CANDIDATE_GENERATION(A^(i-1),P^(i-1))
    P^i ← FREQUENCY_CALCULATION(C^i,ω,f_min)
    A^i ← {D_j | P^i_j=<D_j,L_j>∈P^i}
    i ← i+1
end;
```

```
procedure INITIALIZATION(𝒮,ℰ,F,ω,f_min)
begin
  A¹ ← {E_j | E_j ∈ ℰ∧ f(E_j)≥ f_min}
  P¹ ← A¹
  P² ← FREQUENCY_CALCULATION(F,ω,f_min)
  C² ← CANDIDATE_GENERATION(A¹,P¹)
  P² ← P² ∪ FREQUENCY_CALCULATION(C²,ω,f_min)
  A² ← {D_j | P²_j=<D_j,L_j>∈P²}
  return P²
end;
```

Fig. 2. (a) Main algorithm: Pattern search. (b) Initialization procedure.

types in F, the number of occurrences of each different temporal arrangement are included in a frequency distribution δF_j^2, that is subjected to a clustering procedure [8] in the FREQUENCY_CALCULATION procedure, merging similar arrangements and obtaining the set P^2. Those subsequences of $\mathcal{S}$ where no occurrence of F exists are removed, reducing the search space. Then the set C^2 of pattern candidates of size 2 is built from the frequent event types in P^1, using pairs of event types not extracted from F; frequency distributions δC_j^2 are built from the occurrences of every C_j^2 in $\mathcal{S}$, and after clustering new frequent patterns are added to P^2. An example of the impact of the seed pattern in clustering is shown in Fig. 3: by removing uninteresting temporal arrangements, the intervals inconsistent with the knowledge provided (negative axis) are ignored, and the clustering finds two intervals where only one was previously found. The procedure CANDIDATE_GENERATION in iteration i uses the frequent temporal associations and frequent patterns from step $i-1$ to build the candidate patterns of size i through combination. When $i=2$ the combination step

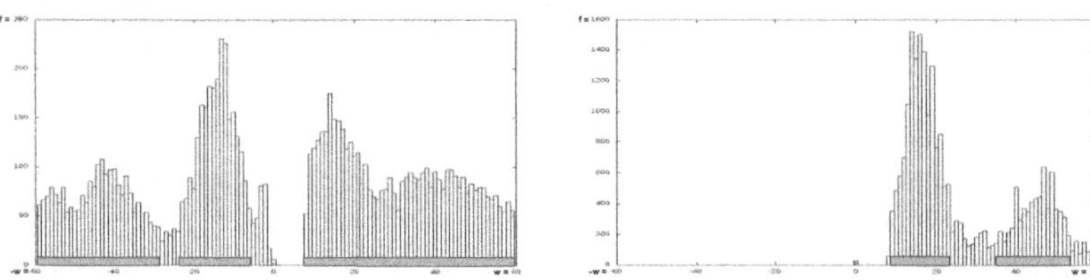

Fig. 3. Clustering of a frequency distribution: without (left) and with (right) seed F

is not performed, as candidates consist of temporal associations of size 2, and there are no known distinct temporal arrangements in the previous level. The FREQUENCY_CALCULATION procedure searches for occurrences of the candidates in all temporal windows in $\mathcal{S}$, providing frequent patterns according to $f_{\min}$.

4 Experimental Results

The data collection used[1] totals over 18000 events (with 8 different event types) and 34 hours of sleep, with sequences containing events in polysomnography tests of patients diagnosed with SAHS. Annotations made by the physician allow to validate the results of the search, verifying that patterns induced correspond to annotated patterns. In this domain, the most basic seed knowledge consists of the definition of episodes. For instance, an airflow limitation must start before it ends. The seed pattern used (Fig. 4) consists of the 8 event types on the records, 4 constraints representing 4 episodes as the previously described, and the implicit constraint that all events occur within the same window. The algorithm requires consistently less processing time than the version without seed, suggesting that the seed effectively helps to reduce the search space. As the window size w increases, so do the number of events and overlapping pattern occurrences in the window, rapidly increasing search time. Some apnea episodes can last 60s, specially in late hours of the night or in long-time SAHS patients, so a window might hold two or more occurrences of an episode. By introducing temporal constraints, seed patterns reduce the number of possible occurrences to those satisfying them, allowing to discard overlapping and reducing the cost. Table 1 shows results with w=80s and $f_{\min}$=30. Figure 4 shows one of the 2 patterns of size 8 found using the seed, corresponding to an apnea episode usual in patients

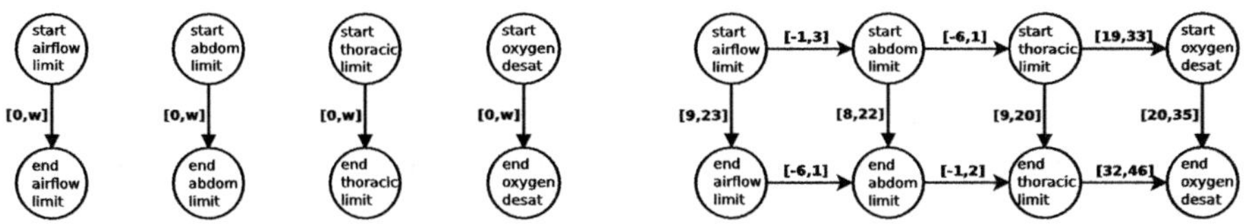

Fig. 4. Seed pattern (left) and pattern found using this seed (w=80s, $f_{\min}$=30)

Table 1. Possible combinations, candidates generated and frequent patterns found

Size	Combinations	Candidates	Freq. Patterns without Seed	Freq. Patterns with Seed
1	8	8	8	8
2	-	-	69	81
3	768	407	347	306
4	81543	737	684	434
5	$4'9 \cdot 10^6$	709	683	352
6	$1'1 \cdot 10^8$	385	379	167
7	$7'5 \cdot 10^8$	108	106	39
8	$8'1 \cdot 10^8$	12	12	2

[1] http://www.gsi.dec.usc.es/datacollections (Section: Apnea)

in an advanced stage of the disease or late in the night; in this case no new event types are added to the seed, but the constraints provided by the user are refined.

5 Conclusions and Future Work

A new Temporal Data Mining technique is proposed, where patterns found are represented with the STP formalism, that allows the user to specify a seed pattern consisting of several events of interest and some temporal constraints between them. This knowledge focuses the search to those patterns that extend the seed by incorporating new event types or by refining the constraints, and allows to prune it in two ways: ignoring those subsequences where no occurrence of the seed is found, and limiting the patterns found to those consistent with the seed, reducing the number of patterns while increasing their interest for the user. Results obtained with both synthetic and real data are promising. Our immediate goal is to evaluate our technique over a larger SAHS database, and over other different collections of temporal data.

Acknowledgments. This work was funded by the Spanish MICINN (TIN2009-14372-C03-03) and by the Xunta de Galicia (08SIN002206PR). M. R. Álvarez is funded by an FPU grant from the Spanish MEC (AP2008-02593).

References

1. Agrawal, R., Srikant, R.: Mining sequential patterns. In: Proc. 11th Int. Conf. on Data Engineering, pp. 3–14. IEEE Computer Society Press, Los Alamitos (1995)
2. Álvarez, M.R., Félix, P., Cariñena, P., Otero, A.: A data mining algorithm for inducing temporal constraint networks. In: Hüllermeier, E., Kruse, R., Hoffmann, F. (eds.) IPMU 2010. LNCS (LNAI), vol. 6178, pp. 300–309. Springer, Heidelberg (2010)
3. Dechter, R., Meiri, I., Pearl, J.: Temporal constraint networks. Artificial Intelligence 49, 61–95 (1991)
4. Dousson, C., Duong, T.: Discovering chronicles with numerical time constraints from alarm logs for monitoring dynamic systems. In: Proc. 16th IJCAI, pp. 620–626 (1999)
5. Garofalakis, M., Rastogi, R., Shim, K.: Spirit: Sequential pattern mining with regular expression constraints. In: Proc. 25th VLDB Conference, pp. 223–234 (1999)
6. Mannila, H., Toivonen, H., Verkamo, A.: Discovery of frequent episodes in event sequences. Data Mining and Knowledge Discovery 1(3), 259–289 (1997)
7. Pei, J., Han, J., Mortazavi-Asl, B., Wang, J., Pinto, H., Chen, Q., Dayal, U., Hsu, M.: Mining sequential patterns by pattern-growth: the prefixspan approach. IEEE Trans. on Knowledge and Data Engineering 16(11), 1424–1440 (2004)
8. Yager, R., Filev, D.: Approximate clustering via the mountain method. IEEE Trans. on Systems, Man and Cybernetics 24(4), 1279–1284 (1994)

A Rule-Based Method for Specifying and Querying Temporal Abstractions

Martin J. O'Connor, Genaro Hernandez, and Amar Das

Stanford Center for Biomedical Informatics Research
Stanford, CA 94305, U.S.A.
martin.oconnor@stanford.edu

Abstract. The Knowledge-Based Temporal Abstraction (KBTA) method is a well-established mechanism for representing and reasoning with temporal information. Implementations to date have been somewhat heavyweight, however, and custom tools are typically required to build abstraction knowledge and query the resulting abstractions. To address this shortcoming, we created a lightweight method that allows users to rapidly specify KBTA-based temporal knowledge and to immediately construct complex temporal queries with it. The approach is built on the Web Ontology Language (OWL), and its associated rule and query languages, SWRL and SQWRL. The method is reusable and can serve as the basis of a KBTA implementation in any OWL-based system.

1 Introduction

The Knowledge-Based Temporal Abstraction (KBTA; [1]) method provides a principled means for reasoning with temporal information in knowledge-based systems. It allows users to build a formal specification of a domain's temporal knowledge and the types of temporal inferences that can be made with it. There are variety of KBTA-based tools for the acquisition and querying of temporal information. A particular focus of tool development activity is to support querying and visualizing of temporal abstractions. Tools such as KNAVE and KNAVE II [2] allow users to express queries on temporal data and provide a rich set of visualization for displaying the results of those queries.

Despite the power of these tools, they suffer from query-related limitations. Generally, the set of temporal abstractions for an application is pre-specified, and the possible queries are restricted to them. Generating a query with a new abstraction requires the use of a separate acquisition module to describe it. The new abstraction must then be incorporated into the application. Furthermore, working with the acquisition module may also require specialist knowledge. Thus, new types of queries cannot be immediately generated and executed. As a result, current KBTA tools are not suited for generating *ad hoc* queries. This weakness is primarily a result of a disconnect between the way that knowledge in KBTA systems is specified and how it is queried. This situation, in turn, is a reflection of weak temporal querying support typically provided by ontology-based systems. Because of this poor support, queries require custom modules to implement temporal abstractions specified using the KBTA method.

M. Peleg, N. Lavrač, and C. Combi (Eds.): AIME 2011, LNAI 6747, pp. 255–259, 2011.

There is a need for a lightweight approach to representing and querying information specified using the KBTA method. This approach should support a seamless integration of the specification and querying steps in the KBTA method, so that abstractions can be defined interactively and executed immediately. In addition, it should be reusable and easily adaptable for use in new tools. This paper outlines such an approach. We used the Ontology Web Language (OWL; [3]) in association with the Semantic Web Rule Language (SWRL; [4]) and the SWRL-based OWL query language SQWRL [5] to provide lightweight yet expressive mechanisms to rapidly specify and query KBTA knowledge.

2 Background

The KBTA method provides a principled, knowledge-driven computational mechanism for performing temporal abstraction. This task involves taking raw time-stamped data and using domain knowledge to generate high-level summaries of the data. The KBTA method specifies a set of basic knowledge entities to describe temporal abstractions, and a set of inference mechanisms to generate abstractions.

There are five core conceptual entities specified by the method. Each one is associated with a subject in a particular domain. They are: (1) *Primitive parameters*, which represent raw measurable data; (2) *Events*, which model actions rather than measurable data; (3) *Contexts*, which represent an interpretation of a subject's state; (4) *Abstract Parameters*, which model information derived from primitive parameters or other abstract parameters; and (5) *Patterns*, which represent value and temporal constraints defined over parameters, events, and contexts.

These five entities are used by KBTA's inference mechanisms, which are: (1) *Temporal Context Formation*, which creates temporal contexts; (2) *Contemporaneous Abstraction*, which takes a parameter occurring at a point in time and generates a contemporaneous abstract parameter from it; (3) *Temporal Inference*, which provides several mechanisms for combining similar propositions occurring over different time intervals; (4) *Temporal Interpolation*, which provides a similar mechanism for combining similar propositions that may be temporally disjoint; (5) *Temporal Pattern Matching*, which creates intervals based on complex temporal patterns.

In general, KBTA implementations use an ontology language to represent knowledge entities, and inference mechanisms are encoded with external (often, rule-based) tools. A shortcoming of this approach is that knowledge specification and inference mechanisms are decoupled. Thus, dynamic specification of new temporal abstractions and queries is not generally possible. These shortcomings reflect the fact that the underlying ontology languages are not always sufficiently expressive to implement KBTA inference mechanisms. For example, the Frames-based ontology language used in RÉSUMÉ [6] systems did not have a general-purpose rule or query language. However, more recent description-logics-based languages such as OWL have rule-based extensions with strong formal underpinnings. In particular, SWRL and SQWRL can be used to express knowledge-level queries directly on OWL ontologies. These technologies can be used to implement a reusable, end-to-end, declarative implementation of the KBTA method.

3 Representing and Reasoning with Time in OWL

A variety of approaches have been proposed to represent temporal information in RDF and OWL [7]. The valid-time model predominates [8]. In it, a piece of information—often referred to as a *fact*—can be associated with instants or intervals denoting the times that the fact is held to be true. Facts have a value and one or more valid-times. Conceptually, this means that every fact is held to be true during the time(s) associated with it. Previously, we developed an OWL ontology to encode this model. The core fact class is represented by the OWL class `temporal:Fact`. This class is associated with the property `temporal:hasValidTimes`, which holds the time(s) during it is held to be true. A `temporal:ValidTime` class has subclasses `temporal:ValidInstant` and `temporal:ValidInterval` that represent its valid times.

We used SWRL's mechanism for creating user-defined methods to define a library implementing Allen's temporal operators [9]. When using these operators in conjunction with the temporal model, SWRL and SQWRL can express complex temporal criteria. For example, the following is a SQWRL query to select patients who took drugs for more than a week during the first three months of 2008:

```
Patient(?p) ^ hasTreatment(?p, ?t) ^ hasDrug(?t, ?d) ^
temporal:overlaps(?t, "2008-1", "2008-3") ^
temporal:duration(?d, ?t, temporal:weeks) ^ swrlb:greaterThan(?d, 1)
→ sqwrl:select(?p)
```

We extended SQWRL's collection and aggregation operators to incorporate the temporal model, thus permitting the expression of temporal queries with aggregate operations. For example, a query to return the first three Didanosine (DDI) treatments for each patient, together with dosage information, can be written:

```
Patient(?p) ^ hasTreatment(?p, ?tr) ^
hasDrug(?tr, DDI) ^ hasDose(?tr, ?dose) °
temporal:makeSet(?trs, ?tr) ^ temporal:groupBy(?trs, ?p) °
temporal:firstN(?f3tr, ?trs, 3) ^ temporal:equals(?f3tr, ?tr) →
sqwrl:select(?p, DDI, ?dose)
```

Here, treatments are inserted into a set (`?trs`) and grouped by patients (`?p`); `temporal:firstN` then selects the first three treatments from each grouped set.

4 Implementing the KBTA Method Using OWL and SWRL

We used SWRL's temporal model and operators to provide a completely declarative approach to defining and executing abstractions using the KBTA method. Our first step was to develop an OWL ontology representing the five core conceptual entities required by the method. The KBTA ontology defines four core classes. They are `kbta:Context`, `kbta:Event`, `kbta:PrimitiveParameter`, and `kbta:AbstractParameter`. They represent contexts, events and the two types of parameters. The ontology also defines the class `kbta:Subject`, which can be associated with these entities using the properties `kbta:hasContext`, `kbta:hasEvent`, and `kbta:hasParameter`. Primitive parameters are derived from the temporal ontology's `temporal:Fact` class, and thus can be associated with values and a temporal extent and manipulated by SWRL's temporal operators. The ontology also can also specify catenable, downward hereditary, and temporal interpolation characteristics for these parameters. Next, we developed an approach that uses SWRL and SQWRL to execute the five KBTA inference mechanisms.

Temporal Context Formation. This mechanism takes parameters, events, or contexts associated with a subject and generates a new context for them when specific criteria are met. These criteria can easily be expressed in SWRL. New contexts can be generated by defining a custom `kbta:makeContext` built-in. In its basic form, this built-in takes two parameters: the first is an unbound variable that will be bound during rule execution to the new generated context. The second is an existing parameter, context, or event from which the context will take its valid-time periods. The `kbta:makeContext` built-in also takes optional parameters to explicitly supply a new interval for the generated context so that new contexts can be temporally offset. For example, the following rule uses this built-in to generate a failing regimen context for a patient who has a mutation test with 24 weeks of the of a treatment regimen:

```
Patient(?p) ^ hasRegimen(?p, ?r) ^ hasMutation(?p, ?m) ^
temporal:contains(?r, ?m) ^ temporal:hasFinish(?r, ?fr) ^
temporal:duration(?d, ?m, ?fr, temporal:Weeks) ^
swrlb:lessThan(?d, 24) ^ kbta:makeContext(?c, ?r) →
FailingRegimen(?c) ^ hasFailingRegimen(?p, ?c)
```

Here, a patient is a subclass of `kbta:Subject;` `hasRegimen` and `hasMutation` are subproperties of `kbta:hasParameter`. They are associated with regimens and mutations, which are interval- and instant-based parameters. `FailingRegimen` is a context, and `hasFailingRegimen` is a sub-property of `kbta:hasContext`. If a patient meets the specified temporal criteria, the system generates a new context. It is classified as a failing regimen, and is associated with the patient.

Contemporaneous Abstraction. Like contexts, abstract parameters are generated from parameters, events, or contexts. We defined a built-in called `kbta:makeAbstraction` to generate new abstractions. It generates a new abstraction from an existing parameter, event or context. The following is a rule that uses it to generate a 'high' viral load abstraction for patients with a viral load greater than 2.0:

```
Patient(?p) ^ hasViralLoad(?p, ?v) hasViralValue(?v, ?vv) ^
swrlb:greaterThan(?vv, 2.0) ^
kbta:makeAbstraction(?a, ?v) →
ViralAbstraction(?a) ^ hasValue(?a, High) ^
hasViralAbstraction(?p, ?a)
```

Here, a viral load is a primitive parameter with an associated floating point viral load value; `ViralAbstraction` is an abstract parameter with `High` as a possible value.

Temporal Inference. The temporal inference mechanism requires combining facts with temporally adjacent or overlapping intervals, a process known as coalescing. SQWRL's collection operators have been extended to support coalescing. The operators have a native understanding of the KBTA ontology describing the facts placed in collections. Thus, catenable parameters, events, or contexts placed into a SQWRL collection are automatically coalesced. The following is an example query using this approach to find all patients with treatment durations longer than 2 months:

```
Patient(?p) ^ hasTreatment(?p, ?t) °
sqwrl:makeSet(?ts, ?t) ^ sqwrl:groupBy(?ts, ?p) °
temporal:duration(?d, ?ts, temporal:Months) ^ swrlb:greaterThan(?d, 2)
→ sqwrl:select(?p)
```

Here, SQWRL's set construction operator groups all treatments for each patient and coalesces adjacent or overlapping treatments with the same treatment values.

Temporal Interpolation. SQWRL's collection operators were also modified to consider the KBTA-described semantics of facts placed in collections. If facts in a collection meet minimal distance criteria, they can be combined.

Temporal Pattern Matching. As shown in previous examples, the SWRL temporal library can be used to meet the requirements of this mechanism. Combined with SQWRL collection operators' native understanding of the KBTA ontology, these operators allows the expression of essentially arbitrary temporal criteria.

5 Discussion

While current KBTA-based tools support robust querying and visualization of temporal data, the abstraction specification process is generally decoupled from the querying mechanism. Thus, specifying new temporal abstractions dynamically is not generally possible. This paper has outlined a method that integrates the specification and querying components of the KBTA method. The approach allows rapid specification and immediate execution of temporal abstractions. Our approach allows temporal queries be represented directly at the knowledge level, thus facilitating analysis that is much more rapid than is possible with other tools.

Acknowledgements. This research was supported in part by grant 1R01LM009607 from the National Library of Medicine.

References

1. Shahar, Y.: Context-Sensitive Temporal Abstraction of Clinical Data. In: Intelligent Data Analysis in Medicine and Pharmacology. Kluwer Academic Publishers, Boston (1997)
2. Klimov, D., Shahar, Y., Taieb-Maimon, M.: Intelligent visualization and exploration of time-oriented data of multiple patients. Artificial Intelligence in Medicine (2010)
3. OWL Web Ontology Language (2004), `http://www.w3.org/TR/owl-features`
4. SWRL Submission (2004), `http://www.w3.org/Submission/SWRL/`
5. O'Connor, M.J., Das, A.K.: SQWRL: a Query Language for OWL. OWL: Experiences and Directions. In: Fifth International Workshop, Chantilly, VA (2009)
6. Shahar, Y., Musen, M.A.: RÉSUMÉ: a Temporal-Abstraction System for Patient Monitoring. Computers and Biomedical Research 26, 255–273 (1993)
7. Frasincar, F., Milea, V., Kaymak, U.: tOWL: Integrating Time in OWL. In: Semantic Web Information Management: A Model-Based Perspective. Springer, Heidelberg (2010)
8. Snodgrass, R.T.: The TSQL2 Temporal Query Language. Kluwer, Boston (1995)
9. Allen, J.F.: Maintaining Knowledge about Temporal Intervals. Communications of the ACM 26(11), 832–843 (1983)

Web-Based Querying and Temporal Visualization of Longitudinal Clinical Data

Amanda Richards, Martin J. O'Connor, Susana Martins,
Michael Uehara-Bingen, Samson W. Tu, and Amar K. Das

Stanford Center for Biomedical Informatics Research
251 Campus Drive, X215, Stanford, CA, USA
{amandach,martin.oconnor,smartins,mub,swt,das}@stanford.edu

Abstract. We report on work in progress on the development of SWEETInfo (Semantic Web-Enabled Exploration of Temporal Information), a tool for querying and visualizing time-oriented clinical data. SWEETInfo is based on an open-source Web-based infrastructure that allows clinical investigators to import data and to perform operations on their temporal dimensions. The architecture combines Semantic Web standards, such as OWL and SWRL, with advanced Web development software, such as the Google Web Toolkit. User interaction with SWEETInfo creates OWL-based specifications of (1) data operations, such as filtering, grouping, and visualization, and (2) data pipelines for data analyses. Both of these can be shared with and adapted by other users via the Web. Our system meets the functional and nonfunctional specifications derived from the use cases. We will demo how SWEETInfoprovides non-technical users the ability to interactively define data pipelines for such complex temporal analyses.

Keywords: Temporal querying, data visualization, Semantic Web, ontologies, OWL, SWRL, intelligent data analysis, clinical research.

1 Introduction

Investigating thelongitudinal dimensions of patient data iscrucialin clinical research, and central to cohort identification, trend analysis, and outcomes studies. There have been a number of prior approaches for querying, abstracting and visualizing time-oriented data [1-3]; most of these methods are not directly accessible norreadily usable by the clinical research community. To address this need, we have developed a new approach called Semantic Web-Enabled Exploration of Temporal Information (or, SWEETInfo) that allows researchers to interactively import sets of patient data, view their temporal dimensions on a timeline, and perform a series of data transformations based on temporal and non-temporal criteria. Our Web-based application builds upon advances in extending Semantic Web technologies to support temporal representation, querying, and reasoning[4].

2 Design Requirements

Although the ontology-based approach to SWEETInfo is domain independent, we have designed the application to support the needs of clinical researchers. We have

M. Peleg, N. Lavrač, and C. Combi (Eds.): AIME 2011, LNAI 6747, pp. 260–264, 2011.

been particularly motivated by recent and ongoing collaborations with investigators in immune tolerance, HIV drug resistance and breast cancer.

2.1 Functional Specifications

Through our work with clinical investigators, we have identified that the functional specifications for data visualization and manipulationinclude the abilities to:

1. Visualize timeline graphs for individual patients
2. Create pipelines for data manipulation that include operators for filtering patients, grouping patients, creating variables and contexts, and slicing timeline graphs
3. Define criteria for these operators based on non-temporal, temporal, and aggregate conditions
4. View the result of operators by visualizing which patients met the criteria
5. Reuse criteria definitions across different operators and data analyses
6. Share datapipeline with collaborators

The nonfunctionalspecifications include having ready access to the tool and making the user interface simple for those who have little programming expertise.

2.2 Use Cases

The use case for a new user starts with creating a user accountat theSWEETInfo website (sweetinfo.org, to be released in summer 2011). A new user thendefines a new project and imports data for that project. Through a series of steps, the user connects to a relational database, specifies an ID (such as patient), and iteratively definesproject variables by selecting tables and columns in the database. In this data importation process, the user names the variables, determines whether the temporal information is instant or interval based, and associates the appropriate timestamp value(s) from the table. After variable definitions are completed, the user is presented with a *Database Node* and a *View Node* on a data pipeline on the screen.

The data visualization use case allows the user to click on a View Node to visualize the set of visual (patient) objects that are imported from the database or that are the result of an operation node. Figure 1 shows both *Browser View* (multiple visual objects) and *Timeline View* (single visual object) for a View Node. The Timeline View appears when the user clicks on a visual object in the Browser View.

The data operation use case permits the user to click on a View Node and define criteria for one of five operators: (1) Grouping, (2) Filter In/Out, (3) New Variable, (4) New Time Context, or (5) Change Visual Object. Each criterion is specified through one of four tab selections for value, function, timing, and duration based conditions (Figure 2). The user can create a set of constraintsto define an operator by combining thecriteria with logical conjunctions or disjunctions. The user names the constraint set, and can reuse that set of criteriawithin another operator or project. Once an operator is applied, the pipeline spawns a new *Operator Node* and a View Node from that which contains the set of visual (patient) objects that resulted from the operator. The View Node is empty if an operator (such as Filter In) does not return visual objects that met the constraints of the criteria. A user can apply multiple operators to a single View Node, in which case the pipeline will split into branches for each Operator Node. Figure 3 shows a pipeline at the SWEETInfo site that was created for an example data transformation in HIV drug resistance analysis.

3 Web-Based Implementation

We adopted a standard layered Web architecture to support the nonfunctional specifications of SWEETInfo, but had to make a number of customizations because we chose to incorporateSemantic Web technologies. Our implementation differs from most Web applications in that OWL ontologies are used to encode and maintain the application data. We created a custom data access layer to separate completely front-end and back-end components for reasons of performance and modularity.

3.1 Front-End Component

We used Google's GWTsystem with traditional HTML and CSS technologies to createthe front-end component. Because temporal visualization is central to SWEETInfo, the system requires the ability to generate highly detailed graphs. We also wanted full rendering control of the graphs so the user could modify them interactively. Current GWT graph libraries do not offer sufficient flexibility for these types of graphs, so we instead used a GWT mechanism to wrap a JavaScript graphics library called Dojo.

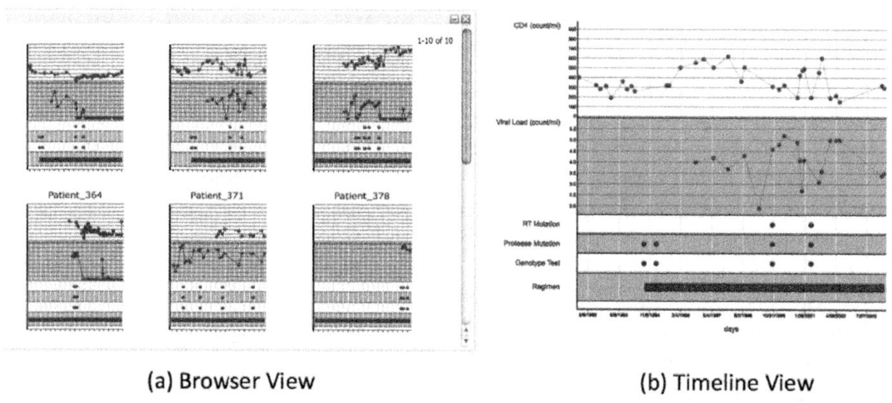

(a) Browser View (b) Timeline View

Fig. 1. (a) In the Browser View window, the user can view a set of patient data that were imported from the database or resulting from a data operation as a set of small graphs. (b) The user can select one graph and view it in more details in Timeline View.

In-browser generation of visual objects for Browser Viewcan becomputationally expensive. We developed an approach to quickly generate visual-object images in the back end. These graphs are fed to the front end as PNGs. When users select a graph for detailed inspection from the Browser View, a highly detailed graph is generated for the Timeline View using the Dojo-based wrapper.

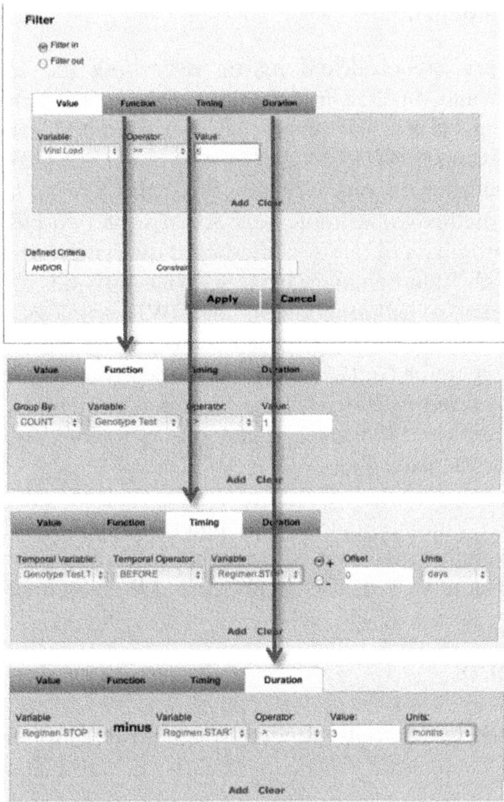

Fig. 2. The user can specify criterion for each of the five data operators (such as the shown Filter dialog box) by selecting among four tabs specifying value, function, timing, and duration conditions. The criterion can be combined logically as a constraint set, which the user names and is able to reuse in other data operators or projects.

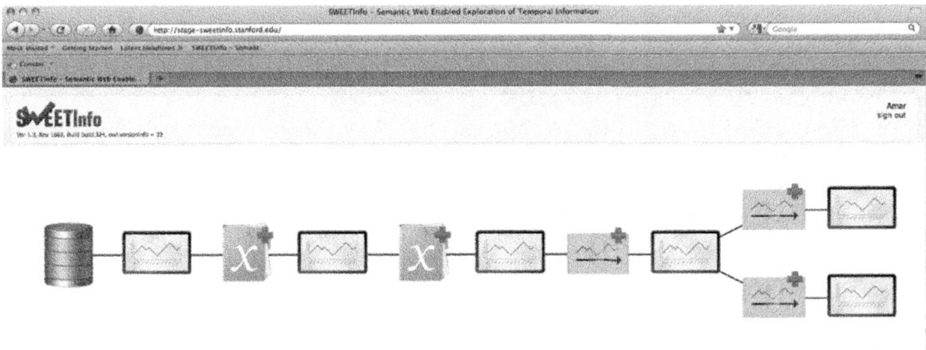

Fig. 3. The main SWEETInfo interface shows a data pipeline that connects a Database Node with subsequent View Nodes and Operator Nodes

3.2 Back-End Component

We chose to use OWLtoencodeand reason over both the application data (user, importation, project and pipeline information) and clinical research data within the back-end component. OWL, however, has very limited temporal operators for manipulating time values. SWRL, OWL's rule language,provides a small set for simple instant-based comparisons. We thus used the SWRL *built-in* mechanism to define a library of methods that implement Allen's interval-based operators [5]. We have created anotherbuilt-in library for rule-based querying called SQWRL (Semantic Query-Enhanced Web Rule Language) [5]. SQWRL provides a set of SQL-like query operators for retrieval of information in an OWL ontology. A Jess rule engine provides OWL, SWRL, and SQWRL-based reasoning within SWEETInfo. After the dialog box for the Operator Node is completed, the criteria specified by the user are saved in the ontology and executed by the back end component as SQWRL queries. The query results are passed to the graph generation module before being rendered by a new View Node on the front end.

Except for ongoing work on the data importation interface, the described components ofSWEETInfoareimplemented and currently functional on our staging site. We are now evaluating our tool with clinical researchers to assess the robustness, completeness and usability of the user interface and Web architecture design.

Acknowledgments

The project described was partially funded by grant R01LM009607from the National Institutes of Health.

References

1. Augusto, J.C.: Temporal reasoning for decision support in medicine. Artificial Intelligence in Medicine 33(1), 1–24 (2005)
2. Stacey, M., McGregor, C.: Temporal abstraction in intelligent clinical data analysis: A survey. Artificial Intelligence in Medicine 39(1), 1–24 (2007)
3. Wohlfart, E., Aigner, W., Bertone, A., Miksch, S.: Comparing information visualization tools focusing on the temporal dimensions. In: 12th International Conference on Information Visualisation, London, UK, pp. 69–74 (2008)
4. O'Connor, M.J., Das, A.K.: A Method for Representing and Querying Temporal Information in OWL. In: Fred, A., Filipe, J., Gamboa, H. (eds.) BIOSTEC 2010. CCIS, vol. 127, pp. 97–110. Springer, Heidelberg (2011)
5. Allen, J.F.: Maintaining Knowledge about Temporal Intervals. Communications of the ACM 26(11), 832–843 (1983)

Careflow Planning: From Time-Annotated Clinical Guidelines to Temporal Hierarchical Task Networks*

Arturo González-Ferrer[1], Annette ten Teije[2], Juan Fdez-Olivares[1], and Krystyna Milian[2]

[1] Department of Computer Science and AI, Universidad de Granada, Spain
[2] Department of Computer Science, Free University Amsterdam, The Netherlands

Abstract. Decision-making, care planning and adaptation of treatment are important aspects of the work of clinicians, that can clearly benefit from IT support. Clinical Practice Guidelines (CPG) languages provide formalisms for specifying knowledge related to such tasks, such as decision criteria and time-oriented aspects of the patient treatment. In these CPG languages, little research has been directed to efficiently deal with the integration of temporal and resource constraints, for the purpose of generating patient tailored treatment plans, i.e. care pathways. This paper presents an AI-based knowledge engineering methodology to develop, model, and operationalize care pathways, providing computer-aided support for the planning, visualization and execution of the patient treatment. This is achieved by translating time-annotated Asbru CPG's into temporal HTN planning domains. The proposed methodology is illustrated through a case study based on Hodgkin's disease.

1 Introduction

Care pathways are increasingly seen as a means to put Clinical Guidelines in practice by interdisciplinary teams; they help to reduce patient uncertainty and delays, to improve resource utilization and enhance efficiency savings, and to develop a family-centred care [12]. Specifically, the aim of care pathways is to model a timed process of patient-focused care, by specifying key events, clinical exams and assessments to produce the best prescribed outcomes, within the limits of the resources available, for an appropriate episode of care [1]. While these pathways were not traditionally embedded into IT-supported environments, the new trend is to code organizational arrangements into systems such as scheduling and workflow engines [16]. So, automated guideline-based generation of care pathways is clearly of interest in the clinical domain, but its resolution is not trivial, in particular when considering the existence of temporal constraints.

Indeed, the management of uncertainty and temporal issues is highly relevant in the CPG's domain [2], and some research goals were identified recently,

* Work partially supported by projects P08-TIC-3572 and TIN2008-06701-C03-02. We gratefully acknowledge the assistance and proof-reading by Frank van Harmelen.

M. Peleg, N. Lavrač, and C. Combi (Eds.): AIME 2011, LNAI 6747, pp. 265–275, 2011.

specifically for the treatment of temporal aspects [19]. Concretely, one of these goals is the identification of candidate actions for the care process, highly related to the automated generation of care pathways. Nonetheless, the research in AI has shown that the complexity of temporal inference is strictly related to the expressivity of temporal languages [19]. Specifically, both CPG languages and Planning & Scheduling (P&S) languages have been shown to be very expressive in terms of their temporal constraints representation [19,4], but they provide different capabilities. While CPG languages are very user-friendly for the guideline acquisition phase, one of the main shortcomings of the associated execution engines developed so far [11], is that they do not provide support for the generation of end-to-end tailored treatment plans. On the other hand, traditional P&S languages and techniques have shown their potential for representing and interpreting temporal information, allowing the automated generation of time-annotated plans, the adaptation to custom constraints and the allocation of resources to tasks [6].

Hence, on the basis of the existing similarities between some CPG's representational structure and the Hierarchical Task Network planning paradigm [5,4], we propose in this paper the translation of the knowledge present in a CPG into a corresponding temporal HTN planning domain. Thus, starting from an automated knowledge acquisition process where the CPG temporal information is analyzed and translated into the corresponding HTN domain, and followed by a knowledge-driven process based on P&S techniques, we can obtain a situated plan for the steps to be carried out for the patient's treatment. This way, we can automatically generate a care pathway that can later be deployed into any executable form (e.g. a workflow engine for plan visualization and execution), providing a cornerstone for the development of guideline-based careflow management systems [18].

The paper is structured as follows. Section 2 introduces the languages used and the methodology followed, section 3 describes the representation of temporal patterns in both languages, section 4 shows the rules used for the translation, section 5 shows some results and section 6 offers some conclusions.

2 Materials and Methods

In this section, a brief overview of the CIG and P&S languages used is given, as well as the life-cycle of the methodology presented.

CIG languages: Asbru. Different Computer Interpretable Guideline languages (CIG's) were developed in recent years, with the aim to manage multiple modeling aspects of guidelines [17,11]. Since the translation of temporal patterns is one of our main research aims, the methodology here presented is applied to Asbru[14], given its known capacity to model time-oriented aspects. Furthermore, Asbru follows a hierarchical decomposition of guidelines into networks of component tasks that unfold over time, known as Task Network Model (TNM), that is also followed by the target HTN planning language, described later. Fortunately, many of the existing CIG languages are TNM-based as well, so the methodology could easily be adapted to any other of these languages, since they share the organization of plan components, and they can express multiple arrangements of these components and interrelationships between them [17].

Asbru is an XML-based task-specific, time-oriented and intention-based plan representation language to embody CPG's and protocols as skeletal plans [13]. Each one of these skeletal plans consists of a *plan-body* that can be composed of either *subplans* (a set of steps performed in parallel or sequentially), *cyclical-plan* (repeated several times), *plan-activations* (a call to another plan) or a *user-performed* step (a specific action performed by the user). In addition, time-annotated conditions can be attached for the selection of plans, or the transition of a plan between multiple states. The tightly coupled control loop between the generation and execution of plans (i.e. continual planning [13]), makes Asbru very compelling for the management of CPGs, specifically in high-frequency domains. Even so, our aim is to support low-frequency domains, where the introduction of workflow capabilities could be highly interesting, in order to carry out the human-centered execution of long term care pathways. Also, note that what is relevant for this paper are the powerful knowledge representation capabilities of Asbru, not its execution engine.

Hierarchical Task Network planning: HPDL. The HPDL planning language (described in [4]) is an HTN [5] extension of the well-known planning language PDDL [7]. HTN planning specifications are separated into a planning *domain* (predicates, actions and tasks), designed as a hierarchy of tasks representing compound and atomic activities (see Figure 2), and a planning *problem* where objects, initial states and a set of goals are outlined. In such hierarchical domains, it is possible to describe how every compound task may be decomposed into different subtasks and the order that subtasks must follow, by using different *methods*. These methods include a precondition that must be satisfied by the world state in order for the method to be applicable by the planner.

HTN planning is known to be very useful in real-world applications. A recent study[2] described how different planning paradigms, including HTN, can provide support for the execution of CPG's. Actually, it has shown to be an enabling technology to support clinical decisions and processes in medical treatments[6].

The methodology presented in this paper can be observed in Figure 1. Specifically, we modeled in Asbru the Hodgkin disease guideline, where the goal of an

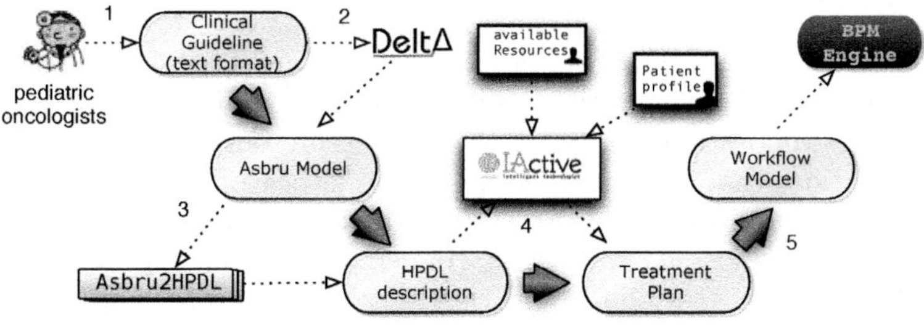

Fig. 1. Methodology life-cycle. Numbers 1-5 represent the multiple steps.

oncologist when planning a treatment, is mainly to schedule chemotherapy, radiotherapy and monitoring of a patient. Even so, Asbru guidelines are conceived to be directly executed, but they are not conceived to support the automated generation of patient-focused care pathways. For this reason, we translate the Asbru model into a corresponding HTN planning domain, enabling, by means of a knowledge-driven process, the automated generation of these care pathways. The pathways can then be deployed in the form of a *careflow*, thus offering an ubiquitous, user-friendly access (e.g. mobile or PDA-based) to a workflow engine, providing a communication channel for the care team. This facilitates the execution of every step in the pathway, checking, through customized triggers correctly embedded into the workflow engine, that the steps are carried out following the temporal patterns initially specified in the original guideline [8].

Note that Asbru models can be translated into HPDL domains because of the structural similarities between them: a) Asbru skeletal plans are equivalent to HPDL compound tasks or primitive actions, b) both share a hierarchical structure c) both are able to represent several different task ordering schemas, and d) both are powerful and expressive for the representation and interpretation of temporal constraints. The next section is devoted to the representation of such constraints, while the steps depicted in Figure 1 are analysed in section 5.

3 Analysis of Temporal Knowledge

The aim of this section is to show how to represent Asbru's temporal contraints with HPDL, in order to introduce the translation algorithm presented later in section 4. The representation with HPDL of Asbru's multiple task ordering schemas (parallel, sequential, unordered or any-order), commonly known as basic *workflow patterns* [15], has been already studied in [4], and also for the translation of business process models in [9]. Therefore, our analysis is focused specifically on time annotations, synchronization or delays among tasks and repetitive or cyclical temporal patterns.

Time annotations. Asbru time annotations are used to constrain the temporal occurrence of plan elements (including the plans themselves). A time annotation can include three time ranges, constraining start and end times and the duration of the interval. These constraints are defined as time shifts relative to a reference point, enabling to easily define them relative to an event not known at plan creation time (e.g. the start of a plan). The plan starts in a specific *starting interval* [ESS, LSS] and finishes in a *finishing interval* [EFS, LFS]. Furthermore, its duration has to be within the *duration interval* [minDur, maxDur].

Asbru time annotations can be equivalently represented with the HPDL temporal annotations that are described in [4]. In the case of HPDL, every primitive action (or task) a_i has two time points $start(a_i)$ and $end(a_i)$. Therefore, given a time-annotated Asbru skeletal plan T (remember that an Asbru model is compound of several skeletal plans, and that these skeletal plans are equivalent to HPDL tasks or actions), we can express it with an equivalent HPDL task or action T' by using special time-point variables `?start`, `?end` and `?duration`:

`[ESS,LSS]` for T can be expressed in HPDL with `(and (>= ?start ESS) (<= ?start LSS))`, `[EFS,LFS]` can be expressed as `(and (>= ?end EFS) (<= ?end LFS))`and, finally, `[minDur,maxDur]` as `(and (>= ?duration minDur)(<= ?duration maxDur))`.

A more complex issue is the management of the reference time points that can appear in an Asbru model: a fixed point in time, a reference to a plan activation, or a set of cyclical time points. We focus first on the last two.

Time-annotated reference to plan activation. This mechanism allows us to synchronize the timeline of skeletal plans. For example, to synchronize a plan B with the start of a plan A, B can refer to "A entering activated state", while synchronizing with the end of a plan A could be done with a reference to "A leaving complete state". Furthermore, a delay can be added with respect to the referenced plan. These are known as plan-pointers in Asbru, and they can be similarly represented by means of so-called *temporal landmarks*[4] in HPDL. These landmarks are asserted in the current state, and later on, they may be recovered and posted as deadlines to other tasks in order to synchronize two or more activities. This is done by means of *deductive inference tasks* of the form `(:inline <p><c>)`, fired when the expression <p> is satisfied by the current treatment state, providing additional bindings for variables or asserting/retracting literals into the planner's knowledge base, depending on the expression <c>. Figure 2(a) shows the definition of a compound task representing the parallel execution of four drug administration cycles. This task is executed sequentially two times, where the second is delayed 28 days since the start of the first one.

```
(:task CommonInit
 :parameters(?p - patient)
 (:method boys
  :precondition()
  :tasks(
    (CYCLE-OPPA ?p)
    ((and (>= ?start (cstart OPPA))
    (= ?duration (* 28 24)) ) (Delay OPPA))
    ((>= ?start (last-completed OPPA))
    (CYCLE-OPPA ?p))))
)
(:task CYCLE-OPPA
 :parameters(?p - patient)
 (:method only
  :precondition()
  :tasks(
    (:inline () (assign (cstart OPPA) ?start))
    [(GenericCycle ?p AdminVCR OPPA 1.5 0)
     (GenericCycle ?p AdminPRD OPPA 60 0)
     (GenericCycle ?p AdminPRC OPPA 100 0)
     (GenericCycle ?p AdminADR OPPA 40 0)
    ])))
```

(a)

```
(:task GenericCycle
 :parameters (?p-patient ?c-Ciclo ?cq-CicloQ ?dose ?N)
 (:method prepare
  :precondition (and (< ?N (NRep ?c ?cq))(not (started ?c ?cq))
                (fromStart ?c ?cq ?d)(bind ?N 0))
  :tasks  ((:inline () (assign (last_iter_end ?c) ?start))
           (:inline () (started ?c ?cq))
           (GenericCycle ?p ?c ?cq ?dose ?N))
  )
  (:method loop
   :precondition (and (started ?c ?cq) (< ?N (NRep ?c ?cq))
                 (RepDur ?c ?cq ?d)
                 (fromStart ?c ?cq ?d))
   :tasks((:inline (or
         (and (inBetween ?c ?cq 0)(bind ?K (NRep ?c ?cq)))
         (and (not (inBetween ?c ?cq 0))(bind ?K (+ ?N 1)))))())
         (GenericCycle ?p ?c ?cq ?dose ?K))
   )
   (:method stop
    :precondition (>= ?N (NRep ?c ?cq))
    :tasks ((:inline () (not (started ?c ?cq)))))
)
```

(b)

Fig. 2. (a) use of temporal landmarks and parallel execution of several cycles for drug administration, (b) outline of a recursive HPDL generic cyclical task

Cyclical time annotations. Besides temporal annotations, Asbru also has specific temporal semantics for cyclical plans, called *cyclical time annotations.* The difference with the former is a more complex specification for the reference time point consisting of a *time point*, an *offset* and a *frequency*. Also, a *times-completed* condition can be specified in order to determine the number of repetitions for the plan. We explain next how to represent cyclical tasks with

HPDL (see Figure 2(b)). To that end, we have used a high-level formalism, developed by Anselma et. al [3]. Concretely, this formalism shares some similarities with Asbru cyclical time annotations and it can be represented in HPDL as well. The following primitives are considered at the moment:

1. **fromStart**(min, max). Represents a delay between the start of the timespan where actions are to be included and the beginning of the first repetition. It is similar to Asbru's `<offset>`. In HPDL we add a predicate `(fromStart ?t ?c ?o)`, encoding that task *t* has offset *o* with respect to the start of cycle *c*.
2. **inBetween**(min, max). Represents a delay between the end of each repetition and the start of the next one. It is similar to Asbru's `<frequency>` element. In HPDL we can add a predicate `(inBetween ?t ?c ?f)`, encoding that task *t* has a repetition frequency of *f*, within cycle *c*.
3. **NRep**. Represents the number of repetitions to be carried out. It is similar to Asbru's `<times-completed>` element. In HPDL we can add a function `(NRep ?t ?c)`, encoding that task *t* repeats *n* times, within cycle *c*.
4. **RepDur**. Represents the time that each repetition takes. It is similar to Asbru's `<duration>` element. In HPDL we can add a predicate `(RepDur ?t ?c ?lt)`, encoding that task *t* within cycle *c* has a duration *lt*.

These HPDL predicates and functions are used in order to represent cyclical plans, by using them in the definition of a cyclical task (see Figure 2(b)), that is instantiated with initial state values, as explained in the next section. Thus, we have shown that main Asbru time annotations can be modelled in HPDL.

4 Mapping Asbru to HPDL

This section shows that the Asbru time modeling constructs have a counterpart HTN representation, supported by the Anselma et. al formalism [3]. We describe a knowledge engineering method to extract a corresponding HTN domain from a typical CPG, using a specific subset of the Asbru language:

Objects and Types. The data model of both languages is very similar. While HPDL types are arranged as a hierarchy where "object" is the upper node, and described in a section called `''(:types"`, Asbru types are defined by means of the element `scale-def`. Thus, we translate every qualitative `scale-def` as an HPDL type, so that each of its `qualitative-entry`'s is declared as a constant in the domain and a corresponding object of that type in the problem.

Skeletal plans. For every Asbru "plan", starting in the root node and traversing the Asbru domain definition hierarchically, use the plan name for the definition of a corresponding HPDL compound task (if it contains plan activations) or durative action (if it is a leaf node, usually "user-performed") in the planning domain. If the plan has any "argument" in its definition, translate it as a HPDL task parameter (e.g. "?d - drug"). In addition, apply the next rules:

1. If the "plan-body" is composed of "subplans" of type *"sequentially"* and it is a sequence of "plan-activations", translate them as a sequence of tasks calls, by enclosing them with `( )`.
2. If it is composed of "subplans" of type *"parallel"*, translate them as a parallel execution of tasks calls, by enclosing them with `[ ]`.
3. If it is composed of an "if-then-else" block, where an argument is evaluated and different plan-activations are carried out for every argument value, this will be translated as several HPDL *task methods*, where every method precondition is the one defined on every "if" statement, and the method body is a call to the corresponding HPDL task (the "plan-schema" activated).

Time annotations in plan activations. When a plan activation is time-annotated, using a reference to a plan-pointer as explained previously, we can express the shifts regarding the pointed plan by using a Delay task in HPDL. For example, every earliest starting-shift can be translated as a Delay from the reference-point specified (the start or end of another skeletal plan) (Figure 3). Thus, if the "instance-type" attribute is 'last' and "state" is 'completed', we will add to the HPDL task referenced by the plan-pointer a temporal landmark (e.g.`(assign (last-completed ?planname) ?end)`). Similarly, if "state" is 'activated', we can define a temporal landmark (e.g. `(assign (last-start ?planname) ?start)`). These landmarks are used in the definition of the Delay task used (Figure 3).

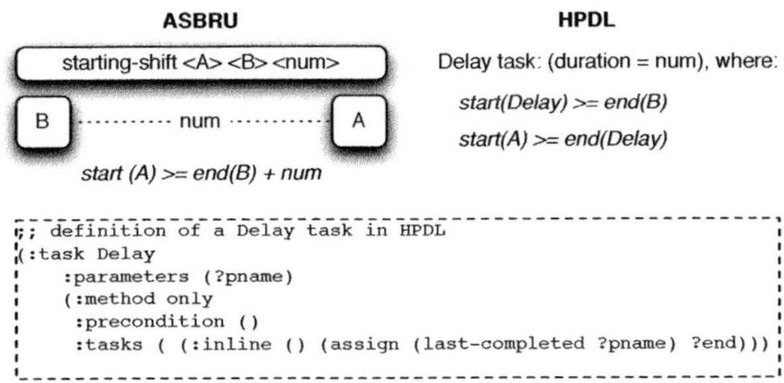

Fig. 3. Expressing delays in Asbru and HPDL

Cyclical Plans. Finally, when a plan is defined with a "cyclical-plan-body", we considered that it is declared with at least some arguments: *freq, nrep, fromstart, mindur, maxdur, partof.* Furthermore, we include *drug* and *dose*, since they are described in the Hodgkin CPG. Thus, on the one hand, the cyclical plan can be translated as a HPDL task similar to the one declared in Figure 2(b). On the other hand, we extract several predicate instances (following the temporal formalism explained in the previous section) from these arguments values found in every call to the cyclical plan, so that those instances are serialized into the HTN problem definition, and used correspondingly in the definition of the HPDL cyclical task (see Figure 2(b)). For example, we will extract the predicate (NRep Prednisona OPPA 15), from a call where *nrep*=15, *drug*=prednisona and *partof*=OPPA, in order to express that the drug is administered 15 times within the chemotherapy cycle named OPPA.

5 Results

In order to show the contribution of our method, we carried out the multiple steps of the life-cycle shown in Figure 1 for the Hodgkin protocol. A schema of the treatment workflow process indicated in such protocol, as well as the temporal patterns to administrate every chemotherapy cycle are outlined in [6].

So, looking at Figure 1, the clinical guideline is firstly described in natural language (70 pages of text) starting from the oncologist's experience (1). Then, it is modeled with DELT/A (the Document Exploration and Linking Tool), obtaining an XML-based Asbru model of the CPG (2). Afterwards, a translation to HPDL is necessary (3). We developed a Java tool to that end named Asbru2HPDL (available at `http://gitorious.org/asbru2hpdl`), that carries out two basic steps: (a) the acquisition of the knowledge present in the Asbru CPG by parsing it into a memory structure (a set of java classes), (b) the serialization of this memory structure into an HPDL domain and problem (section 4 is devoted to describe this step). Following with the life-cycle, the IACTIVE planner[1] takes the HPDL domain and problem as input and generates a tailored care pathway for the patient (4). This plan can either be visualized as a Gantt diagram or translated into a workflow instance that can be executed in a BPM engine (5), ideal for environments where doctors have to carry out the treatment in a collaborative way. This last step can be done in order to provide an execution model of the plan, given that the planner does not include yet an embedded execution and monitoring engine. This is being developed at the moment of writing this paper.

Thus, we obtain a planning domain which includes a high-level task goal, subsequently decomposed by the planner following the strategy and temporal constraints declared in the HTN domain, previously translated from the original CPG. Even so, the workflow specified in an oncology treatment protocol does not include details related to which human and material resources are involved in the therapy planning process, so it is necessary to represent and manage them in order to truly support clinical processes and decisions within a specific institution. Fortunately, capacity and availability dates of discrete resources may be represented in HPDL, using a generalization of timed initial literals [4]. Thus, we add to this domain: a) an initial state representing information that describes the patient profile (e.g. (sex Alice M), (group Alice Group3)), and b) resource constraints, mainly related to the oncologists' availability schedule (e.g. (between "08/11/2010 00:00:00" and "09/11/2010 00:00:00" (available John))). Having this information, the planner can find a solution for the problem of obtaining a plan tailored to a patient profile, while respecting the available resources [6].

[1] It has already been used to automatically generate oncology treatment plans [6].

Although we tried to obtain a treatment plan using directly the only freely available Asbru interpreter, we found several problems. The interpreter is prepared to run in high-frequency domains where a set of time-annotated input parameters have to be injected into the engine, and several extra conditions (mainly filter and complete-conditions) have to be attached for every skeletal plan for it to run correctly. Even so, the resulting care plan cannot be restricted to available resources, its visualization is very unfriendly for the doctors, and so inappropriate for the goal we pursue: to offer IT support in order to improve the current manual planning stage of the care process.

Consequently, we have used Asbru in order to obtain an intermediate computational representation of the CPG, something very useful for our approach, given the difficulty of directly using traditional P&S languages for modeling a CPG. So, once the Asbru representation of the guideline is translated into an HTN planning domain, and later interpreted by the planner, we obtain the sequencing of the clinical tasks, tailored to patient and available resources. We can observe next the contribution of our methodology applied to our case study, obtaining a personalized patient careflow where the decisions about the treatment are automatically carried out: i) supporting on the CPG control-flow information and the patient profile, ii) respecting the temporal patterns for drug administration, and iii) allocating the resources on the basis of their availability schedule. The output of the planner is similar to the following fragment, for the treatment of patient *Alice*, showing the following information: start and end dates of step, duration of drug administration, iteration, the oncologist in charge (Paul or John), the drug administered, the patient, and the dose.

```
...
22/11/2007; 22/11/2007; Duration:1.0; It14 John AdminPRD; Alice gets dose: 60.0
08/11/2007; 23/11/2007; Duration:360.0; It0 John AdminPRC; Alice gets dose: 100.0
08/11/2007; 09/11/2007; Duration:24.0; It0 John AdminADR; Alice gets dose: 40.0
22/11/2007; 23/11/2007; Duration:24.0; It1 Paul AdminADR; Alice gets dose: 40.0
06/12/2007; 07/12/2007; Duration:24.0; It0 Paul AdminVCR; Alice gets dose: 1.5
...
```

A more user-friendly visualization of the plan can be found online at `http://tratamientos.iactive.es` (just select a profile, e.g. "Maria Casares", a start date, then click the button "Generar Plan", to obtain the plan as a Gantt diagram). The optional translation into a workflow model was described in [8].

Note also that our methodology could be extrapolated to other clinical protocols, since we have shown how to deal with the patterns usually managed in CPG's, i.e. multiple task ordering schemas, delays, synchronizations and cycles. Moreover, it could be adapted to use a different CPG language. Undoubtedly, formalizing the guideline (step 2) will remain a difficult task, since it was manually done, but the protocol we modeled was very well structured and the decisions to be taken on each profile were accurately described in the guideline text, so it was straightforward to use the DELT/A tool for its formalization. Nonetheless, several knowledge acquisition tools were developed to help with this task (e.g. *DeGeL* [10]) that could be integrated in the methodology to facilitate this step.

6 Conclusions

We presented in this paper an AI-based knowledge engineering methodology to develop, model, and operationalize care pathways, thus providing an evidence-based Decision Support System for oncology treatments, and illustrating it with Hodgkin's disease. This is carried out starting from the medical knowledge existing in a previously defined CPG, represented in Asbru. Thus, by means of a translation into an HTN planning domain, and through deliberative reasoning, we achieved a solution for the sequencing and scheduling of the tasks involved in the specific protocol, developing a patient-focused computerized care pathway that respects the patient profile, the available resources and the protocol temporal patterns. As future work, we want to test our framework with a real use case in the hospital (i.e. extracting and integrating the patient profile directly from his/her electronic health record) since the oncologists that participate in the *Oncotheraper* project [6] have validated our results. Further tests with a different disease protocol could be also carried out, in order to check the portability of our method.

References

1. Alexandrou, D., Skitsas, I., Mentzas, G.: A holistic environment for the design and execution of self-adaptive clinical pathways. IEEE Trans. Inf. Technol. Biomed. 15(1), 108–118 (2011)
2. Anselma, L., Montani, S.: Planning: supporting and optimizing clinical guidelines execution. In: Computer-based Medical Guidelines and Protocols: a Primer and Current Trends, pp. 101–120. IOS Press, Amsterdam (2008)
3. Anselma, L., Terenziani, P., Montani, S., Bottrighi, A.: Towards a comprehensive treatment of repetitions, periodicity and temporal constraints in clinical guidelines. Artificial Intelligence in Medicine 38(2), 171–195 (2006)
4. Castillo, L., Fdez-Olivares, J., García-Pérez, Ó., Palao, F.: Efficiently handling temporal knowledge in an HTN planner. In: 16th ICAPS, pp. 63–72 (2006)
5. Erol, K., Hendler, J., Nau, D.S.: HTN planning: Complexity and expressivity. In: 20th AAAI Conference, pp. 1123–1128. AAAI Press, Menlo Park (1994)
6. Fdez-Olivares, J., Castillo, L., Cózar, J., García Pérez, O.: Supporting clinical processes and decisions by hierarchical planning and scheduling. Computational Intelligence 27(1), 103–122 (2011)
7. Fox, M., Long, D.: PDDL2.1: an extension to PDDL for expressing temporal planning domains. Artificial Intelligence Research 20(1), 61–124 (2003)
8. González-Ferrer, A., Fdez-Olivares, J., Sánchez-Garzón, I., Castillo, L.: Smart Process Management: Automated Generation of Adaptive Cases based on Intelligent Planning Technologies. In: 8th BPM (Demonstration Track), pp. 28–33 (2010)
9. González-Ferrer, A., Fdez-Olivares, J., Castillo, L.: From business process models to hierarchical task network planning domains. Knowl. Eng. Rev. (accepted, 2011)
10. Hatsek, A., Young, O., Shalom, E., Shahar, Y.: DeGeL: a clinical-guidelines library and automated guideline-support tools. In: Computer-Based Medical Guidelines and Protocols: A Primer and Current Trends, pp. 203–212 (2008)
11. Isern, D., Moreno, A.: Computer-based execution of clinical guidelines: a review. International Journal of Medical Informatics 77(12), 787–808 (2008)

12. Kelsey, S.: Managing patient care: are pathways working? Practice Development in Health Care 4(1), 50–55 (2005)
13. Miksch, S., Seyfang, A.: Continual Planning with Time-Oriented, Skeletal Plans. In: Proceedings of ECAI (2000)
14. Miksch, S., Shahar, Y., Johnson, P.: Asbru: a task-specific, intention-based, and time-oriented language for representing skeletal plans. In: 7th Workshop on Knowledge Engineering: Methods & Languages, pp. 1–25 (1997)
15. Mulyar, N., van der Aalst, W., Peleg, M.: A pattern-based analysis of Clinical Computer-interpretable Guideline modeling languages. J. Am. Med. Inform. Assoc. 14(6), 781–787 (2007)
16. Panella, M., Vanhaecht, K., Sermeus, W.: Care pathways: from clinical pathways to care innovation. International Journal of Care Pathways 13(2), 40–50 (2009)
17. Peleg, M., Tu, S., Bury, J., Ciccarese, P., Fox, J., Greenes, R.A., Hall, R., Johnson, P.D., Jones, N., Kumar, A., Miksch, S., Quaglini, S., Seyfang, A., Shortliffe, E.H., Stefanelli, M.: Comparing computer-interpretable guideline models: A case-study approach. J. Am. Med. Inform. Assoc. 10(1), 52–68 (2003)
18. Quaglini, S., Stefanelli, M., Cavallini, A., Micieli, G., Fassino, C., Mossa, C.: Guideline-based careflow systems. Artif. Intell. Med. 20(1), 5–22 (2000)
19. Terenziani, P., German, E., Shahar, Y.: The temporal aspects of clinical guidelines. Studies In Health Technology And Informatics 139, 81–100 (2008)

An Archetype-Based Solution for the Interoperability of Computerised Guidelines and Electronic Health Records

Mar Marcos[1,⋆], Jose A. Maldonado[2,⋆⋆], Begoña Martínez-Salvador[1], David Moner[2], Diego Boscá[2], and Montserrat Robles[2]

[1] Universitat Jaume I, Castellón, Spain
[2] ITACA Institute, Universidad Politécnica de Valencia, Spain

Abstract. Clinical guidelines contain recommendations based on the best empirical evidence available at the moment. There is a wide consensus about the benefits of guidelines and about the fact that they should be deployed through clinical information systems, making them available during consultation time. However, one of the main obstacles to this integration is still the interaction with the electronic health record. In this paper we present an archetype-based approach to solve the interoperability problems of guideline systems, as well as to enable guideline sharing. We also describe the knowledge requirements for the development of archetype-enabled guideline systems, and then focus on the development of appropriate guideline archetypes and on the connection of these archetypes to the target electronic health record.

1 Introduction

Clinical guidelines contain recommendations about different aspects of clinical practice in relation to a specific clinical condition. These recommendations are based on the best empirical evidence available at the moment. For this reason, the use of guidelines has been promoted as a means to control variations in care, reduce inappropriate interventions and deliver more cost-effective care, among other things. Despite some discrepancies, there is a wide consensus on the benefits of guidelines. There is also consensus about the fact that guidelines should be deployed through clinical information systems, and that they should be made available to medical professionals during consultation time [1]. Current guideline systems include reminder systems as well as increasingly more complex systems representing significant parts of guideline procedural knowledge. Whatever is the case, there must be some interaction with the clinical information system in

⋆ This research has been supported by Universitat Jaume I through project P11B2009-38, and by the Spanish Ministry of Education through grant PR2010-0279.

⋆⋆ This research has been supported by the Spanish Ministry of Science and Innovation under Grant TIN2010-21388-C02-01, and by the Health Institute Carlos III through the RETICS Combiomed, RD07/0067/2001.

M. Peleg, N. Lavrač, and C. Combi (Eds.): AIME 2011, LNAI 6747, pp. 276–285, 2011.

general, and with the electronic health record (EHR) in particular, to obtain all the necessary information.

Over the last decade, clinical guidelines have been one focus of research in the areas of Artificial Intelligence and Medical Informatics. Significant contributions in these areas include a variety of languages for the representation of guidelines (see [2], [3] for a review). Recently the focus of attention is shifting from the representation of guidelines to the integration of guideline systems in realistic healthcare settings [4]. Despite these efforts, the interaction with the EHR remains as one of the main obstacles for the interoperability of guideline systems within clinical information systems [5]. An important problem is the lack of standardisation as regards data. There have been several initiatives, involving standardization bodies, to define a generic EHR architecture for the communication of health data. However, its use is not directly supported in the current guideline representation languages.

One of the main contributions of recent EHR architectures is the dual model methodology [6] for the description of the structure and semantics of health data. The dual model methodology distinguishes a reference model and archetypes. A reference model is represented by a stable and small object-oriented model that describes the generic and stable properties of health record information (such as folder, document, section, and audit). The generality of the reference model is complemented by the particularity of archetypes. Archetypes are detailed, reusable and domain-specific definitions of clinical concepts (such as Apgar score, discharge report, and primary care EHR) in the form of structured and constrained combinations of the entities of the reference model. Their principal purpose is to provide a powerful way of managing the description, creation, validation and querying of EHRs. From a data point of view, archetypes are a means for providing structural and terminology-based semantics to data instances that conform to some reference model.

In a previous paper we propose the utilisation of openEHR archetypes in the framework of guideline representation languages [7]. We view computerised guidelines (CGs) as objects with archetype-enabled fragments in specific points where interactions should occur, e.g. patient data queries and/or physician order generation. In this paper we take a further step and present an archetype-based approach to make the interoperability of CGs and EHRs possible. We also describe the knowledge requirements for the development of archetype-enabled CGs, and then focus on the development of a set of CG archetypes and on the connection of these archetypes to the EHR. The latter steps are illustrated with examples from a guideline for chronic heart failure.

2 Approach

We are concerned with the use of archetypes (openEHR or other) within CGs as a mechanism for the interaction with the EHR, and also as a way to make possible the shared use of CGs. In our view, shared use (and reuse) of CGs is a crucial issue because guideline recommendations are valid in a more or less wide scope (national or international) which implies that usually they have to be implemented in different healthcare institutions, possibly with some adaptations. Our interest in reuse is not limited to CG procedures but also covers the models of relevant clinical concepts in the CG.

We are also concerned with technical solutions to implement this approach. Technical implementation requires a platform for the access to the EHR data via archetypes, in the likely case the EHR system does not support archetypes natively. Additionally, a software for the execution of CGs (CG engine) supporting the use of archetypes is required. For the former, we plan to use the data integration engine of the LinkEHR Normalization Platform [8] (see section 4 for more details). With respect to the CG engine, the programming work to adapt an existing engine so that it supports data access via archetypes is underway.

In addition, the view of archetype-enabled CGs has several requirements as regards knowledge modelling:

1. it is necessary to design a collection of archetypes suitable for the decision tasks carried out in the guideline.
2. it is necessary to ensure that the guideline model (CG) is compliant with these archetypes.
3. it must be ensured that the connection with the target EHR (or clinical databases) via the designed archetypes is feasible.

With respect to (1.), to increase the chances of reuse it is important that the guideline archetypes are designed considering the available archetypes and standards. Requirement (2.) is also crucial since CGs are often modelled without regard to the interaction with the EHR, which hinders interoperability. Here again, CGs should be modelled taking into account EHR standards and available archetypes all along. Finally, requirement (3.) involves the definition of a series of mappings relating the archetyped concepts from (1.) to the corresponding data items in the target EHR. Because guidelines often operate on data abstracted from lower-level EHR data, these mappings may relate one archetype to several data items (or even archetypes), e.g. by means of logical abstractions. The rest of the paper is mainly devoted to the requirements (1.) and (3.).

Since the seminal work on the Arden syntax [9], different authors have sought the integration of EHR systems with decision support systems in general and with guideline systems in particular. The KDOM framework [10] and the MEIDA architecture [11] are remarkable examples of recent work dealing with this problem using standards. Overall, our approach is similar to the ideas of these latter platforms. A distinctive feature of our work lies in the utilisation of the full-fledged archetype framework instead of the simplified versions of HL7 RIM used in MEIDA and KDOM, for the definition of the virtual health record (VHR).

From a data model perspective, the utilisation of archetypes brings about several advantages over previous initiatives. First, the VHR/data models we work with are of a higher level (clinical concept level instead of reference model one) and can contain semantic descriptions (by means of terminology references). Second, archetypes allow dealing with VHRs based on different EHR architectures (e.g. CEN/ISO EN13606, openEHR or HL7 CDA), due to their deliberate independence of the reference model. Third, no matter what VHR is used, data access via archetypes operates in such a way that data instances of the VHR are actual instances of the underlying reference model. Last but not least, clinicians are the main actors in the development of archetype models, which ensures both the medical and the technical validity thereof.

From the perspective of integration architecture, the use of archetypes in theory makes possible the direct access to EHR data without any kind of wrapper mechanism, provided that the EHR system natively supports archetypes and uses archetype models compatible with the CG ones (which ensures e.g. that the value for systolic blood pressure will be always located in the same path within the blood pressure archetype, be it specialised or not).

3 Knowledge Resources

A guideline for chronic heart failure. We have worked with the guideline for the diagnosis and treatment of chronic heart failure (CHF) developed by the European Society of Cardiology (ESC) [12]. According to the ESC, there are at least 10 million patients with heart failure in the countries it represents. The prognosis of heart failure is poor, hence the importance of a correct patient management. The guideline had been previously modelled in the PROforma guideline representation language.

The ESC CHF guideline is a 26 page document containing recommendations for the diagnosis, assessment, and treatment of CHF, for use in clinical practice. An evidence-based approach has been applied in the elaboration of the guideline, except for the diagnosis part, which is based on consensus. The guideline has text format but nevertheless contains several explanatory figures and tables. A section on descriptive terms in heart failure as well as a few tables with definitions have been particularly useful for the purposes of our work.

The openEHR Clinical Knowledge Manager. We have used as archetype source the openEHR Clinical Knowledge Manager[1] (CKM), which is a web-based repository allowing for archetype search, browse and download. Archetypes in the CKM have been created by independent domain experts, mainly clinicians and computer scientists, and then they have been released to the community as open source and freely available content. Before publication, archetypes undergo an iterative review process to ensure that they cover as many use-cases as possible and thus constitute a sensible maximal data set (with a high reuse potential).

According to openEHR the main categories for the description of clinical concepts are observation, evaluation, instruction and action. This categorisation is related to the way in which information is created during the care process: an *observation* is created by an act of observation, measurement, or testing; an *evaluation* is obtained by inference from observations, using personal experience and/or published knowledge; an *instruction* is an evaluation-based instruction to

[1] See `http://www.openehr.org/knowledge/`.

be performed by healthcare agents; and an *action* is a record of the interventions that have occurred, instruction-related or not. The number and specificity of available archetypes differs significantly among and within categories. E.g. within observation, there exist very specific archetypes such as *Apgar score* and *body weight*, while other archetypes like *imaging test* are rather generic.

4 Software Tools and Methods

The LinkEHR platform. The LinkEHR platform The LinkEHR Normalization Platform[2] is a set of tools and modules that allow: i) the creation of an archetype-based customizable view over a set of heterogeneous and distributed EHR data sources [8]; ii) the editing of archetypes based on different reference models (standards) as long as an XML Schema is available [13] (several reference models have been tested successfully: EN13606, openEHR, HL7 CDA, CDISC and CCR); and iii) the specification of declarative mappings between archetypes and data sources, and from these mappings, the automatic generation of XQuery scripts which translate source XML data into XML documents that are archetype compliant.

LinkEHR employs archetypes for both the semantic description of legacy EHRs and the publication of existing clinical information in the form of standardized EHR extracts. Since health data reside in the underlying EHR systems, it is necessary to define some kind of mapping information that links entities in the archetype to data elements in data repositories (e.g. elements and attributes in the case of XML sources). Basically, these mappings specify how to create archetype instances from the content of the data sources.

Mapping methods in LinkEHR. At the schema level, the above mentioned mappings require an explicit representation of how the source schema (legacy EHR data schema) and target schema (archetype) are related to each other. The effort required to create and manage such mappings is considerable. The common case is to write intricate and non-reusable software to perform the required transformations. This is even more complex with archetypes, since they are used to model generic concepts without any consideration regarding the internal architecture of the EHR. LinkEHR allows the definition high-level non-procedural mapping specifications that consist in a set of correspondences between entities of archetypes and source schemas. Two types of correspondences are supported: value and structural correspondences. The former specify how to calculate atomic values, whereas the latter may be used to control the generation and grouping of elements in the target.

Value correspondences are defined by a set of pairs, consisting of a transformation function that specifies how to calculate a value in the target from a set of source values, and a filter indicating the conditions that source data must satisfy to be used in the transformation function. The simplest kind of transformation function is the identity function which copies a source value into a target value.

[2] See `http://www.linkehr.com`.

But quite often it is necessary to specify arbitrary complex functions. For this purpose, the tool comes with a variety of functions such as type conversion, and mathematical, logical, string, date and time functions. The example in Table 1 illustrates a simple correspondence transforming gender codes. It transforms the local gender code in the path `/patient/gender` of an XML EHR extract (source data) into a normalized code (to be stored in the target data). Note that the order is relevant and only the first applicable function is used.

Table 1. A mapping transforming the gender codes from an XML source

Filter	**Function**
/patient/gender='M' OR /patient/gender='m'	0
/patient/gender='W' OR /patient/gender='w'	1
/patient/gender=0 OR /patient/gender=1	/patient/gender
true	9

5 Archetypes for Guideline Interoperability

Identification of clinical concepts from the guideline As a first step, we have identified the clinical concepts necessary to support CHF management and hence requiring archetypes. We have reviewed the ESC guideline with the help of medical experts, who had previously highlighted in the text all the relevant terms, including clinical concepts, tests, interventions, etc. Then we have analysed the identified concepts, using a mind map as a tool, making explicit the relationships among them.

The guideline sometimes refers to rather high-level/abstract concepts. This has been depicted in the mind map by means of abstraction relationships linking the high-level concept to the lower-level EHR ones from which it can be obtained. An example is the concept *ACEI intolerant*[3], which is based on the concepts *cough*, *hypotension*, *renal insufficiency*, *hyperkalaemia*, *syncope*, and *angioedema*. In a few cases there is no definition for the abstract concept in the guideline. Here we have sought additional information to specify the abstraction relationship. As a result the mind map not only includes the concepts in the guideline but also related concepts necessary for the definition thereof. A list of the concepts used in the ESC guideline, together with indications of the most suitable CKM archetypes to store the necessary information, can be found in a previous paper [7].

Design of archetypes from the clinical concepts. From the clinical concepts identified in the previous step we have developed a set of archetypes for use in a CG for CHF management. We have proceeded in a bottom-up way, starting with the concepts directly related to EHR data. As an illustration, in the rest of the section we focus on the archetypes for the concept *cough* and for the more abstract one *ACEI intolerant.* These required the specialisation of generic CKM

[3] ACEI stands for angiotensin-converting enzyme (ACE) inhibitors.

archetypes, concretely openEHR-EHR-CLUSTER.symptom.v1 in the case of *cough* and openEHR-EHR-EVALUATION.adverse.v1 in the case of *ACEI intolerant.*

Due to the generality of CKM archetypes (they are designed to be used in a wide range of scenarios), many entities (attributes or types) may not be relevant to all the potential usages. When defining our set of archetypes the principal task has been the selection of relevant entities and associated terminologies. For instance, in the case of openEHR-EHR-CLUSTER.symptom-cough (a specialisation of openEHR-EHR-CLUSTER.symptom.v1), we have only retained the entities to hold the information about the type, character, duration and severity of cough. For coding the type of cough, we have chosen to use SNOMED-CT. For coding the cough severity, we have considered the use of a local terminology as defined in the original CKM archetype. Figure 1 shows the overall structure of the archetype openEHR-EHR-CLUSTER.symptom-cough.

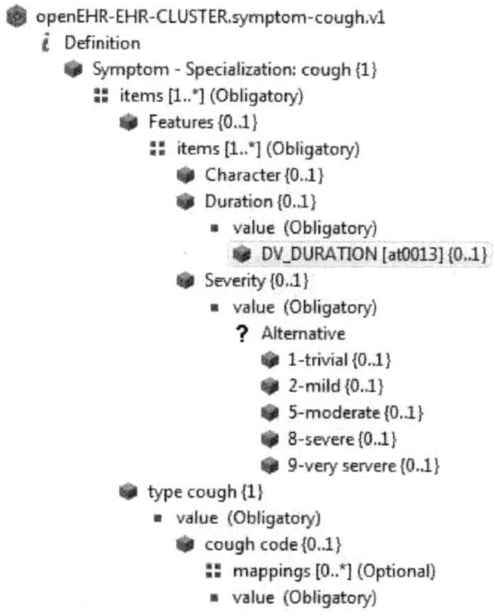

Fig. 1. Overall structure of the archetype openEHR-EHR-CLUSTER.symptom-cough

Mapping of archetypes to a clinical database. Unlike archetype definition, mapping specifications are particular to each EHR setting. In the mapping examples we describe next, we assume particular database features. The first mapping examples are related to the cough severity as defined in the archetype openEHR-EHR-CLUSTER.symptom-cough (see Severity in Figure 2). The severity is modelled by a DV_ORDINAL, which is a data type used to model finite scores where there is an implied ordering. This type contains two attributes: value, that represents the ordinal (position) in the enumeration of values, and symbol, that is the textual representation of the value. See the left hand side of Figure 2 for the definition of a DV_CODED_TEXT. According to the generic archetype, our archetype defines five levels of severity, namely: trivial (value=1), mild (value=2), moderate (value=5), severe (value=8) and very severe (value=9). Let us suppose that the source database offers its data as XML documents, and that it uses a severity scale ranging from 1 to 9 (source path is `/root/severity`) that needs to be mapped to the five-level scale used in the archetype. At least two mappings need to be defined for this scale mapping: one for the attribute holding the textual representation of the local code (mapping **a** in Figure 2), and one for the attribute holding the ordinal (mapping **b** in Figure 2).

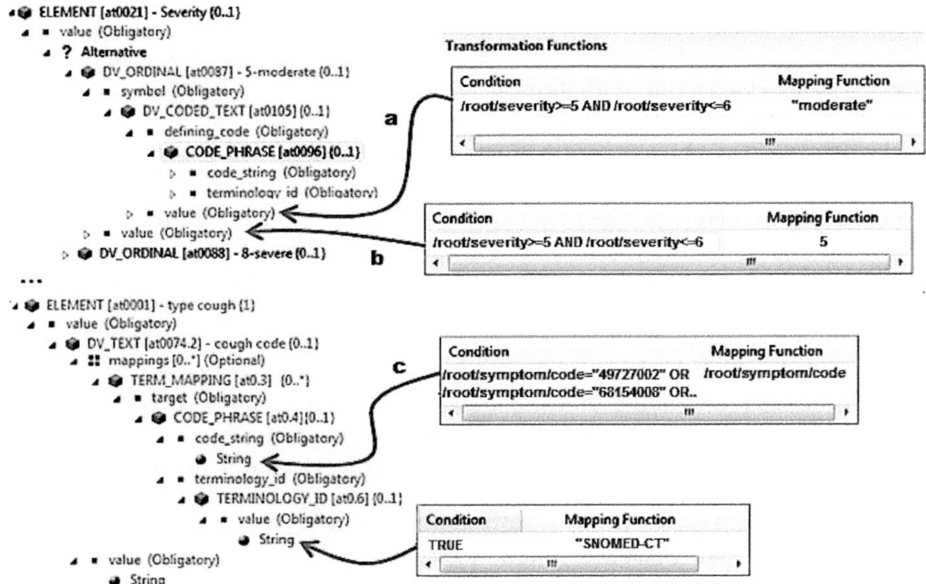

Fig. 2. Mappings for the archetype `openEHR-EHR-CLUSTER.symptom-cough`

A different kind of mapping is related to the attribute holding the cough coded value. Let us assume that the source database uses a SNOMED-CT coding (source path is `/root/symptom/code`), and that the same coding is employed in the target data. Obviously, only those symptom codes related to cough must be used in the mapping, such as cough (SNOMED-CT::49727002), and chronic cough (SNOMED-CT:: 68154008). This terminological mapping appears in Figure 2 as mapping **c**.

Another possibility is using archetypes as sources, which allows the definition of more abstract concepts. A simple example is described next, which uses the archetype `openEHR-EHR-CLUSTER.symptom-cough` as source. Among other things, a patient that has either severe or very severe cough, including dry cough (SNOMED-CT::11833005), chronic cough (SNOMED-CT::68154008), or non-productive cough (SNOMED-CT::409596002), can be considered ACEI intolerant. The following expression uses the entities in `openEHR-EHR-CLUSTER.symptom-cough` to define a condition to be used as one of the filters in the mapping of openEHR-EHR-EVALUATION.adverse-ACEI_intolerant:

```
  --dry, chronic or non-productive cough
(/items[at0001]/value[at0074.2]/mappings[at0.3]/target[at0.4]/code_string=11833005 OR
 /items[at0001]/value[at0074.2]/mappings[at0.3]/target[at0.4]/code_string=68154008 OR
 /items[at0001]/value[at0074.2]/mappings[at0.3]/target[at0.4]/code_string=409596002) AND
  --severe or very severe cough
(/items[at0034]/items[at0021]/value[at0088]/value = 8 OR
/items[at0034]/items[at0021]/value[at0092]/value = 9)
```

6 Conclusions and Future Work

There is a general consensus about the fact that clinical guidelines should be deployed using some computer support and that this support should be integrated within the clinical information system, to take full advantage of their potential benefits. However, currently one of the main obstacles to this integration is the interaction with the EHR. With the aim of solving the interoperability problems of guideline systems, we propose the utilisation of archetypes as a canonical data representation of the concepts used in a CG. The utilisation of archetypes has several advantages with respect to previous initiatives, among others the possibility of dealing with VHRs described in terms of clinical concepts, possibly based on different EHR architectures.

The approach is built around the development of a collection of guideline-specific archetypes, taking into account the (medically valid) clinical models in existing archetype repositories. It implies the proper utilisation of CG archetypes within the guideline (guideline-archetype adjustment), as well as the specification of a series of mappings relating the archetypes to the corresponding data in the target clinical databases (archetype-database mapping). Despite the overload of developing the necessary archetypes and mappings, the resulting CG procedure and data models should have a high potential for reuse.

Another contribution of our work is the development of a set of archetypes for use in a real-world guideline, including sample archetype-database mappings. For these tasks we have used the LinkEHR data integration platform. Archetype editing with LinkEHR has been straightforward, after identifying the relevant CKM archetypes and determining the necessary adaptations (including links to terminologies). LinkEHR tools are also well suited for the definition of the archetype mappings in our sample guideline (terminological and abstraction ones).

As future work, we will proceed with the technical implementation of our approach, which requires the adaptation of an existing CG engine to support data access using archetypes. Also with the aim of validating the approach, we will tackle the development of archetypes for other clinical guidelines to determine if LinkEHR mapping methods are sufficient or, on the contrary, additional functionalities are required. At a different level, we intend to investigate ontological frameworks for the data model mappings we are dealing with, including conceptual models allowing for reasoning e.g. about how different data models relate.

References

1. Sonnenberg, F., Hagerty, C.: Computer-Interpretable Clinical Practice Guidelines. Where Are We and where Are We Going? IMIA Yearbook of Medical Informatics, 145–158 (2006)
2. Peleg, M., Miksch, S., Seyfang, A., Bury, J., Ciccarese, P., Fox, J., Greenes, R., Hall, R., Johnson, P., Jones, N., Kumar, A., Quaglini, S., Shortliffe, E., Stefanelli, M.: Comparing computer-interpretable guideline models: A case-study approach. J. Am. Med. Inform. Assn. 10, 52–68 (2003)
3. de Clercq, P.A., Blom, J.A., Korsten, H.H.M., Hasman, A.: Approaches for creating computer-interpretable guidelines that facilitate decision support. Artif. Intell. Med. 31, 1–27 (2004)
4. Panzarasa, S., Quaglini, S., Cavallini, A., Micieli, G., Marcheselli, S., Stefanelli, M.: Technical Solutions for Integrating Clinical Practice Guidelines with Electronic Patient Records. In: Riaño, D., ten Teije, A., Miksch, S., Peleg, M. (eds.) KR4HC 2009. LNCS, vol. 5943, pp. 141–154. Springer, Heidelberg (2010)
5. Chen, R., Georgii-Hemming, P., Åhlfeldt, H.: Representing a Chemotherapy Guideline Using openEHR and Rules. In: Proc. of the 22nd Int. Conf. of the European Federation for Medical Informatics (MIE 2009), pp. 653–657. IOS Press, Amsterdam (2009)
6. Beale, T., Heard, S.: Architecture Overview (April 2007), `http://www.openehr.org/releases/1.0.2/architecture/overview.pdf`
7. Marcos, M., Martínez-Salvador, B.: Towards the Interoperability of Computerised Guidelines and Electronic Health Records: An Experiment with openEHR Archetypes and a Chronic Heart Failure Guideline. In: Riaño, D., ten Teije, A., Miksch, S., Peleg, M. (eds.) KR4HC 2010. LNCS, vol. 6512, pp. 101–113. Springer, Heidelberg (2011)
8. Angulo, C., Crespo, P., Maldonado, J.A., Moner, D., Pérez, D., Abad, I., Mandingorra, J., Robles, M.: Non-invasive lightweight integration engine for building EHR from autonomous distributed systems. Int. J. of Med. Inform. 76(S3), 417–424 (2007)
9. Hripcsak, G., Ludemann, P., Pryor, T.A., Wigertz, O.B., Clayton, P.D.: Rationale for the Arden Syntax. Comput. Biomed. Res. 27, 291–324 (1994)
10. Peleg, M., Keren, S., Denekamp, Y.: Mapping computerized clinical guidelines to electronic medical records: Knowledge-data ontological mapper (KDOM). J. Biomed. Inform. 41(1), 180–201 (2008)
11. German, E., Leibowitz, A., Shahar, Y.: An architecture for linking medical decision-support applications to clinical databases and its evaluation. J. Biomed. Inform. 42(2), 203–218 (2009)
12. The Task Force for the Diagnosis and Treatment of Chronic Heart Failure of the ESC: Guidelines for the diagnosis and treatment of chronic heart failure: executive summary (update 2005). Eur. Heart J. 26, 1115–1140 (2005)
13. Maldonado, J., Moner, D., Boscá, D., Fernández, J., Angulo, C., Robles, M.: LinkEHR-Ed: A multi-reference model archetype editor based on formal semantics. Int. J. of Med. Inform. 78(8), 559–570 (2009)

Variation Prediction in Clinical Processes

Zhengxing Huang, Xudong Lu*, Chenxi Gan, and Huilong Duan

College of Biomedical Engineering and Instrument Science of Zhejiang University.
The Key Laboratory of Biomedical Engineering, Ministry of Education, China
lxd@vico-lab.com

Abstract. For clinical processes, meaningful variations may be related to care performance or even the patient survival. It is imperative that the variations be predicted timely so that the patient care "journey" can be more adaptive and efficient. This study addresses the question of how to predict variations in clinical processes. Given the assumption that a clinical case with low appropriateness between its specific patient state and its' applied medical intervention is more likely to be a variation than other cases, this paper proposes a method to construct an appropriateness measure model based on historical clinical cases so as to predict such variations in future cases of clinical processes. The proposed method is demonstrated on a real life data set from the Chinese Liberation Army General Hospital. The experimental results confirm the given assumption and indicate the feasibility of the proposed method.

1 Introduction

Clinical processes, as a unique type of patient-linked process (i.e., diagnostic and therapeutic procedures to be carried out for a specific patient), are becoming an important issue in healthcare domain [1–4]. In clinical practice, there are many factors and uncertainties affecting the execution of clinical processes. These uncertainties can result from inter-observer variability, inaccurate evaluation of the patient and some deficiencies in grading scales [3, 4]. As a result, the patient care "journey" may not go towards the expected direction, and slightly different from the predefined medical intervention or procedure. In such cases, the variations happen inevitably in clinical process execution.

Clinical process variation is usually conceptualized in terms of process outcomes, and a well-defined body of knowledge has developed that takes this perspective [5]. In clinical practice, for example, length of stay (LOS), mortality, and infection rate, etc., are commonly used measures of clinical process variations [6, 7]. From the outcome perspective, clinical process variation is conceptualized as reliability (the standard deviation of some output parameter) and accuracy (changes in the mean value over time relative to some target) [6]. Accuracy and reliability of outputs are enormously important because they directly affect the performance of clinical processes.

* Corresponding author.

M. Peleg, N. Lavrač, and C. Combi (Eds.): AIME 2011, LNAI 6747, pp. 286–295, 2011.

As valuable as these measures are, they restrict the attention to the analysis of clinical process variations, not the forecast and foster/prevention of these variations. From the operational perspective, timely identification of a patient's care outcome is indeed desirable. Meaningful variations may be related to care performance or even the patient survival. If these variations can be predicted timely, the patient care "journey" could be more adaptive and efficient. As a matter of fact, the variation prediction in clinical process execution is of increasing interest to medical staff and hospital managers, who prefer mindful and timely adjustment of patient care in case of variations being predicted.

In this study, we address the question of how to predict variations in clinical process execution. We present a clinical process-aware information system model. Based on this model, medical interventions can be evaluated by calculating their information entropies. Then, the appropriateness of a specific clinical case can be calculated. Note that each case consists of a specific patient state as the precondition/problem and a specific medical intervention as the consequence/answer. It is assumed that cases with lower appreciativeness are more likely to be variations than others. Further, we use real life data from the Chinese Liberate Army General Hospital to evaluate the proposed method.

2 Preliminaries

In this section we introduce some basic concepts needed for the remainder of the discussion. We discuss rough set theory, and clinical processes, so as to set up a necessary context for describing the proposed method.

2.1 Rough Set Theory

In rough set theory (RST) [8], an information system is a quadruple $IS = \langle O, A, V, f \rangle$, where O is a non-empty finite set of objects; A is a non-empty finite set of attributes; V is the union of attribute domains, i.e., $V = \bigcup_{a \in A} V_a$, where V_a denotes the domain of attribute a; and $f : O \times A \rightarrow V$ is an information function so that for any $a \in A$ and $x \in O$, $f(x, a) \in V_a$. Each subset $B \subseteq A$ of attributes determines a binary relation $IND(B)$, called indiscernibility relation, defined as follows:

$$IND(B) = \{(x, y) \in O^2 | \forall a \in B, f(x, a) = f(y, a)\} \tag{1}$$

Given any $B \subseteq A$, relation $IND(B)$ induces a partition of O, which is denoted by $O/IND(B)$, where an element from $O/IND(B)$ is called an equivalence class or elementary set. For every element $x \in O$, let $[x]_B$ denote the equivalence class of relation $IND(B)$ that contains element x. Let $B \subseteq A$, the B-lower and B-upper approximation of X, $X \subseteq O$, is defined respectively as $\underline{X}(B) = \{x \in O | [x]_B \subseteq X\}$ and $\overline{X}(B) = \{x \in O | [x]_B \bigcap X \neq \emptyset\}$.

An important method of attributes reduction is based on the difference of dependency [8]. Dependency of attributes can be defined in the following way: for

A and B, B depends on A in degree γ_B, $\gamma_A(B) = \frac{|POS_A(B)|}{|O|}$, where $POS_A(B) = \bigcup_{X \subseteq O/IND(B)} \underline{X}_A$ called a positive region of the partition $O/IND(B)$ with respect to A, is the set of all elements of O that can be uniquely classified to blocks of the partition $O/IND(B)$, by means of A. If $\gamma_A(B) = 1$, B depends totally on A and the decision table is consistent. If $0 < \gamma_A(B) < 1$, B depends partially on A and the decision table is partial inconsistent, and if $\gamma_A(B) = 0$, B is totally independent on A and the decision table is completely inconsistent. Given $a \in A$, the significance of attribute a is defined as

$$\gamma_a(B) = \gamma_A(B) - \gamma_{A-\{a\}}(B) \tag{2}$$

If $\gamma_a(B) = 0$, then attribute a can be removed from the set of conditional attributes.

2.2 Clinical Processes

A clinical process consists of several sets of medical interventions in sequence [2–4, 9] and one set of medical interventions can be seen as a basic process fragment [10]. Note that a medical intervention consists of a set of clinical activities and each activity represents a specific order. In general, a clinical process is described as an interconnected hierarchical model including the top-level outcome flow and the medical intervention level along a care time-line. During the execution of a specific clinical process instance, medical staff evaluate the patient state, propose a set of possible causes of the clinical problems, and then identify a possible set of solutions. Furthermore, medical staff selects existing or design new medical interventions. The clinical activities of those interventions will be scheduled, resulting in the execution of actions. The executions of these clinical activities will often change the patient state, which in turn urges the process itself to be adaptive as well.

3 Variation Prediction in Clinical Processes

3.1 Clinical Process-Aware Information System

Formally, a clinical process-aware information system can be described as follows:

Definition 1 (Clinical Process-aware Information System). Let $CPAIS = \langle O, S, T, A, V, f \rangle$ be a clinical process-aware information system, where O is a non-empty finite set of completed cases of medical interventions, each case corresponds to an execution of a specific medical intervention; S is a non-empty finite set of patient states, $S \in \mathbb{P}(A \times V)$; T is a non-empty finite set of medical interventions; A is a non-empty finite set of patient features; V is the union of patient feature domains, i.e., $V = \bigcup\{V_a | a \in A\}$, where V_a denotes the domain of the feature a; and $f : O \times A \rightarrow V$ is an information function which associates an unique value of each feature of every case belong to O, i.e., $\forall a \in A$ and $o \in O$, $f(o, a) \in V_a$.

Table 1. An example of clinical process-aware information system

Case	Age($year$)	Random blood glucose(%)	HbA1C(%)	Diagnosis duration($year$)	BMI(kg/m^2)	Medication Intervention
o_1	55($\geq$ 55)	12.8($\geq$ 11.0)	8.40($\leq$ 8.44)	13($\geq$ 10)	32.4($\geq$ 30)	Tablet-Insulin treatment
o_2	60($\geq$ 55)	10.5($\leq$ 11.0)	8.32($\leq$ 8.44)	6($\leq$ 10)	27.7($\leq$ 30)	Tablet treatment
o_3	66($\geq$ 55)	12.7($\geq$ 11.0)	8.42($\leq$ 8.44)	15($\geq$ 10)	32.1($\geq$ 30)	Tablet-Insulin treatment
o_4	55($\geq$ 55)	12.6($\geq$ 11.0)	8.27($\leq$ 8.44)	2($\leq$ 10)	22.4($\leq$ 30)	Tablet-Insulin treatment
o_5	56($\geq$ 55)	11.1($\geq$ 11.0)	8.30($\leq$ 8.44)	12($\geq$ 10)	30.3($\geq$ 30)	Tablet-Insulin treatment
o_6	60($\geq$ 55)	12.1($\geq$ 11.0)	8.50($\geq$ 8.44)	12($\geq$ 10)	32.0($\geq$ 30)	Tablet-Insulin treatment

The *CPAIS* is founded on the assumption that, in the universe of discourse associated with every case of medical intervention, some cases are characterized by the same set of patient features are indiscernible because of insufficient information. Any set of all indiscernible cases is called an elementary set and forms a basis granule of knowledge about the universe. For example, Table 1 shows an example decision table with a set of cases $O(o_1, \cdots, o_6)$ contained in the rows of the table. The columns denote a set of patient features A (*age*, *Random blood glucose*, *HbA1C*, *Diagnosis duration* and *BMI*) of these cases and medical interventions T. As mentioned above, a specific clinical case consists of a specific patient state and a specific medical intervention. For example, the case o_1 consists of a specific patient state described as {('age', '55'), ('Random blood glucose', '12.8'), ('HbA1C', '8.40'), ('Diagnosis duration', '13'), ('BMI', '32.4')} and a specific medical intervention 'Tablet-Insulin treatment' which is applied in the condition of that patient state.

For the patient features in Table 1, all cases can be formed in different elementary sets for specific medical interventions according to the differences of the patient features. For example, it formes four elementary sets $\{o_1, o_3, o_5\}$, $\{o_2\}$, $\{o_4\}$ and $\{o_6\}$. This means that cases $\{o_1, o_3, o_5\}$ are indiscernible, while the other cases are characterized uniquely with all available patient states. Based on the definitions above, we propose a variation prediction service in clinical process-aware information system.

A schematic of our variation prediction service is provided in Figure 1. Generally, a set of historical clinical cases and a set of medical interventions serve as the input of the module for significant patient feature selection in order to index specific medical interventions. Note that there are an amount of patient features regularly recorded in clinical information systems. Some features are redundant and irrelevant for the selection and the application of specific medical interventions. The feature-selection module can eliminate these redundant and irrelevant patient features and select significant ones to index specific medical interventions. The medical interventions indexed by a set of significant features and the historical clinical cases are then used to construct the prediction model, which is finally used to serve the request of an incoming partial case for the variation prediction on possible next medical intervention to execute. In this request, the patient state information of that partial case is sent to the prediction service. Based on the inputs, the prediction service measures the appropriateness between the patient state and the medical intervention next to execute, then provides the clinical process-aware information system a prediction result, i.e., whether the variation would happen or not.

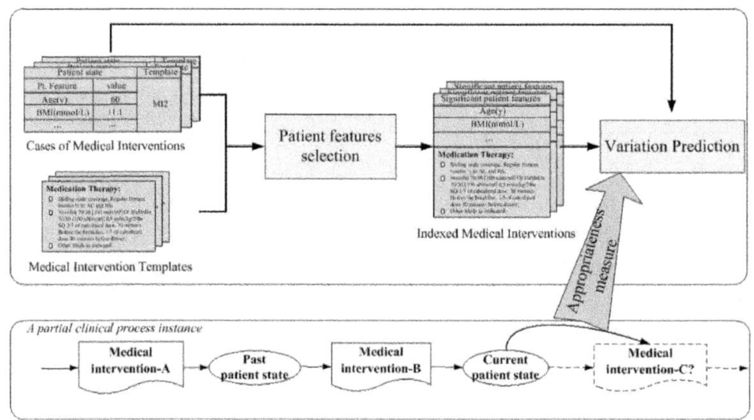

Fig. 1. The methodology of variation prediction in clinical processes

3.2 Significant Patient Feature Selection to Index Specific Medical Interventions

As mentioned above, medical interventions, as basic alternatives, can be selected and applied in considering specific patient states in clinical process execution. Thus, it is important to discover the dependencies between these medical intervention and these patient states. Intuitively, the selection of a medical intervention t, $t \in T$, depends totally on a set of patient features B which is able to describe the specific patient state, $B \subseteq A$. If the values of features from B uniquely determine the condition of t's selection. In other words, t depends totally on B, if there exists a functional dependency between values of B and t. Formally, such a dependency can be defined as:

$$\gamma_B(t) = \frac{|POS_B(t)|}{|O|}, \tag{3}$$

Note that if $\gamma_B(t) = 1$, then the selection of t depends totally on B, and if $\gamma_B(t) < 1$, we say that the selection of t depends partially (to degree $\gamma_B(t)$) on B. If $\gamma_B(t) = 0$, then the selection of t is independent with B.

Furthermore, we consider the question whether we can remove some irrelevant features from A for the selection of t. Let A be a set of patient features and T be a set of medical interventions. We will say that $Red(t) \subseteq A$ is a t-reduct (reduct with respect to $t \in T$) of A, if $Red(t)$ is a minimal subset of A such that

$$\gamma_A(t) = \gamma_{Red(t)}(t), t \in T \tag{4}$$

3.3 Variation Prediction in Clinical Processes

In this study, we propose an information entropy based variation prediction method. In particular, we give the definition of medical intervention information entropy as follows:

Definition 2 (Medical Intervention Information Entropy). Given a clinical process-aware information system $CPAIS = \langle O, T, S, A, V, f \rangle$, where O is a non-empty finite set of cases of medical interventions, T is a non-empty finite set of medical interventions, S is a non-empty finite set of patient states, A is a non-empty finite set of patient features, and $Red(t) \subseteq A$ is a t-reduct (reduct with respect to $t \in T$) of A. Let $IND(Red(t))$ be the indiscernibility relation on O determined by $Red(t)$, and $O/IND(Red(t)) = \{Red(t)_1, Red(t)_2, \cdots, Red(t)_m\}$ denote the partition of O induced by $IND(Red(t))$. The information entropy $E(Red(t))$ of medical intervention t is defined as:

$$E(Red(t)) = -\sum_{i=1}^{m} \frac{|Red(t)_i|}{|O/IND(Red(t))|} log_2 \frac{|Red(t)_i|}{|O/IND(Red(t))|} \tag{5}$$

where $\frac{|Red(t)_i|}{|O/IND(Red(t))|}$ denotes the probability of any case $o \in O/IND(Red(t))$ being in equivalence class $Red(t)_i$, $1 \leq i \leq m$.

In particular, for a specific $s \in S$ and a specific $t \in T$, let $o = (s, t)$ be a partial clinical case. Let $E_o(Red(t)) = -\frac{|[o]_{Red(t)}|}{|O/IND(Red(t))|} log_2 \frac{|[o]_{Red(t)}|}{|O/IND(Red(t))|}$ denote the information entropy of medical intervention t in $[o]_{Red(t)}$ from $O/IND(Red(t))$, where $[o]_{Red(t)}$ is the equivalence class of o under relation $O/IND(Red(t))$. The appropriateness $appr(s,t)$ under relation $IND(Red(t))$ is defined as:

$$appr(s,t) = 1 - \frac{E_{(o)}(Red(t))}{E(Red(t))} \tag{6}$$

where $o = (s, t)$ and $E(Red(t))$ denotes the information entropy of medical intervention t, $t \in T$.

The aim of variation prediction is to predict a specific medical intervention which behaves in an unexpected way or has abnormal properties under a specific patient state. Appropriateness can be deemed as a kind of normal property. Therefore, in this study, we may consider a specific case imposed a specific medical intervention, of which appropriateness is low, as behaving in an unexpected way or featuring abnormal properties when comparing with other cases which selected different medical interventions.

Formally, for a specific $s \in S$ and a specific $t \in T$, if $1 - appr(s,t) > \alpha$, then the case $o = (s,t)$ is called a clinical process variation, where $1 - appr(s,t)$ represents the inappropriateness factor of the patient state s and the medical intervention t.

Taking Table 1 as example, let $t=$ 'Tablet-Insulin treatment', $a_1=$ 'Age', $a_2=$ 'Random blood glucose', $a_3=$'HbA1C', $a_4=$'Diagnosis duration' and $a_5=$ 'BMI'. The $POS_A(t) = \{\{o_1, o_3, o_5\}, \{o_4\}, \{o_6\}\}$, thus $\gamma_A(t) = \frac{|\{\{o_1,o_3,o_5\},\{o_4\},\{o_6\}\}|}{|O|} = \frac{5}{6}$.

For each patient feature, the dependency is calculated as $\gamma_{a_1}(t) = \gamma_A(t) - \gamma_{A-\{a_1\}}(t) = \frac{5}{6} - \frac{|\{\{o_1,o_3,o_5\},\{o_4\},\{o_6\}\}|}{|O|} = 0$. Similarly, we compute that $\gamma_{a_2}(t) = 0$, $\gamma_{a_3}(t) = \frac{2}{3}$, $\gamma_{a_4}(t) = 0$, and $\gamma_{a_5}(t) = \frac{1}{3}$. Thus, the patient features a_3 and a_5 are significant to index the medical intervention 'Tablet-Insulin treatment'. $E_{o_1}(\{a_3, a_5\}) = E_{o_3}(\{a_3, a_5\}) = E_{o_4}(\{a_3, a_5\}) = E_{o_5}(\{a_3, a_5\}) = -\frac{4}{5}log_2\frac{4}{5} = 0.258$ and $E_{o_6}(\{a_3, a_5\}) = -\frac{1}{5}log_2\frac{1}{5} = 0.464$.

Correspondingly, we can obtain that $appr(o_1) = appr(o_3) = appr(o_4) = appr(o_5) = 1 - \frac{0.258}{0.464+0.258} = 0.644$, and $appr(o_6) = 1 - \frac{0.464}{0.464+0.258} = 0.356$.

Suppose $\alpha = 0.6$. Hence, the inappropriateness factor of o_1 is $1 - appr = 0.356 < \alpha$, therefore, o_1 has low probability to be a variation. Analogously, we can obtain that o_3, o_4, and o_5 has low probability to be variations as well. And $1 - appr(o_6) = 0.644 > \alpha$, thus, o_6 could be a variation. It means if the medical intervention 'Tablet-Insulin treatment' is applied in the condition of patient state {('age', '60'), ('Random blood glucose', '12.1'), ('HbA1C', '10.50'), ('Diagnosis duration', '12'), ('BMI', '32.0')}, variations might happen in that case.

4 Experiment

4.1 Experiment Design

The experiments are set in the environment of the department of endocrinology of the Chinese Liberate Army General Hospital. The overview of the experimental flowchart is illustrated in Figure 5, which mainly involves five steps:

1. For this experiment, 140 pieces of referral Electronic Patient Records (EPRs) of geriatric type 2 diabetes patients were selected from the whole between 2006-2009 by experienced medical staff. Each piece of referral EPR represents an whole instance of a specific patient clinical process in hospital. Based on the data set, it is able to extract/define a set of medical intervention templates which are applied in patients' clinical processes. It can extract clinical instances of these medical interventions from the data set as well, and each instance represents an application of a specific medical intervention. As results, we extracted 842 clinical cases from 140 pieces of EPR. Meanwhile, we select 47 patient features based on medical staff's recommendation. For each clinical case, we extracted the values of those features. The patient state consists of these features with their values and describes the problem of a specific clinical case, whose solution is the applied medical intervention. In this step, the attending of medical staff plays an important role in designing medical intervention templates. After discussion with medical staff, we define 11 medical intervention templates for the treatment of geriatric type 2 diabetes patients.
2. Based on the results of the first step, we extract the set of significant patient features to index the specific medical intervention as described in Section 3.2. These significant patient features are used in the variation prediction process.

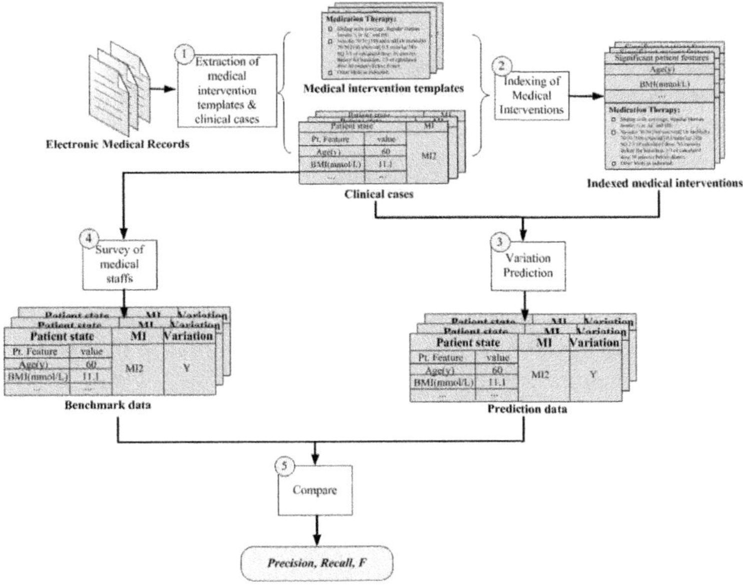

Fig. 2. The flowchart of the experiment

3. Based on the set of clinical cases extracted from EPR and the set of medical interventions which are indexed by the set of patient features, it is able to predict if the variation would happen in a specific clinical case, as described in Section 3.3. Each predicted case consists of a specific patient state, a label of the applied medical intervention and a predicted value. If the variation is predicted to happen, the predicted value is "Y", otherwise it is "N". Note that we use a parameter α to represent the threshold value of variation prediction. Thus, one can study α's impact on the results and then choose the best value of α to predict variations in clinical process execution.
4. As to the benchmark data, we asked medical staff to point out variations of clinical cases. Each benchmark case consists of a specific patient state, a label of the applied medical intervention and a benchmark value. If variation is pointed out in a specific clinical case, the benchmark value is "Y", otherwise, it is "N". In this experiments, the number of the benchmark cases in which variations are pointed out by medical staff are 305 among 842, i.e., the variation rate is 36.2%.
5. The last step is the comparison between the prediction results and the benchmark. The matrixes "Recall", "Precision" and "F" are calculated, where $Precision = \frac{|P \cap B|}{|P|}$, $Recall = \frac{|P \cap B|}{|B|}$, and $F = 2 \cdot \frac{Precision \cdot Recall}{Precision + Recall}$, where P denotes the set of predicted clinical cases in which the predicted value is "Y"; B denotes the set of benchmark cases in which in which the benchmark value is "Y"; and $P \cap B$ denotes the set of common cases contained in both P and B.

4.2 Results and Analysis

In the proposed approach, the parameter α is the threshold value. In this experiment, we study α's impact on the results of the experiments. Figure 5(A) shows the impact of α on the number of predicted cases and common cases (contained in both P and B). We observe that the value of α impacts the prediction results. As to the trends of the number of the predicted cases with α changing, we could see that the number of the predicted cases decreases when α becomes bigger and flattens out when the α exceeds 0.8. In the condition of $\alpha = 0.8$, the number of the predicted clinical cases with variations is 280, i.e., the predicted variation rate is about 33.2%. In particular, there are 292 common cases between the predicted ones and the benchmark ones in the condition of $\alpha = 0.7$, and it is almost equal with the benchmark value.

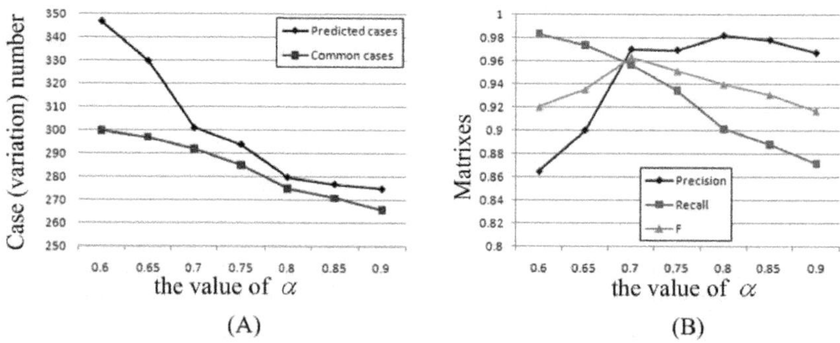

Fig. 3. (A) Impact of parameter α on variation prediction; (B) Impact of parameter α on *precision*, *recall*, and F

Figure 5(B) shows the impacts of α on *precision*, *recall* and F. We observe that the value of α impacts the prediction results significantly. With α increases, *precision* increases at first, but when α surpasses a certain threshold, *precision* holds a steady state with further increases in the value of α; With α increases, *recall* decreases; With α increases, F increases at first, but when α surpasses a certain threshold, F decreases with further increases in the value of α. From Figure 5(B), we observe that, the "F" achieves the best performance when α is around 0.7, while smaller values like $\alpha = 0.6$ or larger value like $\alpha = 0.9$ can potentially degrade the performance.

5 Conclusion

Variations in clinical processes are believed to influence productivity, quality, flexibility, and a host of other aspects of patient care plan design and management. In this paper, we address the question of how to predict variations in clinical process execution. We test the performance of the proposed method, investigate the sensitivities of some importance parameters as to the evaluation matrixes. The experiments results indicate the efficiency of the proposed method.

Clinical impact assessment for the proposed method is in progress. We are having further discussion with clinical experts for improvements, and evaluating the proposed method in comparison of the Rule-based ones. Moreover, we are working with developers on embedding this technique into Electronic Medical Record (EMR), which is supposed to provide practitioner reminders and alerts as well as availability of complete and accurate data for clinical staff, so as to achieve high quality of clinical process execution and prevent medical errors with an adaptive mechanism for clinical process execution.

For future research we envision to answer a practical question, that is not how to limit variations through increased controls, but how to foster 'good' variations (that results in improved patient care performance for example) and limit 'bad' variations (that results in decreased patient satisfaction for example). This could be followed by more formal analysis of an amount of clinical processes in order to document and systematically measure the extent of variations and to explore the appropriateness of these variations in different clinical situations.

References

1. Peleg, M., Gutnik, L.A., Snow, V., Patel, V.L.: Interpreting procedures from descriptive guidelines. Journal of Biomedical Informatics 39(2), 184–195 (2006)
2. Lenz, R., Reichert, M.: IT support for healthcare processes-premises, challenges, perspectives. Data & Knowledge Engineering 61(1), 39–58 (2007)
3. Huang, Z., Lu, X., Duan, H.: Supporting adaptive clinical treatment processes through recommendations. Computer Methods and Programms in Biomedicine (2010) (accpeted)
4. Huang, Z., Lu, X., Duan, H.: Using recommendation to support adaptive clinical pathways. Journal of Medical Systems (2010) (accpeted)
5. Chu, S., Cesnik, B.: Improving clinical pathway design: lessons learned from a computerised prototype. International Journal of Medical Informatics 51(1), 1–11 (1998)
6. Okita, A., et al.: Variance analysis of a clinical pathway of video-assisted single lobectomy for lung cancer. Surgery Today 39 (2009)
7. van de Klundert, J., Gorissen, P., Zeemering, S.: Measuring clinical pathway adherence. In: Journal of Biomedical Informatics (2010) (in press, corrected proof)
8. Pawlak, Z.: Rough sets. International Journal of Computer and Information Sciences 11, 341–356 (1982)
9. Adlassnig, K.P., Combi, C., Das, A.K., Keravnou, E.T., Pozzi, G.: Temporal representation and reasoning in medicine: research directions and challenges. Artificial Intelligence in Medicine 38(2), 101–113 (2006)
10. Peleg, M., Tu, S.W.: Design patterns for clinical guidelines. Artificial Intelligence in Medicine 47(1), 1–24 (2009)

A Constraint Logic Programming Approach to Identifying Inconsistencies in Clinical Practice Guidelines for Patients with Comorbidity

Martin Michalowski[1], Marisela Mainegra Hing[2], Szymon Wilk[3], Wojtek Michalowski[2], and Ken Farion[4]

[1] Adventium Labs, Minneapolis MN 55401, USA
martin.michalowski@adventiumlabs.org
[2] University of Ottawa, Telfer School of Management, Ottawa Canada
{wojtek,mhing}@uottawa.ca
[3] Poznan University of Technology, Institute of Computing Science, Poznan Poland
szymon.wilk@cs.put.poznan.pl
[4] Children Hospital of Eastern Ontario, Ottawa Canada
farion@cheo.on.ca

Abstract. This paper describes a novel methodological approach to identifying inconsistencies when concurrently using multiple clinical practice guidelines. We discuss how to construct a formal guideline model using Constraint Logic Programming, chosen for its ability to handle relationships between patient information, diagnoses, and treatment suggestions. We present methods to identify inconsistencies that are manifested by treatment-treatment and treatment-disease interactions associated with comorbidity. Using an open source constraint programming system (ECLiPSe), we demonstrate the ability of our approach to find treatment given incomplete patient data and to identify possible inconsistencies.

Keywords: Clinical practice guideline, comorbidity, Constraint Logic Programming.

1 Introduction

This paper describes methodological research on developing a guideline model based on Constraint Logic Programming (CLP) [1] that allows for the semi-automatic adaptation of a guideline to a patient-specific situation characterized by the need to treat multiple diseases concurrently (*comorbidity*). A clinical practice guideline (CPG) represents systematically developed statements to assist physician decision-making, aiming to improve quality of care and reduce practice variations. CPGs were originally intended to help with managing a patient who has a single medical condition. While the population is aging and medical care involves increasingly complex cases, there is clearly a need to adapt guidelines for management of patients with comorbidity.

M. Peleg, N. Lavrač, and C. Combi (Eds.): AIME 2011, LNAI 6747, pp. 296–301, 2011.

The use of CPGs at the point of care is limited and a number of barriers have been identified [2,3]. One particular barrier is that the CPG seldom allows for customization to a patient-specific situation, especially in light of comorbidity. This shortcoming can be addressed by creating a computer executable model of the guideline that can be easily manipulated and tailored to a specific patient. In our research we consider simplified intervention CPGs that were developed to assist physicians in one-time disease management and that are used in a primary care organization on the in-patient population. The executable CPG model is build using the constraint logic programming (CLP) paradigm and we developed an approach to identify potential inconsistencies if multiple CPG models need to be evaluated concurrently. This places our work in the broad category of reasoning in medicine [4] and our attempt to deal with inconsistencies shares some similarities with conflict resolution methods in automated reasoning [5].

This paper is organized as follows. First we describe CLP methodology and show how we use this framework in the context of CPGs. Next we describe how we model a single CPG as a CLP and show how a model for comorbid condition is created. We then outline how such a combined model can introduce inconsistencies and present methods for resolving them. We continue by presenting a case study and summarizing our contributions.

2 Methods

CLP is a form of constraint programming that combines logic programming (LP) with a constraint satisfaction problem (CSP) by embedding constraints within the body of clauses in a logic program. Formally, a logic program is seen as logical theory made up of a set of rules called *clauses* that relate the truth value of a literal (an n-ary predicate where the n terms can be either a variable, constant, or a n-ary function) to the value of a collection of other literals. Executing a logic program entails asking for the truth value of a certain statement called the goal. CLP unifies LP and constraint satisfaction problems (CSPs) [1] by using logic programming as a constraint programming language to solve a CSP.

We use CLP over finite domain constraints because the constraints we represent are over binary (true/false). In the CLP representation of a guideline, a variable is associated with an action or decision step from a CPG (i.e., take oral cortiosteriods (OC) or complicated ulcer symptoms experienced (CUS)). Than, an instance of a variable is $OC :=$ true or $CUS :=$ false. A constraint describes the relationship between variables and is represented in the body of a clause in the logic program. For example $\neg OC \wedge CUS$ means a patient cannot take oral cortiosteriods when experiencing ulcer symptoms. Solving the CLP model entails assigning a value to each variable such that no constraints are violated. As such, the solution task can be approached in three different ways: (1) model checking (to determine whether the problem has a solution), (2) search to find a single solution, or (3) search to find all solutions. In this research, we solve the CLP model by searching to find a single solution.

3 Modeling and Combining Multiple CPGs

We start with generating a CLP model for a CPG along with an associated knowledge base ($\mathcal{K}$) containing external information about adverse interactions between patient's conditions. Second, for a patient with comorbidity all individual models relevant to a patient's condition are combined into a single CLP model and this combined model is solved. A solution includes a set of valid actions and when one doesn't exist, we identify the inconsistencies.

3.1 Modeling a Single CPG

We start with a flowchart CPG representation that is converted to a decision graph from which logical rules are derived (each possible path in the decision graph becomes a rule). These rules are used to generate a CLP model of the guideline. For the sake of brevity we will describe in detail only the last step of this modeling process (details of the former steps are presented in [6]). As a working example, we use a peptic ulcer condition. The starting point for the modeling process is the set of logical rules generated from the AIHA[1] Peptic Ulcer in Adults CPG.

We augment a CPG with information from a knowledge base representing external knowledge not included in the guideline. Drug interactions that are established from the Epocrates database[2] are examples of knowledge that affects the realization of a patient's treatment plan. An external knowledge base is represented as a set of clauses. Given the set of logical rules representing a CPG and a set of clauses representing an external knowledge base associated with the given CPG, we map them into a CLP model. All variables in the CLP model correspond to the predicates in the rules. We refer to this model as a *CLP-CPG model* and one for peptic-ulcer is shown in Figure 1.

$$\mathcal{V} = (CUS, SC, CNSAID, NSAID, PET, PHPT, ET, OD, OC, IC)$$
$$\mathcal{CL} = \left\{ \begin{array}{c} CUS \rightarrow SC \equiv true \\ \neg CUS \wedge CNSAID \rightarrow \neg NSAID \equiv true, \\ \neg CUS \wedge \neg CNSAID \wedge PET \rightarrow SC \equiv true, \\ \neg CUS \wedge \neg CNSAID \wedge \neg PET \wedge PHPT \rightarrow ET \equiv true, \\ \neg CUS \wedge \neg CNSAID \wedge \neg PET \wedge \neg PHPT \rightarrow OD \equiv true, \\ \neg OC \equiv true,\ \neg NSAID \equiv true,\ \neg(ET \wedge IC) \equiv true \end{array} \right\}$$

Fig. 1. CLP-CPG model of the peptic-ulcer CPG

A rule-based model of the CPG always has a feasible assignment of values because the original CPG, by definition, always provides diagnosis and a treatment recommendation when presented with valid patient information. Moreover, the clauses introduced by the external knowledge base do not affect feasibility, thus

[1] www.aiha.org

[2] www.epocrates.com

by transitivity, a CLP-CPG model will also always provide a solution given a valid instantiation of variables. However, when combining CLP-CPG models to create a combined CLP model representing multiple CPGs, we can no longer guarantee the existence of a solution.

3.2 Combining Multiple CPGs

In a combined CLP-CPG model, the set of variables is simply the superset of variables in the individual models and the set of constraints is the union of constraints from each model. In cases where there are no shared variables between single models, solving the combined model is equivalent to solving each CLP-CPG independently. In the case of a combined model with variables present across multiple constraints, this dependence results in a solution that is constrained by the interaction of multiple CPGs.

There are several challenges associated with the concurrent use of CPGs and here we focus on those that involve inconsistencies. The inconsistencies can occur at two levels. One is related to drug interactions when combining different medications and the other is related to drug-disease interactions [7] where a certain medication can exacerbate symptoms of a condition. Thus, when combining multiple CLP-CPG models to account for comorbid condition, it is necessary to identify inconsistencies if they exist. We call such inconsistencies *points of contention (POC)*.

Formally, a POC is defined as follows:

Definition 1. *A POC is a set of variables T in the combined CLP-CPG model whose domains are annihilated (reduced to the empty set) during search, resulting in no found solution.*

A POC occurs when given a patient's state one CPG explicitly identifies a class of actions that are inadmissible according to some actions defined by another CPG. When considering a combined CLP-CPG model, we are also able to identify a POC that is not evident from consulting only the CPGs themselves but becomes apparent when external knowledge is introduced. The first step to eliminating a POC is to check whether it is due to a variable's value assigned during search for a solution or due to a variable with a value predefined according to available patient information. In the first case we use standard backtrack search to find a valid solution representing a course of feasible actions. If backtracking does not produce a solution or the POC is caused by a variable's predefined value, the problem becomes more difficult. Our approach is to present the physician with a partial solution along with the identified POC. The partial solution includes assignments of values to variables not included in the POC and the POC itself provides information that is used by the physician in making treatment decisions. We use backmarking [1], available as part of the ECLiPSe[3] solver, as a method to generate a partial solution.

[3] www.eclipseclp.org

3.3 A Case Study

To illustrate our proposed approach, we generated CLP-CPG models from asthma and peptic ulcer CPGs using the process described in Section 3.1. We solve the combined CLP-CPG model using the ECLiPSe system. We constructed various real-world scenarios for patients with comorbidity involving asthma exacerbation and peptic ulcer by assigning different initial values to variables. Due to a lack of space, we only summarize our results below.

For scenarios with no POC, we were able to return a valid solution that assigned values to unbounded variables. For the scenarios where no solution was found, we were able to identify the source of the inconsistency (POC). To our knowledge this is the first time inconstancies in concurrently used CPGs were automatically identified and flagged for further action by the physician.

The considered CPGs were quite simple. More complex CPGs may result not only in a larger number of variables, but also a larger number of constraints. Additionally the nesting and temporal dimension of a complex CPG can become issues that produce more variables. However, CLPs are solved for millions of variables and constraints in practice therefore these issues will not present a computational problem.

4 Discussion and Future Work

The approach presented in this paper is one of the few attempts to use CPG models as an active support tool that provides solutions for incomplete patient information and helps a physician identify inconsistencies in two (or more) CPGs for a patient with comorbidity. In our future work we will focus on representing more complex CPGs and developing external knowledge bases representing comprehensive interactions. We are exploring several ideas for improving the technique of revising CPGs according to identified POCs by using domain knowledge, thus significantly diminishing the need for revisions made by the physician.

Acknowledgements. Research described in this paper was funded by grants from the Natural Sciences and Engineering Research Council of Canada. The third author acknowledges support of the Polish Ministry of Science and Higher Education. The authors would like to thank Professor Brian Rowe, M.D. from the University of Alberta Hospital for help with interpreting clinical practice guidelines.

References

1. Dechter, R.: Constraint Processing. The MIT Press, Cambridge (1989)
2. Cabana, M.D., Rand, C.S., Powe, N.R., Wu, A.W., Wilson, M.H., Abboud, P.A.C., Rubin, H.R.: Why don't physicians follow clinical practice guidelines? a framework for improvement. Journ. of the American Medical Assoc. 282, 1458–1465 (1999)
3. Latoszek-Berendsen, A., Tange, H., van den Herik, J., Hasman, A.: From clinical practice guidelines to computer-interpretable guidelines. Methods of Information in Medicine 49(6), 550–570 (2010)

4. Horvitz, E.: Automated reasoning for biology and medicine. In: Advances in Computer Methods for Systematic Biology: Artificial Intelligence, Databases, and Computer Vision (1993)
5. Charles, J., Petrie, J.: Revised dependency-directed backtracking for default reasoning'. In: AAAI 1987, pp. 167–172 (1987)
6. Hing, M.M., Michalowski, M., Wilk, S., Michalowski, W., Farion, K.: Identifying inconsistencies in multiple clinical practice guidelines for a patient with co-morbidity. In: Proc. of KEDDH 2010, pp. 447–452 (2010)
7. Lindblad, C., Hanlon, J., Ross, C., Sloane, R., Pieper, C., Hajjar, E., Ruby, C., Schmader, K.: Clinically important drug-disease interactions and their prevalence in older adults. Clinical Therapeutics 28(8), 1133–1143 (2006)

Towards the Formalization of Guidelines Care Actions Using Patterns and Semantic Web Technologies

Cédric Pruski[1], Rodrigo Bonacin[1,2], and Marcos Da Silveira[1]

[1] CR SANTEC, Centre de Recherche Public - Henri Tudor, 2A rue Kalchesbrück, L-1852 Luxembourg
{cedric.pruski,marcos.dasilveira}@tudor.lu
[2] CTI Renato Archer, Rodovia Dom Pedro I, km 143,6, 13069-901, Campinas, SP, Brazil
rodrigo.bonacin@cti.gov.br

Abstract. Computer Interpretable Guidelines (CIG) have largely contributed to the simplification and dissemination of clinical guidelines. However, the formalization of CIG contents, especially care actions, is still an open issue. Actually, this information, which is the heart of the guideline, is still expressed as free text and therefore prevents the development of intelligent tools for assisting physicians defining treatments. In this paper, we introduce a framework for formalizing care actions using natural language processing techniques, Semantic Web technologies and medical standards.

Keywords: CIG, Natural Language Processing, Ontologies, Semantic Web.

1 Introduction

If CIGs have drastically improved the simplification and dissemination of clinical guidelines, there are still open issues. Actually, the expression of care actions denoting elements of the CIGs that intend to recommend something to be performed by health professionals is often done by using free text. In consequence, these expressions offer limited possibilities to be exploited in an efficient way by computers which in turn prevent the development of decision support tools for assisting healthcare professionals building the most appropriate treatment plans for their patients. In addition, there still exists a gap between some guidelines' specification framework and the application of the designed CIGs, mainly when patient's data is required [1]. Actually, existing medical information systems are using standard approaches like Health Level 7 (HL7), for building patients' health record (PHR) and stored it in the system. However, the current CIG execution tools are not able to automatically exploit this information because the connection between data and guidelines is not explicitly provided or in some cases this link is CIG specification language dependent [1].

This paper proposes, on the one hand, an approach to formalize care actions using linguistic patterns [2], [3] and Semantic Web technologies and, on the other hand, a (semi-)automatic way to build the link between the resulting formalization of the guidelines and the PHR. This is done through the consistent use of standards like the

M. Peleg, N. Lavrač, and C. Combi (Eds.): AIME 2011, LNAI 6747, pp. 302–306, 2011.

Unified Medical Language System (UMLS) and the Reference Information Model (RIM). Our approach is part of the global iCareflow framework [4]. It is guideline specification language independent and aims at deriving computer interpretable guidelines to personalized careflows using logic rules and Semantic Web technologies, and can be used in complement to the approach presented in [5].

The remainder of the paper is structured as follows: Section 2 introduces the conceptual framework for the formalization of care actions including the definition of the approach's elements. We wrap up with concluding remarks and outline future work in Section 3.

2 The Medical Action Formalization Framework

The Medical Action Formalization Framework (MedAForm) is basically the element of the iCareflow approach [4] that deals with the formalization of care actions contained in CIGs. This section is devoted to the description of the concepts composing the MedAForm framework.

2.1 Care Action Formalization

Our approach is performed in two steps (Fig 1): First, the care actions are extracted from CIGs and associated with standard vocabularies; second, these actions are associated to a standard data model via the generation of an ontology.

In the first step the text describing the care actions is used as input. This text, coming from a CIG independently of its specification language, is split into linguistic tokens in order to map them to a model representing medical knowledge like UMLS. It produces a set of *Actions Information* according to pre-defined selection's rules. It is basically all elements of the text that match elements of the knowledge model together with its associated formal concept inferred using the medical knowledge during the mapping process.

In the second step, the actions information is compared with a set of pre-defined patterns in order to identify the pattern group that each action belongs to. The output consists of an instance of a *reference model* (e.g. RIM), which serves as a link between the formalized guidelines and the patient health record for personalization and execution purposes in our global approach [4].

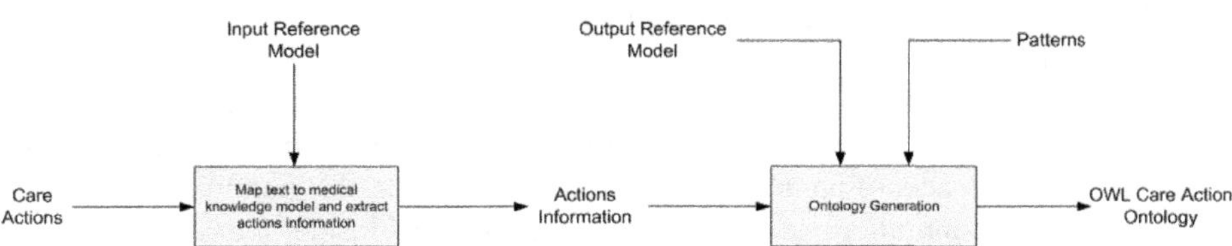

Fig. 1. The MedAForm Approach

The implementation of our approach is carried out through the definition and the use of patterns, ontology, and logic rules under the SWRL format which are described in the forthcoming sections.

2.1.1 Linguistic Pattern Matching

The selection of the pattern is done in a semi-automatic way. The initial set of patterns has been inspired by [3] and enriched after analyzing over 200 care actions extracted from guidelines implemented in SAGE [6] and PRO*forma* [7]. The goal is to generate an OWL ontology corresponding to the formal representation of the care actions contained in the guidelines, for adaptation purpose. The set of patterns we proposed contains information coming from the reference medical knowledge model and from the output model (see Fig. 1) in addition to the linguistic elements. The proposed set of patterns follows the format below:

(LinguisticElement, PatternOntology, Rules)

The *LinguisticElement* contained in the pattern indicates the type of action we are facing (i.e. a substance administration therapy, a radiological act, etc.). It is usually a verb which acts as a key to find the most appropriate pattern regarding the care action given as input. According to our study, 20 verbs cover more than 50% of the care actions and 5 verbs cover 24% of the selected actions information, hence we define:

$$\text{Linguistic element}=\left\{\begin{matrix}\text{Use, Give, Refer, Control, Set, Discharge, Account,}\\ \text{Return, Direct, Base, Treat, Supply,...}\end{matrix}\right\}$$

The *PatternOntology* denotes the OWL ontology that contains concepts and relations to represent the care action given as input at a high level of abstraction. The ontology is populated with individuals whose labels are defined using the terms composing the care action, which have been mapped to the knowledge model. This ontology is common to all patterns and aligned with the UMLS semantic network.

Rules denotes a set of SWRL rules. It enables the definition of equivalent concepts of *PatternOntology* to concepts of the ontology representing the output reference model and which makes it possible to link the guideline with the patient's data.

Example: Consider the following care action *"Give oral activated charcoal 50g"* that has been extracted from the Tallis[1] set of guidelines.

In the above example, the left part corresponds to the *Pattern Ontology* describing the care action in the UMLS model (classes of this ontology are equivalent to those of the UMLS semantic network). The linguistic element is *Give*, boxes associated with circles represent the classes of the care action and boxes associated with diamonds denote individuals. These are created using the information extracted by the linguistic analyzer implemented at information extraction step (see Fig. 1). Their label corresponds to the terms of input care action user wants to formalize. The red arrows illustrate the mapping function defined through SWRL Rules. Since the set of rules to apply is selected according to the linguistic element of the pattern, there are no ambiguities and contradictions in the used rules. Elements inside of dashed lines serve as input to refine the representation of the action in the output model. In this example, sets in dashed line explain the construction of the SWRL rules[2].

---

[1] `http://www.cossac.org/tallis`

[2] In Fig. 2, only two rules are mentioned for readability reasons.

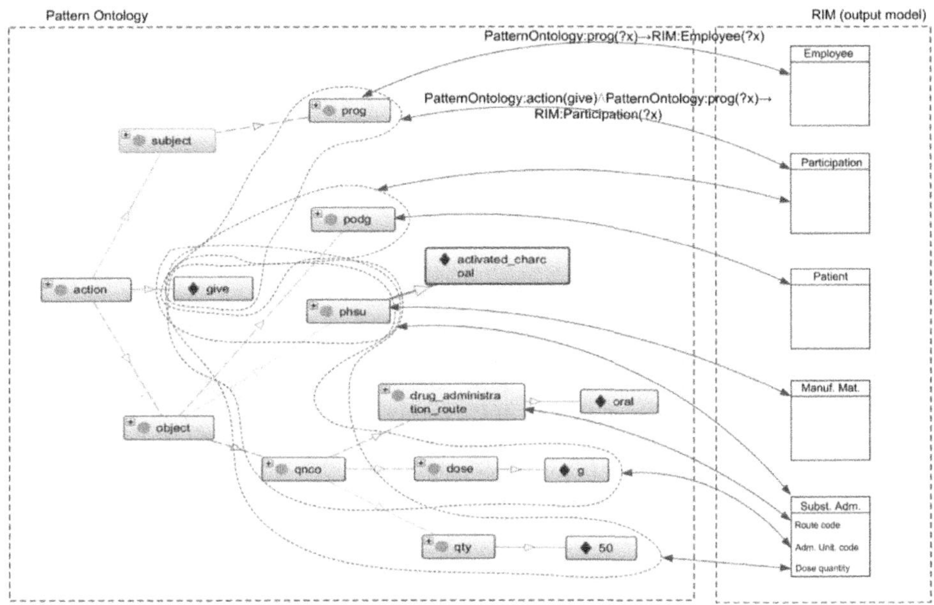

Fig. 2. Illustrative Example

At run time, the selection of the pattern is done in a semi-automatic way. The system starts by matching the *linguistic elements* of the existing patterns and those of the care actions. If several elements are detected, ambiguities are removed in a cyclic way by using the *PatternOntology*. As the *PatternOntology* is aligned with the medical knowledge model to extract the information from the care action, the system maps the classes of the *PatternOntology* with the information extracted based on the medical knowledge model. The system stops if the information can no longer be exploited. If several patterns remain, the user selects the most appropriate one.

2.1.2 Ontology Generation

Patterns serve as basis for the building of the ontology representing the initial guideline. The classes of the generated ontology are mapped to classes or a set of classes of the *PatternOntology*. The resulting ontology is expressed in OWL for homogeneity reasons. Then it is populated by individuals, inferred from using the individuals of the *PatternOntology* in combination with the SWRL rules.

In the example of Fig. 2, the instance of the class "Manuf. Mat." is "activated charcoal". It has been inferred from using the following SWRL rule:

PatternOntology:phsu(?x)→RIM:ManufMat(?x)

3 Conclusion

In this paper we have presented an approach to formally describe care actions in a way that can be linked to patients' medical records. The introduced framework, which is guideline specification language independent, implements linguistic patterns, Semantic Web technologies and is compatible with well-accepted standards. In our future tasks we will first consider creating a repository for linguistic patterns and we will improve the interface of the tool for facilitating both the capture of care actions and the construction of new linguistic patterns.

References

1. Peleg, M., Keren, S., Denekamp, Y.: Mapping Computerized Clinical Guidelines to Electronic Medical Records: Knowledge-Data Ontological Mapper (KDOM). Journal of Biomedical Informatics 41, 180–201 (2008)
2. Essaihi, A., Michel, G., Shiffman, R.N.: Comprehensive Categorization of Guideline Recommendations: Creating an Action Palette for Implementers. In: Proc. AMIA Symp. (American Medical Informatics Association), Washington D.C., pp. 220–224 (2003)
3. Serban, R., ten Teije, A., van Harmelen, F., Marcos, M., Polo-Conde, C.: Extraction and use of linguistic patterns for modelling medical guidelines. Artif. Intell. Med. 39, 137–149 (2007)
4. Bonacin, R., Da Silveira, M., Pruski, C.: From Medical Guidelines to Personalized Careflows: the iCareflow Ontological Framework. In: The 23rd IEEE International Symposium on Computer-Based Medical Systems. IEEE Computer Society, Perth (2010)
5. Kaiser, K., Akkaya, C., Miksch, S.: How can information extraction ease formalizing treatment processes in clinical practice guidelines?: A method and its evaluation. Artificial Intelligence in Medicine 39, 151–163 (2007)
6. Beard, N., Campbel, J.R., Huff, S.M., Leon, M., Mansfield, J.G., Mays, E., McClay, J.C., Mohr, D.N., Musen, M.A., O'Brien, D., Rocha, R.A., Saulovich, A., Scheitel, S.M., Tu, S.W.: Standards-Based Sharable Active Guideline Environment (SAGE): A Project to Develop a Universal Framework for Encoding and Disseminating Electronic Clinical Practice Guidelines. In: Proc. AMIA Symp., p. 973 (2002)
7. Fox, J., Johns, N., Rahmanzadeh, A.: Disseminating medical knowledge: The PROforma approach. Artificial Intelligence in Medicine 14, 157–181 (1998)

Exploiting OWL Reasoning Services to Execute Ontologically-Modeled Clinical Practice Guidelines

Borna Jafarpour, Samina Raza Abidi, and Syed Sibte Raza Abidi

NICHE Research Group, Computer Science Deapartment, Dalhousie University
{borna,abidi,sraza}@cs.dal.ca

Abstract. Ontology-based modeling of Clinical Practice Guidelines (CPG) is a well-established approach to computerize CPG for execution in clinical decision support systems. Many CPG computerization approaches use the Web Ontology Language (OWL) to represent the CPG's knowledge, but they do not exploit its reasoning services to execute the CPG. In this paper, we present our CPG execution approach that leverages OWL reasoning services to execute CPG. In this way, both CPG knowledge representation and execution semantics are maintained within the same formalism. We have developed three different OWL-based CPG execution engines using OWL-DL, OWL 2 and SWRL. We evaluate the efficacy of our execution engines by executing an existing OWL based CPG. We also present a comparison of the execution capabilities of our three CPG execution engines.

Keywords: Clinical Guidelines, Semantic Web, Execution Engine, OWL.

1 Introduction

To operationalize Clinical Practice Guidelines (CPG) in clinical care settings there exist a variety of methods to computerize the paper-based CPG in terms of computer interpretable format and then to execute the computerized CPG through clinical decision support systems. A few approaches to mention are PRO*forma*, GLIF, and EON.

Semantic Web technologies offer (a) knowledge representation languages for authoring ontologies that encapsulate the knowledge regarding a specific topic and (b) reasoning services that can be used to perform reasoning on the modeled knowledge.

Although OWL, as a knowledge modeling language, is extensively used to represent the CPG knowledge [3], [5], [6], the reasoning potential of OWL is not properly exploited to execute the OWL-based CPG models. There are a few semantic web based execution engine that use Semantic Web Rule Language (SWRL) to execute CPG that are modeled using OWL [1], [2]. However, these execution engines are closely tied to a specific CPG and are not generic enough to be applied to other guidelines.

In this paper, we explore the use of OWL reasoning services to develop generic execution engines that can execute CPG modeled in OWL. We present three generic OWL-based CPG execution engines based on OWL-DL, OWL 2 and OWL-DL + SWRL. We present a comparison of the executional capabilities of our CPG

M. Peleg, N. Lavrač, and C. Combi (Eds.): AIME 2011, LNAI 6747, pp. 307–311, 2011.

execution engines. We also compare their execution performance by executing a CPG modeled in an OWL-based CPG ontology [6].

2 OWL-Based Execution of Clinical Practice Guidelines

As per our approach, to execute an ontologically modeled CPG through OWL-based reasoning services, it is necessary to preprocess the OWL-based CPG in order to supplement it with additional OWL constructs to further enhance the executional semantics to the OWL-based CPG. This extension of the original OWL-based CPG to an *extended* OWL-based CPG is required to (a) address the Open-World (OWA) and Non-unique Naming Assumptions (NNA) adopted by OWL reasoners, (b) handle preconditions, (c) provide a richer data-type expressivity for performing mathematical and logical operations on patient data, (d) handle loops and (e) handle state transitions. The nature of the extensions to the original OWL-based CPG is determined by the requirements of the target CPG execution engine.

Our CPG execution engine is composed of a program that uses an API to load, save and manipulate the CPG ontology and an OWL reasoner. Our execution engine program performs queries to find *Active* tasks and inserts triples in the ontology to record (a) the completion of tasks, (b) any output/recommendation/decision generated by tasks. All the execution activities—such as finding the next tasks, checking preconditions, state transitions—are undertaken by the OWL reasoner within the CPG ontology. We use Pellet as the reasoner and Jena as the API to load, manipulate and save OWL files in this project. TURTLE syntax is used to demonstrate the OWL constructs used in this paper.

2.1 OWL-DL Based CPG Execution Engine

Our first CPG execution engine uses OWL-DL which is the most expressive yet decidable species of OWL. However, this CPG execution engine does not support the handling of loops and mathematical functions. We explain below how we extended the original OWL-based CPG ontology to address the below issues so that the OWL reasoners can effectively execute the CPG:

State Transitions. Our execution is governed by a state transition model which consists of five different states: *Inactive*, *Active*, *Completed*, *Discarded*, *WaitingForSubsteps* (Wfss). To handle the desired state transitions, specific OWL triples are added to the ontology. For instance, the state transition rule "A composite task is completed if all of its sub tasks (denoted by *hasTask* property) are completed" is implemented by assertion of the following triple set:

```
[a owl:Restriction; owl:onProperty :hasTask;
owl:allValuesFrom :Completed]rdfs:subClassOf :Completed.
```

Preconditions. Handling precondition satisfaction criteria of "all" or "any" can be easily implemented using *owl:allValuesFrom* and *owl:someValuesFrom,* respectively. However, handling "any *k*" rules needs Qualified Cardinality Restriction (QCR) expressivity which is not supported in OWL. Our workaround is to create *n!/(n-k)!k!* intermediate nodes which represent different combination of *k* out of *n* preconditions. A combination point is satisfied when all of its assigned preconditions are satisfied (*owl:allValuesFrom*) and a task has a satisfied criterion when at least one of its combination points is satisfied (*owl:someValuesFrom*). This method may create a large number of intermediate nodes which can slow down the reasoning process.

Open-World Assumption and Non-unique Naming Assumption. The OWA states that from the absence of a statement, a reasoner cannot infer that it is true. NNA states that it is possible that two names refer to the same entity. For instance, if task *t1* has two subtasks *t11* and *t12* which are *Completed*, we expect the OWL reasoner to infer that *t1* is *Completed* as well. However, because of the abovementioned assumption, this is will not happen and we need to assert that *t1* has exactly two subtasks (because of OWA) and they are not referring to the same task with different names (because of NNA) to draw the desired conclusion.

```
:t1 a [a owl:Restriction owl:onProperty :hasTask owl:cardinality 2]".
:t11 owl:differentFrom :t12
```

2.2 OWL 2 Based CPG Execution Engine

OWL 2 is the new version of OWL, and its advantage for CPG execution purposes is that it (a) supports QCR that allow to efficiently handle "any *k* out of *n*" precondition satisfaction criteria, and (b) offers datatype expressivity to handle user defined ranges when comparing numeric values of datatype properties. The OWL 2 CPG execution engine builds on the OWL-DL execution algorithm and state transition strategy, with additional methods to (a) handle preconditions more effectively and (b) perform numeric comparisons to evaluate preconditions. Preconditions are handled more effectively because there is no longer the need to create *n!/(n-k)!k!* intermediate nodes. We illustrate the OWL 2 based improvements to address the following issues:

Preconditions. To handle satisfaction criterion of "any *k* out of *n*", we iterate over the tasks and create three OWL classes for each *k* that we encounter during processing: (i) *Task_Preconditions_**Required**_k*: shows the minimum number of preconditions that should be satisfied in order to say that the task's criterion is satisfied. The task with the criterion "any *k*" is set as an instance of this class (during preprocessing) (ii) *Task_Preconditions_**Satisfied**_k* whose members are the tasks that have at least *k* preconditions satisfied at that point in time (During execution). Note that this does not signify the exact number of preconditions that the task needs to be satisfied in order for it to be deemed as being complete. It uses the QCR capability of OWL 2 in the following way:

```
:Task_Preconditions_Satisfied_k a
[a owl:Restriction; owl:onProperty :hasPrecondition;
owl:onClass :SatisfiedPrecondition; owl:minQualifiedCardinality k].
```

(iii) An intersection of these two classes which represents the tasks that are waiting for *k* preconditions and have at least *k* satisfied precondition and should be regarded as tasks with satisfied precondition criterion.

Datatype Expressivity. To handle a precondition (*p1*) such as "older than 18" we need to compare the age of the patient against a data range. Our solution is to create three classes for each comparison: (a) *Precondition_**Should**_GT_18* whose instances are assigned during preprocessing, (b) *Precondition_**Has**_GT_18* whose instances are entities with a value larger than 18 for their *hasAge* property and are assigned via the data ranges capability of OWL 2 during execution and (c) intersection of the above mentioned classes which is a subclass of *TaskSatisfiedPrecondition*.

2.3 OWL-DL + SWRL Based Execution Engine

OWL 2 has the following limitations for the purposes of CPG execution: (a) no ability to handle loops because of the lack of a mathematical function for incrementing a counter; (b) limited data type expressivity. For instance, it cannot compare two property values that are entered during execution (e.g. is first blood work measurement showing a value greater than that of the second one?).

To address these shortcomings, we have developed an execution engine that leverages SWRL Comparison and Math built-ins to enhance the functionalities of the OWL-DL based execution engine. These SWRL rules are added to the OWL-DL based execution engine during preprocessing. To account for decidability issues that may arise as a result of using SWRL we have developed a DL-Safe [4] solution for handling loops. Data type expressivity and loops are handled in the following fashion:

Datatype Expressivity. OWL-DL and OWL 2 are not capable of comparing two property values from two different objects. This can be necessary for comparisons of two values that are entered during execution of the guideline. We used SWRL rules and its built-ins for this mean. For instance, the built in *swrlb:greaterThan* is used to handle all "*GreaterThan*" comparison criteria in the CPG.

```
hasNumericValue(?v1,nv1) ^ hasNumericValue(?v2, ?nv2)  ^
hasComparisonCriteria(?comparison, greaterThan) ^
swrlb:greaterThan(?nv1, ?nv2) → SatisfiedPrecondition(?p)
```

Loops. Using a single value and a single rule to keep the record of iteration is not DL-Safe because the OWL reasoner uses the new value to fire the rule infinitely. This causes undecidability in the ontology. We use SWRL built-in *swrlb:add* to manage a counter for *for* loops and impement a DL-Safe solution by defining two datatype properties: *hasItrNum* that holds the iteration number and is set 0 at the beginning and *hasItrNumCopy* that holds a copy of the *hasItrNum*'s value. The loop handling rules operate as follows: (i) When the first task of the loops is *Completed*, value of *hasItrNum* is copied to *hasItrNumCopy*, and (ii) When the last task of the loop is *Completed*, 1 is added to *hasItrNumCopy* and its value is copied to *hasItrNum*. Loop is terminated when we reach the maximum number of iterations.

3 Discussion and Comparison

We tested and measured performance of our execution engines by execution of the CPG for Congestive Heart Failure and Atrial Fibrillation explained in [6] and through a range of clinical scenarios that were developed by medical experts. Same experts validated the correctness of the generated recommendations based on the CPG under execution. We also developed a graph traversal based execution engine [5] which is included in the speed and executional capabilities comparison of Table 1. Basic Execution Tasks are what OWL-DL offers.

Table 1. Capabilities (± : somewhat supported, +: supported, -: not supported) and performance (1 is the fastest) of the CPG execution approaches

	Graph Traversal	OWL-DL	OWL 2	SWRL
Basic Execution Tasks	+	+	+	+
QCR	+	-	+	+
DataTypeExpressivity	+	-	±	+
Rules	-	-	-	+
Reasoning	-	+	+	+
Loops	+	-	±	+
Speed	1	2	3	4

Table 1shows that from a speed perspective, graph traversal based approaches seem to be superior to semantic web approaches. However, it should be noted that the graph traversal based execution approaches do not directly support reasoning (based on intermediate results and inputs), handling of a range of relations (such as functional, transitive, causal, etc) and exceptions—given the complexity of CPG and the criticality of the knowledge processing expected in clinical setting these functionalities are important to have in a CPG execution engine. From an implementation perspective, graph based approach create a tight coupling between the CPG ontology, the execution engine, and technologies that are used in it which makes the execution engine tied to specific technologies. On the contrary, semantic web approaches allow for the execution semantics to be represented separately, such that the reasoner can establish the necessary linkages between the domain knowledge and the execution semantics, which results in flexibility to choose technologies to execute the guidelines. Hence, we argue that OWL based approaches for CPG execution provide a comprehensive and sound execution environment.

References

1. Arguello Casteleiro, M., Des, J., Prieto, M.J., et al.: Executing Medical Guidelines on the Web: Towards Next Generation Healthcare. Knowl-Based Syst. 22, 545–551 (2009)
2. Casteleiro, M.A., Des Diz, J.J.: Clinical Practice Guidelines: A Case Study of Combining OWL-S, OWL, and SWRL. Knowl-Based Syst. 21, 247–255 (2008)
3. Daniyal, A., Abidi, S.R., Abidi, S.S.R.: Computerizing Clinical Pathways: Ontology-Based Modeling and Execution. Stud. Health Technol. Inform. 150, 643–647 (2009)
4. Motik, B., Sattler, U., Studer, R.: Query Answering for OWL-DL with Rules. Web Semant. 3, 41–60 (2005)
5. Din, M.A., Abidi, S.S.R., Jafarpour, B.: Ontology Based Modeling and Execution of Nursing Care Plans and Practice Guidelines. In: 13th World Congress on Medical Informatics. IOS Press, Cape Town (2010)
6. Abidi, S.: Ontology-Based Knowledge Modeling to Provide Decision Support for Comorbid Diseases. In: Riaño, D., ten Teije, A., Miksch, S., Peleg, M. (eds.) KR4HC 2010. LNCS, vol. 6512, pp. 27–39. Springer, Heidelberg (2011)

Guideline Recommendation Text Disambiguation, Representation and Testing

Silvana Quaglini[1], Silvia Panzarasa[2], Anna Cavallini[3], and Giuseppe Micieli[3]

[1] Dept. of Computer Science and Systems, University of Pavia
[2] CBIM, Pavia
[3] IRCCS Foundation "C. Mondino", Pavia

Abstract. This paper describes a knowledge acquisition tool for translating a guideline recommendation into a computer-interpretable format. The novelty of the tool is that it is addressed to the domain experts, and it helps them to disambiguate the natural language, by decomposing the recommendation into elements, eliciting tacit and implicit knowledge hidden into a recommendation and its context, mapping patient's data, available from the electronic record, to standard terms and immediately testing the formalised rule using past cases data.

Keywords: clinical practice guidelines; compliance; knowledge acquisition; formalization.

1 Introduction

In previous papers, we described both our real-time decision support systems (DSSs), based on workflow technology, the so-called "Careflow Management Systems-CfMS" [1], and the off-line module RoMA (Reasoning on Medical Actions), for non-compliance detection and classification [2]. Both systems require the transformation of the knowledge contained in the guideline (GL) recommendations text into formal rules interpretable by a computer system.

The field of medical knowledge acquisition and representation has been extensively explored since the first appearance of medical expert systems in the 1970's [3, 4] until the latest GL-based DSS [5, 6, 7,8]. Representation formalisms have been analyzed and compared in relation to their capabilities of capturing the main patterns of tasks present in a GL and of mapping with the EPR [9].

The knowledge conversion process is a critical point: if errors occur, they are cause of frustration for users, that are annoyed with useless or, even worse, inappropriate advises. This may cause abandoning the DSS. That's why big attention must be put on proper interpretation and formalization of GLs, even if it is a very time-consuming task that requires a strong, continuous collaboration among professionals of different categories e.g., domain experts, knowledge engineers, physicians and other healthcare practitioners, and sometime patients [10]. To develop a collaboration network among these subjects, an architecture is needed.

The use case described in this paper will refer to an integrated system for stroke management, where data are collected in two databases with two different purposes: an electronic medical record, storing detailed data in a Stroke Unit, and a stroke

M. Peleg, N. Lavrač, and C. Combi (Eds.): AIME 2011, LNAI 6747, pp. 312–316, 2011.

registry, collecting summary discharge data from 41 regional centers. All these centers adopt the same GLs, called SPREAD (Stroke Prevention and Education Awareness Diffusion)[11]. The intent of this article is not to describe yet a new formalism for representing GLs, nor a new language for writing GL rules, but to present a tool (FORMA) for making the knowledge conversion process more agile for the domain expert, facilitating his interaction with other subjects involved and supporting all the phases for the disambiguation of the natural language.

2 The Solution Proposed

Typically, formalizing a recommendation starting from a narrative text involves various and non-banal kinds of reasoning, to be developed in different steps: 1) identification of relevant knowledge; 2) disambiguation of GL knowledge in order to clarify eligibility conditions (both the inclusion and exclusion criteria) and actions to be done; 3) identification of clinical concepts and their relationships by means of high-level abstractions; 4) mapping the terms in the knowledge base to the terms adopted by the specific institution (through a link with the specific EPR) and 5) modeling of the recommendation through rules, using standard terminology and computational language, such as Structured Query Language (SQL).

Point 4 is very important in order to bridge the gap between the concepts, outlined in step 3 and modeled in step 5, and their actual representation in daily data entry practice. Moreover, an appropriate level of abstraction is desired, to obtain well understood concepts, not tied to a particular EPR implementation. Abstractions, from a cognitive point of view, are very important, allowing to reason on an higher level and to infer a qualitative clinical status from raw data (e.g. *severe stroke* = NIHSS>5).

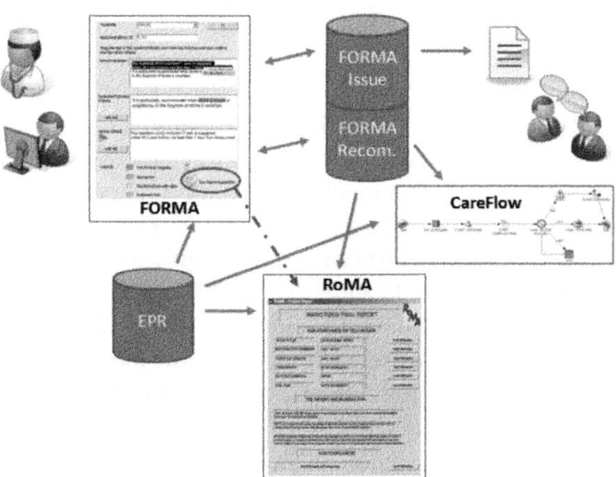

Fig. 1. The architecture of the solution proposed

As described in detail in section 3, the FORMA tool supports the domain expert in the above illustrated steps. Figure 1 shows the architecture of the proposed solution, highlighting the interactions between FORMA and the other systems we implemented.

3 The FORMA Tool

As the first step of the formalization process, the user enters the GL name, the recommendation identifier, and its text in the *recommendation box*, as shown in Figure 2, using keyboard or copy&paste from the GL itself.

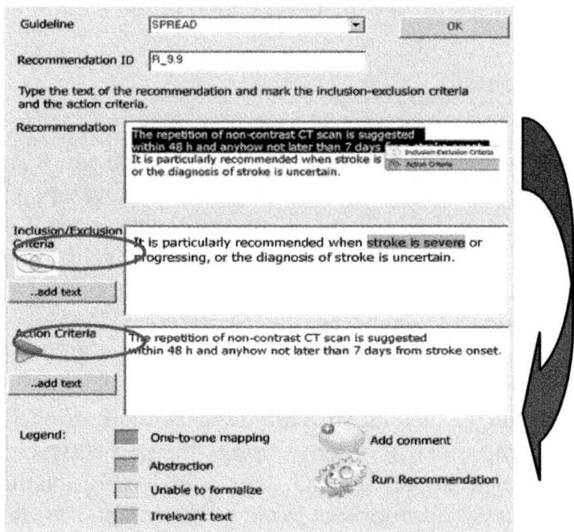

Fig. 2. Form for the entry and mark-up of a recommendation

The text of the recommendation must be analyzed in order to highlight, first of all, the *inclusion-exclusion criteria* and the *action criteria* (action criteria represent either therapeutic action or conclusions reached in case of diagnostic recommendations). The user marks a portion of the text and select the type of criteria to which it refers and the portion of the text is automatically copied into the corresponding section. This step is required for the formalization of the recommendation through the formal rules used by our tools [2]: the inclusion/exclusion conditions constitute the IF part of the rule, while the action criteria represent the THEN part of the rule [8]. For each criteria, the clinical concepts should be identified prior to formalize the recommendation (see legend in Figure 2) by differentiating concepts that can be mapped directly to EPR data items (*one-to-one mapping*), concepts that must be defined by *abstractions*, parts not relevant for the formalization (*irrelevant text*) and portions of text that, while relevant, cannot be formalized exploiting the information actually available in the DB (*unable to formalize*), for example expressions like “clinically stable”, “progressing stroke” or “any clinical condition…”. The user is also allowed to explicitly write down new criteria (see “…add text” in Figure 2) when she/he desires to represent *knowledge* that is *tacit* or *missing* in the original text of the recommendation. These criteria will be formalized as the rest of the recommendation. However, keeping track of these additions is very important: the text of the GLs is periodically revised and, upon the experts consensus, this knowledge can be *officially* added to the GL.

FORMA allows the user storing notes or questions, related to a specific recommendation or medical concept. To include both these comments and additional text, she/he is prompted to specify an *issue type*, selected by a predefined taxonomy, whose main objective is to categorize users' requests to better address them during the discussion with medical experts or the GL periodic revisions.

Once a concept to be formalized has been individuated, the corresponding rule is defined using an expression language and standard terminology. We decided to used SNOMED CT (Systematized Nomenclature of Medicine Clinical Terms). An abstraction can be found within SNOMED as a unique concept, or it can be defined as a relation between different concepts (for example "*stroke is severe*" will be defined by two concepts linked by the relationship "*has_severity*".

The concepts highlighted in the recommendations are mapped with the data item used in the EPR and the abstraction is then defined through a production rule which is automatically translated into SQL with clauses like "WHERE *column* OPERATOR *value*".

When all the information needed to formalize a recommendation has been entered, the user can run it using the connection to the real patients database (button "Run recommendation" in Figure 2). A direct link to RoMA is in fact available, which allows a quick test of the recommendation formalization, on a single patient or on a set of patients data. As a matter of fact, it is difficult, during formalization, to take into account the whole variability of a patient status, and the possibility to see what RoMA detects, or does not detect, as a non-compliance, is very important in order to elicit further hidden or tacit knowledge or discover formalization errors.

All information entered into the FORMA graphical user interface are stored in a database, that serves two purposes:

- to store information about the GL recommendations formalization that will be used both by the CfMS and ROMA. In this way, through a single interface, it is possible to manage the two systems, thus facilitating the maintenance, consistency and updating of recommendations
- to produce reports related to the specific recommendation or the whole GL, highlighting the knowledge added by the operator, unclear concepts, the medical concepts used in the formalization, the corresponding EPR data used, and all the comments/questions inserted. These data may be useful for the SPREAD community of practice and GL revision. .

4 Conclusions and Future Development

This paper has described a knowledge acquisition tool for translating GL recommendations written in natural language into a computer-interpretable format. The distinguishing feature of FORMA, for example in comparison with [8], is its capability to report possible problems encountered during the interpretation, and to elicit/report possible doubts about personal interpretations. FORMA was developed using our past experience in DSS for stroke management and in the formalization of SPREAD GL. In the last SPREAD meeting, FORMA has been proposed to be used "officially" within this medical community, exploiting its functionality from the initial analysis of the text to the recommendations' test phase, and using the results obtained during the periodic revisions of the GL, that occurs every two years. As future development, a recommendation ontology will be developed to better support the user during the formalization, providing the system with automated checking of the rules' completeness. The ultimate goal would be to have, for each type of recommendation, a template of the minimum information set needed for its proper implementation.

References

1. Panzarasa, S., Maddè, S., Quaglini, S., Pistarini, C., Stefanelli, M.: Evidence-based careflow management systems: the case of post-stroke rehabilitation. Journal of Biomedical Informatics 35, 123–139 (2002)
2. Panzarasa, S., Quaglini, S., Cavallini, A., Marcheselli, S., Stefanelli, M., Micieli, G.: Computerised Guidelines Implementation: Obtaining Feedback for Revision of Guidelines, Clinical Data Model and Data Flow. In: Bellazzi, R., Abu-Hanna, A., Hunter, J. (eds.) AIME 2007. LNCS (LNAI), vol. 4594, pp. 461–466. Springer, Heidelberg (2007)
3. Musen, M.A.: An overview of knowledge Acquisition. In: David, J.M., Krivine, J.P., Simmons, R. (eds.) Second Generation Expert Systems, pp. 405–427. Springer, New York (1993)
4. Lanzola, G., Quaglini, S., Stefanelli, M.: Knowledge-Acquisition Tools for Medical Knowledge-Based Systems. Methods of Information in Medicine 34, 25–39 (1995)
5. Serban, R., Puig-Centelles, A., ten Teije, A.: Incremental guideline formalization with tool support. Artificial Intelligence Applications and Innovations IFIP International Federation for Information Processing 204, 106–118 (2006)
6. Terenziani, P., Montani, S., Bottrighi, A., Molino, G., Torchio, M.: Applying artificial intelligence to clinical guidelines: the GLARE approach. Studies in Health Technology and Informatics 139, 273–282 (2008)
7. Peleg, M., Sagi, K., Denekamp, Y.: Mapping Computerized Clinical Guidelines to Electronic Medical Records: Knowledge-Data Ontological Mapper (KDOM). Journal of Biomedical Informatics 41(1), 180–201 (2008)
8. Shiffman, R.N., Michel, G., Essaihi, A.: Bridging the guideline implementation gap: a systematic approach to document-centered guideline implementation. J. Am. Med. Informatics Assoc. 11, 418–426 (2004)
9. Peleg, M., Tu, S., Bury, J., Ciccarese, P., Fox, J., Greenes, R.A., Hall, R., Johnson, P.D., Jones, N., Kumar, A., Miksch, S., Quaglini, S., Seyfang, A., Shortliffe, E.H., Stefanelli, M.: Comparing computer-interpretable guideline models: a case-study approach. J. Am. Med. Inform. Assoc. 10(1), 52–68 (2003)
10. Sharda, P., Das, A., Cohen, T., Patel, V.: Customizing clinical narratives for the electronic medical record interface using cognitive methods. International Journal of Medical Informatics 75, 346–368 (2006)
11. Gschwandtner, T., Kaiser, K., Miksch, S.: Information requisition is the core of guideline-based medical care: which information is needed for whom? Journal of Evaluation in Clinical Practice, 1–9 (August 2010)
12. SPREAD – Stroke Prevention and Educational Awareness Diffusion. Edition of February 16 (2007), `http://www.spread.it`

A Token Centric Part-of-Speech Tagger for Biomedical Text

Neil Barrett* and Jens Weber-Jahnke

Department of Computer Science, University of Victoria, Victoria, Canada
{nbarrett,jens}@uvic.ca
www.simbioses.ca

Abstract. A difficulty with part-of-speech (POS) tagging of biomedical text is accessing and annotating appropriate training corpora. The latter may result in POS taggers trained on corpora that differ from the tagger's target biomedical text. In such cases where training and target corpora differ tagging accuracy decreases. We present a POS tagger that is more accurate than two frequently used biomedical POS taggers (Brill and TnT) when trained on a non-biomedical corpus and evaluated on the MedPost corpus (our tagger: 81.0%, Brill: 77.5%, TnT: 78.2%). Our tagger is also significantly faster than the next best tagger (TnT). It estimates a tag's likelihood for a token by combining prior probabilities (using existing methods) and token probabilities calculated in part using a Naive Bayes classifier. Our results suggest that future work should reexamine POS tagging methods for biomedical text. This differs from the work to date that has focused on retraining existing POS taggers.

Keywords: part-of-speech, POS, tag, TnT, Brill, Naive Bayes, MedPost, accuracy, biomedical.

1 Introduction

Biomedical texts include information related to human health. Several examples of biomedical texts are research papers, medical reference books and clinical documents. Automated processing of biomedical texts can support effective health tools (e.g. [22]). These tools may enhance research processes (e.g. information search) or directly impact quality of care.

Natural language processing (NLP) is computer processing of human language [11] and may be applied to biomedical texts. As an example, Zingmond and Lenert [22] apply NLP to chest X-ray reports to identify new and expanding neoplasms (abnormal tissue growth) for the purpose of monitoring patient follow-ups. Friedman, Knirsch, Shagina and Hripcsak [8] apply NLP to discharge summaries to determine the severity of a patient's community acquired pneumonia.

* This research was funded by the Natural Sciences and Engineering Research Council of Canada.

M. Peleg, N. Lavrač, and C. Combi (Eds.): AIME 2011, LNAI 6747, pp. 317–326, 2011.

Part-of-speech (POS) tagging assigns tags to tokens, such as assigning the tag *noun* to the token *paper*. POS tags and tagging are components of NLP. POS tags supply information about words and surrounding words. For example, POS tags indicate which type of word, such as a noun or a verb, will occur in the vicinity of a tagged word [11]. POS tags affect word pronunciation in text to speech systems [11]. They also improve information retrieval from textual documents, such as the retrieval of names, times, dates and other named entities [11]. POS tags and tagging are an important component of NLP, including NLP of biomedical texts [5,20].

POS taggers are typically trained on linguistically annotated corpora created by human experts. A difficulty with POS tagging of biomedical text is accessing and annotating appropriate training corpora. The latter may result in POS taggers trained on corpora that differ from the tagger's target biomedical text.

In general (see Section 2 for details of previous research), training POS taggers on non-biomedical corpora and applying these trained taggers to biomedical corpora results in an approximate 10% decrease in tagging accuracy. Tagging accuracy is the tagger's ability to assign the correct POS tag to a token. Even in cases where a tagger is trained on one biomedical corpus and applied to a different biomedical corpus a decrease in tagging accuracy can occur [5]. There may be situations where linguistically annotating a corpus for training purposes is infeasible (e.g. financial cost). In such situations it would be beneficial to develop POS tagging methods that perform well across differing corpora.

In this paper, we present a POS tagger that is more accurate than two frequently used biomedical POS taggers when trained on a non-biomedical corpus and evaluated on the MedPost corpus [19]. Our algorithm is also significantly faster than the best tagger of the two frequently used biomedical taggers. Given our work, we suggest how to reduce the difference in accuracy observed when training and application corpora differ.

This paper is organized as follows. Section 2 discusses related work. Our tagger is presented in Section 3. It is evaluated using the method presented in Section 4, with results appearing in Section 5. We discuss these results and their implications to POS tagging of biomedical text in Section 6. Section 7 concludes this paper.

2 Background

Biomedical POS taggers are constructed by retraining existing taggers on biomedical corpora or by supplementing an existing tagger with a biomedical lexicon. In most cases, transformation based or Hidden Markov Model (HMM) taggers are used. These taggers are briefly explained. For more detail see Jurafsky and Martin [11].

Transformation based taggers, such as the Brill tagger [3], work by successively refining assigned tags. Each refinement applies a more specific rule with the goal of assigning a more appropriate tag. Transformation rules may be specified, or learned from templates and training corpora. An example template is: change tag A to B when the preceding word is tagged Z. This rule is applied in the following example drawn from Jurafsky and Martin [11]. Given the word *race* is more likely to be a noun than a verb and the two fragments "to race tomorrow" and "the race for", a transformation based tagger would first tag *race* as a noun and then apply the rule "change noun to verb when the previous tag is TO (word *to*)". This would result in *race* tagged as a verb in "to race tomorrow" and as a noun in "the race for".

HMM taggers such as TnT [2] work by assigning a tag given previous tags and the current token (word). These are respectively named the prior probability and the token probability. In the simplest case, the prior probability is calculated based on one previous tag, simply $P(tag_i|tag_{i-1})$. A standard approach to estimating prior probabilities combines several prior estimates. The token probability is calculated as the probability that a POS tag predicts a given token, $P(word|tag_i)$. The prior probability and token probability are combined to estimate each POS tag. To tag an entire sequence, these tag likelihoods are integrated into a dynamic programming algorithm often referred to as the Viterbi algorithm.

Using mostly transformation based and HMM taggers, researchers have examined whether existing taggers trained using non-biomedical corpora (e.g. newspaper text) accurately tag biomedical corpora. Table 1 summarizes previous research results. (The reader is cautioned against direct comparison of results because previous research varies in methodology and corpora.) Except for Wermter and Hahn [9], tagging accuracy decreases substantially when a tagger is trained on non-biomedical corpora and applied to biomedical corpora. Tagging accuracy can also decrease in cases where a tagger is applied to biomedical corpora that differ from their biomedical training corpora [5].

To improve tagging of biomedical corpora, existing non-biomedical corpora have been supplemented with manually derived biomedical lexicons, autonomously derived biomedical lexicons, or additional biomedical corpora. Previous research suggests that supplementing an existing corpus with a biomedical one improves tagging more than a lexicon does [21]. Furthermore, a supplemental biomedical corpus can return tagging accuracy to values comparable to those seen when training and testing on non-biomedical corpora [17].

3 Token Centric Tagger

In this section, we describe our token centric POS tagger. Our tagger estimates a tag's likelihood for a token by combining prior probabilities (probabilities given previous tags) and token probabilities (probabilities based on the current token). This is similar to HMM taggers. Our tagger calculates token probabilities for unknown tokens using token features and transitions to using the token itself for known tokens. A difference between our tagger and HMM taggers is that our tagger does not use dynamic programming methods.

We calculate prior probabilities using a method described by Jurafsky and Martin [11]. This method is implemented by the TnT tagger [2]. The method

Table 1. Summary of previous research results (E=English, G=German, N=Norwegian, P=Portugese, ME=Maximum entropy, TL=Tagged lexicon, HDS=Hospital discharge summaries, SPR=Surgical pathology reports, CN=Clinical notes, EHR=Electronic health record, po=Portion of, see research papers for corpora)

Research Paper	Tagger	Lang.	Training Corpus	Testing Corpus	Accuracy (in %)
[4]	Brill	E	Brown, WSJ	HDS	89
[4]	Brill	E	HDS	HDS	96.9
[5]	HMM	E	TB-2	TB-2	96
[5]	HMM	E	GENIA	GENIA	97
[5]	HMM	E	Mayo MED	Mayo MED	92
[5]	HMM	E	TB-2	Mayo MED	88
[5]	HMM	E	TB-2	GENIA	85.1
[5]	HMM	E	TB-2, GENIA	MED	88
[5]	HMM	E	TB-2, GENIA	GENIA	97
[5]	HMM	E	TB-2, Mayo MED	Mayo MED	84.41
[21]	HMM	E	WSJ	Fruit fly	88.7
[21]	HMM	E	WSJ, PennBio, GENIA	Fruit fly	96.4
[21]	HMM	E	WSJ, PennBio, GENIA, po. Fruit fly	Fruit fly corpora	97.9, 98.1
[16]	HMM	E	WSJ, MEDLINE lexicon	GENIA	95.8
[16]	HMM	E	WSJ, MEDLINE lexicon	MedPost	94.63
[6]	HMM + TL	E	MedPost	MedPost	95.1
[19]	HMM + TL	E	MedPost	MedPost	97.43
[12]	ME	E	WSJ	SPR	79
[12]	ME	E	WSJ, SPR	SPR	93.9
[12]	ME	E	WSJ, po. SPR	SPR	81.2, 84, 92.7
[18]	TnT	E	TB		89.76
[18]	TnT	E	TB, CN	CN	94.69
[9]	TnT	G	NEGRA news	FRAMED, medical corpus	95.2
[9]	TnT	G	NEGRA news, TL	FRAMED, medical corpus	96.7
[9]	TnT	G	NEGRA news, Specialist lexicon	FRAMED, medical corpus	96.8
[9]	Brill	G	NEGRA news	FRAMED, medical corpus	91.9
[9]	Brill	G	NEGRA news, TL	FRAMED, medical corpus	93.4
[9]	Brill	G	NEGRA news, TL	FRAMED, medical corpus	93.6
[10]	HMM	N	News	EHR patient data	76.87
[10]	HMM	N	News, 1000 EHR words	EHR patient data	84.46
[10]	HMM	N	1000 EHR words	EHR patient data	79.05
[10]	HMM	N	64000 EHR words	EHR patient data	94.54
[17]	OpenNLP	P	po. MAC-Morpho	po. HDS	75.3
[17]	OpenNLP	P	po. MAC-Morpho, TL	po. HDS	90

calculates prior probabilities given no previous tag (a tag's likelihood given the training data), one previous tag and two previous tags. These prior probabilities are weighted then summed resulting in a prior probability distribution over POS tags.

Our tagger's token probability is calculated in part using a Naive Bayes classifier [11]. Naive Bayes classifiers apply Bayes' theorem to calculate the most likely classification (label or label distribution) given feature values. We selected a Naive Bayes classifier because it is know to be conceptually simple, computationally fast, applicable to many datasets and to classify well [7]. The last three characteristics are particularly important. A Naive Bayes classifier is computationally fast for it generally learns by seeing each value once and generally classifies by considering each label and feature-value pair once. Domingos and Pazzani [7] present compelling evidence supporting robustness of Naive Bayes classifiers. In particular, even when classification features have some degree of dependence Naive Bayes classifiers may perform well. This contradicts the assumption that Bayesian classifiers require independent features to perform well.

Our Naive Bayes classifier differs from a typical implementation by differentiating between finite and infinite discrete features. An example finite feature is *token capitalization* which can assume a true or false value. An example infinite feature is English words. New English words are created regularly.

A typical Naive Bayes classifier assigns a probability of 0 to each class (label) given an unknown discrete feature value. The latter occurs because Naive Bayes classifiers rely on the probability of a feature given a class, $P(\ feature \mid class\ )$, which is 0 if the feature value has never been seen during training. The consequence of this behavior on tagging is erroneous tag likelihoods and incorrect tagging. Our Naive Bayes classifier omits features associated with unknown feature values, basing its classification solely on known feature values and their probabilities. Consequently, our Naive Bayes classifier handles infinite discrete features.

Our tagger uses our Naive Bayes classifier to estimate a probability distribution over POS tags for unknown tokens. Our tagger separates (known) tokens learned from training corpora into frequent and infrequent tokens using a token-frequency threshold value (e.g. 10). Tokens occurring less than the threshold in the training corpora are considered infrequent, the remainder are considered frequent.

A frequent token's probability distribution over POS tags is learned from training corpora whereas an infrequent token's probability distribution is calculated using both our Naive Bayes classifier and a token's learned probability distribution. In other words, the more frequent a token the less our tagger relies on its features. The calculation is as follows:

- Let G be a set of POS tags and $g \in G$.
- Let T be the token-frequency threshold.
- Let t be an infrequent token and t_i represent one of its feature values ($0 \leq i \leq k$ represents k features).
- Let f_c be a function that takes a token and returns the token's frequency (count) learned from the training corpora.

$$P(g|t) = wP_{learned}(g|t) + (1-w)P_{bayes}(g|t_0, \ldots, t_k) \text{ where } w = f_c(t)/T$$

Our Naive Bayes classifier uses the following token features:

1. Numeric - the token represents a number.
2. Capitalized - the token is capitalized.
3. Closed class word - the token is a known closed class word (defined below).
4. Suffix - the feature value is the token's suffix (discrete infinite).
5. Lower case token - the token's lower case string (discrete infinite).

Features 1 and 2 were implemented using regular expressions. Feature 3 is derived from a list of closed class words. Closed class words such as pronouns (e.g. he, all) or prepositions (e.g. between, onto) rarely change as a language evolves [1]. For feature 4, a token's suffix was extracted using the Lancaster stemmer provided in NLTK [13]. NLTK (version 2.0b8) is a natural language processing toolkit written in Python (www.python.org). Feature 5 is simply the token's lower case string.

In general, these features were selected because their values identified a particular subset of the POS tags. For example, the numeric feature identifies numeric values which are typically tagged as noun (NN) or cardinal number (CD). Another advantage of the numeric feature is that it generalizes over all numbers.

We conceptualized closed class words as anchors between small sequences of potentially unknown tokens. Given this conceptualization and that a token's tag can be estimated from prior tags, we expected closed-class words to improve tagging accuracy of unknown text, motivating its inclusion in the feature set.

We set our tagger's frequent-token threshold value to 10. This avoids assigning tags to tokens based on few (e.g. 2 or 3) learned cases when more information is available through the Naive Bayes classifier. Consider the token *aids*. The token may appear in text as *AIDS* (acquired immune deficiency syndrome), *Aids* (a typo) or *aids* (He aids the patient.). Our tagger differentiates between *AIDS* (noun) and *aids* (verb). For infrequent cases such as *Aids*, our tagger relies on our Naive Bayes classifier (e.g. feature 5) so as not to exclude POS tags.

Our tagger runs in linear time relative to the number of tokens. For each token, all POS tags are considered and the most likely POS tag is immediately assigned. This differs from TnT – the best tagger of the two frequently used biomedical taggers. TnT uses a dynamic programming algorithm to assign POS tags and consequently runs in quadratic time relative to the number of tokens.

4 Data and Evaluation

We used publicly available corpora and taggers for our evaluation. This is expected to facilitate comparison of our results with future work.

The training corpus is available through NLTK. NLTK includes a selection of corpora such as a sample (10%) of the Penn Treebank's Wall Street Journal newspaper text (WSJ). We used the latter to train all taggers.

We selected the MedPost corpus [19] as our testing corpus. It contains MEDLINE abstracts. We evaluated our taggers on a version of the corpus with duplicate sentences removed. The goal was to avoid biasing results on accurately or inaccurately tagged duplicate sentences. MedPost contains 6695 unique sentences (182360 tokens).

A difficulty with POS tagging of biomedical text is accessing and annotating appropriate training corpora. The latter may result in POS taggers trained on corpora that differ from the tagger's target biomedical text.

MedPost's POS tags are based on the Penn Treebank's [14], but differ slightly. We ran a script provided in the MedPost download to convert the MedPost POS tags to the Penn Treebank's. Aside from a small set of specific word-bound conversions between tag sets, MedPost is a specialization of the Penn Treebank tag set.

Although the MedPost corpus was primarily used as the testing corpus, we also ran several experiments where a percentage of the MedPost corpus was used during training. This percentage was not omitted during subsequent testing. For example, we trained all taggers using the WSJ text and a random 5% of MedPost. We subsequently tested all taggers using the entire MedPost corpus. Our goal was to better understand how training a POS tagger on a small percentage of the testing corpus affected tagging.

We selected a baseline tagger, Brill's tagger [3] and TnT [2] for comparison to our POS tagger. The baseline tagger assigns the most likely tag to each token based on the likelihoods learned in training. For unknown tokens, it assigns the most likely tag given the entire training corpora (e.g. noun). We picked Brill's tagger and TnT because they have been used in previous research and are available in NLTK (NLTK tagging demos).

We recorded the duration of time required to tag the MedPost corpus (excludes training time). All software was run on an Apple XServe with two 2.26 GHz Quad-Core Intel Xeon processors and 12 GB of ram. All taggers are single threaded and were thus restricted to one processor core. That is, times were not improved through parallelization.

5 Results

Our token centric tagger performed best with an accuracy of 81.0% compared to the Brill tagger (77.5%) and TnT (78.2%) (for complete results see Table 2). Our tagger continued to perform best when a subset of MedPost was added to the training corpus. Confidence intervals for 95% confidence were calculated using the normal approximation method of the binomial confidence interval [15]. All confidence intervals are less than ±0.002, or 0.2%.

6 Discussion

Our token centric tagger is an interesting alternative to existing biomedical taggers. It performed best and did so in relatively little time compared to the next

Table 2. Tagging accuracy and duration (TC=Token Centric, T=Threshold; accuracy is an average of 5 runs when taggers are MedPost trained)

Tagger	Training Corpus	Accuracy (%)	Duration (hour:min:sec)
Baseline	WSJ	76.6	-
Brill	WSJ	77.5	0h:0m:10s
Brill	WSJ + random 1% MedPost	84.7	-
Brill	WSJ + random 5% MedPost	88.8	-
TnT	WSJ	78.2	1h:1m:21s
TnT	WSJ + random 1% MedPost	84.9	-
TnT	WSJ + random 5% MedPost	89.3	-
TC (T=10)	WSJ	81.0	0h:5m:47s
TC (T=10)	WSJ + random 1% MedPost	87.6	-
TC (T=10)	WSJ + random 5% MedPost	90.7	-
TC (T=20)	WSJ	80.9	-
TC (T=20)	WSJ + random 1% MedPost	87.5	-
TC (T=20)	WSJ + random 5% MedPost	90.7	-

best tagger (TnT). With an improvement of 2.8% accuracy over the next best tagger, our tagger correctly tags almost one additional token per sentence (assuming even improvement over the entire corpus then: $(2.8\% \times 182360)/6695 = 0.76$ tokens per sentence).

Our tagger focuses on recognizing each token rather than focusing on the POS tag sequence. This is accomplished by immediately selecting the most likely tag for a given token and using an unknown token's features to predict its POS tag. In contrast, TnT focuses on POS tag sequences. It uses a dynamic programming algorithm to select the most likely sequence of POS tags for a sequence of tokens and has no ability to predict POS tags upon encountering an unknown token.

There are several possible reasons for our tagger's strategy being more effective. Focusing on words may allow our tagger to recover more quickly from errors. With a focus on prior probabilities an incorrect tag is likely to significantly affect subsequent tags and overall tagging accuracy. Alternatively, training and testing corpora may differ significantly in prior probabilities decreasing tagging accuracy for taggers that place greater weight on prior probabilities. Another possible reason for our tagger's effectiveness is its capacity to predict a token's POS tag from its features. Taggers missing this capacity may be at significant disadvantage. Given our experience, it is unlikely that a single reason underlies the difference in tagging accuracy between our tagger and those it was compared to.

We set our tagger's frequent-token threshold value to 10. The threshold's goal is to make use of tagging information available in the Naive Bayes classifier when few token cases are seen in training (e.g. differentiate equally probable tags for a token seen twice). We also ran our tagger with a threshold value of 20. The tagging accuracy did not differ significantly. This suggests that 10 training examples are sufficient to establish a tag distribution that is pragmatically successful in tagging corpora. Although we support our choice of threshold value with some pragmatic evidence, we do not have a strong theoretical justification for it. Our goal is to develop a more elegant solution that omits the threshold value entirely.

Our results concur with previous results in that a small supplemental biomedical corpus can return tagging accuracy to values comparable to those seen when training and testing on non-biomedical corpora.

7 Conclusion

We built and evaluated our token centric POS tagger. When trained on a sample of the Penn Treebank's WSJ corpus and applied to the MedPost corpus, our tagger performed better than two frequently used biomedical text taggers (TnT and Brill). Our tagger also performed best when the training corpus was augmented with a small randomly selected portion of the MedPost corpus.

Our results suggest that future work should reexamine POS tagging methods and algorithms for biomedical text. This differs from the work to date that has focused on retraining existing POS taggers. In particular, future work could concentrate on better understanding the effect of prior versus token probabilities and researching better methods for tagging unknown tokens.

References

1. Akmajian, A., Demers, R.A., Farmer, A.K., Harnish, R.M.: Linguistics: An Introduction to Language and Communication, 5th edn. Massachusetts Institute of Technology (2001)
2. Brants, T.: Tnt: a statistical part-of-speech tagger. In: Proceedings of the Sixth Conference on Applied Natural Language Processing, pp. 224–231. Morgan Kaufmann Publishers Inc., San Francisco (2000)
3. Brill, E.: Transformation-based error-driven learning and natural language processing: A case study in part-of-speech tagging. Computational Linguistics 21, 543–565 (1995)
4. Campbell, D.A., Johnson, S.B.: Comparing syntactic complexity in medical and non-medical corpora. In: Proc. AMIA Symp., pp. 90–94 (2001)
5. Coden, A.R., Pakhomov, S.V., Ando, R.K., Duffy, P.H., Chute, C.G.: Domain-specific language models and lexicons for tagging. J. Biomed. Inform. 38(6), 422–430 (2005)
6. Divita, G., Browne, A.C., Loane, R.: dtagger: a pos tagger. In: AMIA Annu. Symp. Proc., pp. 200–203 (2006)
7. Domingos, P., Pazzani, M.: On the optimality of the simple bayesian classifier under zero-one loss. Mach. Learn. 29, 103–130 (1997), `http://portal.acm.org/citation.cfm?id=274158.274160`
8. Friedman, C., Knirsch, C., Shagina, L., Hripcsak, G.: Automating a severity score guideline for community-acquired pneumonia employing medical language processing of discharge summaries. In: Proc. AMIA Symp., pp. 256–260 (1999)
9. Hahn, U., Wermter, J.: High-performance tagging on medical texts. In: COLING 2004: Proceedings of the 20th international conference on Computational Linguistics, p. 973. Association for Computational Linguistics, Morristown (2004)

10. Huseth, O., Brox Rost, T.: Developing an annotated corpus of patient histories from the primary care health record. In: IEEE International Conference on Bioinformatics and Biomedicine Workshops, BIBMW 2007, pp. 165–173 (November 2007)
11. Jurafsky, D., Martin, J.H.: Speech and Language Processing. Prentice Hall, Englewood Cliffs (2009)
12. Liu, K., Chapman, W., Hwa, R., Crowley, R.S.: Heuristic sample selection to minimize reference standard training set for a part-of-speech tagger. J. Am. Med. Inform. Assoc. 14(5), 641–650 (2007)
13. Loper, E., Bird, S.: Nltk: the natural language toolkit. In: Proceedings of the ACL 2002 Workshop on Effective Tools and Methodologies for Teaching Natural Language Processing and Computational Linguistics, pp. 63–70. Association for Computational Linguistics, Morristown (2002)
14. Marcus, M.P., Marcinkiewicz, M.A., Santorini, B.: Building a large annotated corpus of english: the penn treebank. Comput. Linguist. 19(2), 313–330 (1993)
15. Mendenhall, W., Sincich, t.: Statistics for the Engineering and Computer Sciences. Dellen Publishing Company (1984)
16. Miller, J.E., Torii, M., Vijay-Shanker, K.: Adaptation of pos tagging for multiple biomedical domains. In: Proceedings of the Workshop on BioNLP 2007: Biological, Translational, and Clinical Language Processing, BioNLP 2007, pp. 179–180. Association for Computational Linguistics, Stroudsburg (2007)
17. Oleynik, M., Nohama, P., Cancian, P.S., Schulz, S.: Performance analysis of a pos tagger applied to discharge summaries in portuguese. Stud. Health Technol. Inform. 160(Pt 2), 959–963 (2010)
18. Pakhomov, S., Coden, A., Chute, C.: Creating a test corpus of clinical notes manually tagged for part-of-speech information. In: Proceedings of the International Joint Workshop on Natural Language Processing in Biomedicine and its Applications, JNLPBA 2004, pp. 62–65. Association for Computational Linguistics, Stroudsburg (2004)
19. Smith, L., Rindflesch, T., Wilbur, W.J.: Medpost: a part-of-speech tagger for biomedical text. Bioinformatics 20(14), 2320–2321 (2004)
20. Smith, L.H., Rindflesch, T.C., Wilbur, W.J.: The importance of the lexicon in tagging biological text. Nat. Lang. Eng. 12, 335–351 (2006)
21. Tateisi, Y., Tsuruoka, Y., Tsujii, J.i.: Subdomain adaptation of a pos tagger with a small corpus. In: Proceedings of the HLT-NAACL BioNLP Workshop on Linking Natural Language and Biology, LNLBioNLP 2006, pp. 136–137. Association for Computational Linguistics, Stroudsburg (2006)
22. Zingmond, D., Lenert, L.A.: Monitoring free-text data using medical language processing. Comput. Biomed. Res. 26(5), 467–481 (1993)

Extracting Information from *Summary of Product Characteristics* for Improving Drugs Prescription Safety

Stefania Rubrichi[1], Silvana Quaglini[1], Alex Spengler[2], and Patrick Gallinari[2]

[1] Laboratory for Biomedical Informatics "Mario Stefanelli", Department of Computers and Systems Science, University of Pavia, Pavia, Italy
[2] Laboratoire d'Informatique de Paris 6, Université Pierre et Marie Curie, Paris, France
{stefania.rubrichi,silvana.quaglini}@unipv.it
{alex.spengler,patrick.gallinari}@lip6.fr

Abstract. Information about medications is critical in supporting decision-making during the prescription process and thus in improving the safety and quality of care. The Summary of Product Characteristics (SPC) represents the basis of information for health professionals on how to use medicines. However, this information is locked in free-text and, as such, cannot be actively accessed and elaborated by computerized applications. In this work, we propose a machine learning based system for the automatic recognition of drug-related entities (active ingredient, interaction effects, etc.) in SPCs, focusing on drug interactions. Our approach learns to classify this information in a structured prediction framework, relying on conditional random fields. The classifier is trained and evaluated using a corpus of a hundred SPCs. They have been hand-annotated with thirteen semantic labels that have been derived from a previously developed domain ontology. Our evaluations show that the model exhibits high overall performance, with an average F_1-measure of about 90%.

Keywords: Information Extraction, Conditional Random Fields, Adverse Drug Events, Medication Errors, Summary of Product Characteristics.

1 Introduction

The use of medications has a central role in health care provision, yet on occasion it may injure the person taking them as result of adverse drug events (ADEs). Some ADEs are inevitable and include drug effects that are unwanted, unpleasant, noxious, or potentially harmful, but sometimes they are caused by failures during the medication process, therefore they are not inevitable. Thus, to decrease injury, efforts must be put into reducing errors. Medication errors cut across multiple stages (ordering, dispensing, administration) and occur for a variety of reasons. According to a study on ADEs analysis [7], most errors

M. Peleg, N. Lavrač, and C. Combi (Eds.): AIME 2011, LNAI 6747, pp. 327–337, 2011.

occur in the ordering and administration steps: some of them are due to lack of information about the patient, but more often physicians make many prescribing errors that appear to be due to deficiencies of up-to-date knowledge of the drug and how it should be used. These include incorrect doses, forms, frequencies, and routes of administration, as well as errors in the choice of drug. Moreover, information about the patients' condition (allergies, previous diagnoses), lab results and other medicine they are taking is sometimes incomplete, not easily accessible when it is needed, which leads to prescribing errors as well as inappropriate administration of ordered drugs. Several information technologies can help providers absorb and apply the necessary information. In particular, computerized order entry (CPOE) is viewed to play a key role in helping improve safety standards in the process of medication use, especially when decision support is provided. CPOE with clinical decision support can improve patients' safety and lower medication-related costs. To be effective, the underlying medical knowledge must be captured, adequately represented, and made available to the CPOE system.

In this work we consider the problem of automatic extraction of drug information conveyed in the Summary of Product Characteristics (SPC), focusing on a specific section concerned with drug-related interactions. We formulate the problem in a machine-learning framework, in which we seek to assign the correct semantic label such as InteractionEffect or ActiveDrugIngredient, to each word, or segment of sentence, of the text. We employ a state-of-the-art classifier: linear-chain conditional random fields (CRFs). This classifier discriminates between semantically interesting and uninteresting content through the automatic adaptation of hundreds of engineered text characteristics, taking into account the properties of a document, on both a local (word) and global (sentence) level. We introduce a corpus of a hundred interactions sections in the Italian language that have been annotated with thirteen distinct semantic labels, with respect to a previously implemented ontology. We apply the CRF to our data set and evaluate their overall and individual label results. The classifier achieves an average F_1-measure of about 90%, which is promising for real-world applications.

2 Related Work

Over the last two decades there has been an increase of interest in applying Natural Language Processing (NLP) to biomedical text. More specifically, information extraction (IE) techniques have become an invaluable resource for enriching the content and the utility of electronic clinical systems [11]. Excellent efforts have been documented in the literature on IE from textual clinical documents [14,2,5,4,10], and its subsequent application in summarization, case finding, decision-support, or statistical analysis tasks.

As far as the medications domain is concerned, several studies have addressed the issue of IE. The less recent ones concentrated their analysis on the extraction of specific drug features, such as drug names and dosage. In one example, Evans et al [1] reported a method of extracting drug and dosage data from a collection of discharge summaries. They first draw a conceptual model of drug-dosage information and then identified this information using a semantically driven extraction module. This module combines readily available NLP facilities from the Clarit system with newly created resources, including a set of pattern rules and a lexicon. In another study, Sirohi et al [17] performed a dictionary-based NLP study to determine the effects of using varying lexicon to extract drug names from electronic medical records. These authors have shown how the accuracy of results can be enhanced by refining the drug lexicon. A study by Shah et al [16] derived numerical information about daily dosage from unstructured dosage instructions from a patient records database, using a dictionary to standardize words and phrases. Then they converted the extracted information into structured fields. Lastly, Levin et al [8] implemented a system based on lexicon (RxNorm) and regular expressions (Hints List) to extract and normalize drug names from an anesthesia electronic health record, into a standardized terminology. RxNorm and Hints List concepts were used in the mapping module as references for drug names, and medical abbreviations and jargon, respectively.

Lately, more studies have been geared towards the extraction of a more complete set of drug characteristics. In particular, Gold et al [3] built Merki, a parser which can extract drug names and other relevant information from discharge summaries using a lexicon and a set of parsing rules. Similarly, Xu et al [19] implemented a NLP system, MedEx which extracts medication information from clinical notes. Relying on a more detailed medication representation model, they integrated a semantic tagger and Chart parser to capture drug names and signature information from clinical narratives and then to map it onto structured representation.

On the whole, current works focus on clinical text narrative. However, Pereira et al [12] considered another source of information on medications, namely SPC, and thus addressed the problem of automatic indexing. The authors developed a method to automatically generate a dictionary for use with a French Multi-Terminology Indexing tool. Focusing on medical literature, instead, Segura-Bedmar et al [15] aimed at detecting drug-drug interactions by comparing two different approaches. Initially, they employed a hybrid approach, which combined shallow parsing and pattern matching, then they employed a kernel-based approach that uses Support Vector Machines (SVM) and which achieved better results.

3 Methods

3.1 Framework Outline

In this project we propose to extract drug-related interaction information reported as free-text in SPCs. We follow a named entity recognition (NER) approach. NER is a sub-field of IE and refers to the task of identifying expressions in natural language text denoting certain entities (i.e., Named Entities), such as diseases and drugs, and labeling them with their appropriate type. To do so, we have developed a framework for simultaneously recognizing occurrences of multiple entity classes by using linear-chain CRFs. This supervised machine learning approach predicts the labels of words by using large number of interdependent descriptive characteristics (features) of the input by assigning real-value weight to these features. This can be seen as a way to "capture" the hidden patterns of labels and features, and "learn" what the likely output might be, given these patterns. Our methodology is developed through different steps.

Typically, the first step in most NER tasks is to identify the named entities (labels) that are relevant to the concepts, relations and events described in the text. A system for NER is hence based upon specific knowledge about the domain. Thus, as part of the understanding of the text factual information process, we had previously developed a formal model of drug information conveyed in the SPC. We conducted a manual analysis of SPC text so as to identify the underlying semantic concept classes (i.e. concepts representing drug features) and semantic relationships among those concepts. This analysis has resulted in a domain ontology of medication [13], the formal means of representing domain-specific knowledge. Incidentally, in this study, we focused on drug interactions, then we looked, more specifically, at the twelve concepts that properly model drug interaction findings.

As long as the label prediction is on a word-by-word basis, and decisions are made for one sentence at a time, the first stage of our extraction algorithm consists in splitting the text of SPC interaction section into sentences and then to break those input sentences into tokens. We used full stops and white spaces to determine sentence and token boundaries, respectively. Moreover, in order to account for exceptions, we considered a normalization steps that mainly includes removing all punctuation but colon and brackets, adding white spaces between colon and brackets, and the previous word, removing hyphens if they exist between alphanumeric strings, replacing periods that occur between numbers ("3.4") with commas ("3,4").

After the pre-processing step, we defined a set of binary features that express some descriptive characteristics of the data, for instance "current token is capitalized". Every time a text token takes on the value of a feature, the feature will become active for that token. The stream of tokens has been then converted to features. Finally, the algorithm iterates the tokens in the sentence, and labels proper tokens with semantic labels, by learning correspondence between labels and features.

3.2 Conditional Random Fields

Conditional random fields (CRF) [6] are a probabilistic framework for labeling and segmenting sequential data. The underlying idea is to define a conditional probability $p(y|x)$ distribution over label sequences, given a particular observation sequence x rather than the joint distribution over both label and observation sequences. Based on this formulation, let x^* be a novel observation sequence, the understanding process select the label sequence y^* which maximizes the a posteriori probability:

$$y^* = h_\theta(x^*) = \arg\max_{y \in Y} F(x^*, y, \theta)$$

Let X=$< x_1, x_2, \ldots x_n >$ be a set of an input observation sequences, such as a sequence of words in a text document, whose values are observed. Let Y=$< y_1, y_2, \ldots y_n >$ be some sequence of labels, e.g. Y=<*InteractionEffect*, *ActiveDrugIngredient*,...>, whose values the task requires the model to predict. Linear-chain CRFs define the conditional probability of a label sequence given an input sequence to be a normalized product of potential functions, each of the form:

$$\exp(\sum_j \lambda_j t_j(y_{i-1}, y_i, x, i) + \sum_k \mu_k s_k(y_i, x, i))$$

where $t_j(y_{i-1}, y_i, x, i)$ is a transition feature function of the entire observation sequence and the labels at positions i and $i-1$ in the label sequence; $s_k(y_i, x, i)$ is a state feature function of the label at position i and the observation sequence; and λ_j and μ_k are parameters to be estimated from training data. Intuitively, the weights λ_j and μ_k should be highly positive for features that are correlated with the target label, around zero for relatively uninformative features and highly negative for features that tend to be off in accurate tagging. The parameters are set to maximize the conditional log-likelihood of labeled sequences in training set. As a measure to control overfitting, we use a Gaussian regularizer. Our system uses the MALLET [9] implementation of CRFs. In the next section we will show how to adapt this framework to the specific need of the task at hand, describing in detail the set of features we created to discriminate between semantically relevant and unrelevant content.

3.3 Features

What follows is a report on the set of features we used in our experiments.

Orthographical Features. As a good starting point, our set of machine learning features consisted of the simplest and most obvious feature set: word identity features, that is the vocabulary from the training data. Furthermore, we added features that indicate whether the current token is a digit, which is quite useful for identifying *Posology* entities.

Neighboring Word Features. Words preceding or following a target word may be useful for modeling the local context. It is clear that the more context words analyzed, the better and more precise the results become. However, widening the context window quickly leads to an explosion of the computational and statistical complexity. For our experiments, we estimated a suitable window size of [-3,3]. As an example, consider the sequence "avoid drugs association". The middle token would have features word $t =$ `drugs`, word $t-1 =$ `avoid` and word $t+1 =$ `association`.

Prefix Features. Some prefixes can provide good clues for classifying named entities. In particular, we identified a set of words that occur often with the same label; for example Italian words starting with "effet-" (effect) or "farmacinetic-" (pharmacokinetic) are usually *Interaction Effects*, those starting with "mg-" (mg) or "dos-" (dosage) or "giorn-" (day) have usually been tagged as *Posology*, and so on. Therefore, we also included some prefix features. These features help the system recognize informative substrings. However, short prefixes are too common to be of any help in classification. In our experience, the acceptable length for a prefix varies by words and in many cases the prefix coincides with the word root.

Punctuation Features. Also notable are punctuation features, which contain some special punctuation in sentences. After browsing our corpus we found that colon and brackets features might prove helpful. Given a medication in fact, colon is usually preceded by the interacting substance and followed by the explanation of the specific interaction effects. Additionally, round brackets denotes extra information regarding the words that follow. For each token, the punctuation features test if it is preceded or followed by colon or parenthesis. These features have been used in conjunction with a token window of sentence length. This means that punctuation features for token j contain predicates about the previous $j-n$ tokens and the following $j+m$ tokens, where n and m are the distance between the current token and the beginning and the end of the sentence, respectively.

Dictionary Features. Finally, in order to have this model benefit from domain specific knowledge we added semantic features. Farmadati DataBase is provided with a complete archive of active ingredients. We create a binary feature for each entry in the active ingredient archive. Every time a text token coincides with such an entry, the feature is active, indicating that the token describes an active drug ingredient. For dictionary entries that are multi-token, all words are required to match in the input sequence.

4 Evaluation

4.1 Data Collection

The goal of this work lies in extracting content from SPCs, focusing on drug-related interactions. SPCs represent a source of information for health professionals on how to use medication safely and effectively. SPCs contain the latest evidence-based accurate information for any given medicinal product. Its content is regulated by Article 11 of Directive 2001/83/EC. SPCs of specialty medicines for human use are organized into twelve sections: name, therapeutic categories, active ingredient, excipients, indications, contraindication/side effects, undesired effects, posology, storage precautions, warnings, interactions, and use in case of pregnancy and nursing.

Using SPCs in the Farmadati Italia Database, we created a corpus of one hundred manually annotated interaction sections. This contains all the references about the medicines, the para-pharmaceutical and the homeopathic products found in Italy in addition to the medical devices that can be sold in pharmacies; this database includes around 800.000 recorded products. The interaction sections were derived using BDF (Bancadati Federfarma), a commercially available software, combined with a pre-processing algorithm. BDF (Bancadati Federfarma) software enabled the exporting of the SPCs archive as an ASCII text format file. This file lists the SPC lines of each specialty medicines for human and veterinary use in the database. An alphanumeric code at the beginning of each line specifies the drug and the section it refers to. The pre-processing pass over the exported file allowed us to split it into different files, associated with the corresponding medicine and stating the different sections in each file. Moreover our database may not be properly hyphenated due to some length constraints: we solved this problem using an Italian language lexicon [20].

We split the 100 interaction sections into two sets at random: one for training, which consists of 60 sections and one for testing, which contains 40 sections. In total, there are 745 input sentences for training and 508 input sentences for testing.

4.2 Gold Standard

The gold standard was generated by manual annotation of the data set. The annotation process was performed by a biomedical engineer with domain knowledge. Semantic annotation is used to establish links between the entities in the text and their semantic descriptions or concept classes. We used the following thirteen semantic labels, according to the ontology-based model described above: *ActiveDrugIngredient, AgeClass, ClinicalCondition, DiagnosticTest, DrugClass, IntakeRoute, OtherSubstance, InteractionEffect, Posology, PharmaceuticalForm, PhysiologicCondition, RecoveringAction, None*. The label *None* has been given to indicate elements that are not relevant for this research.

Leveraging the established ontology, we mapped its elements to the SPCs' text content. We carefully inspected all the corpus lines distinguishing the different senses with respect to the ontology; we then annotated each word in the extracted SPC interaction sections with the corresponding class in the ontology. Active ingredients tagging was performed by a look-up of terms in Farmadati active ingredients archive. A review of the data has been used to validate and, when necessary, correct the annotations.

As an example, consider the following sentence (translated from Italian):

$\langle$**Enoxaparin**$\rangle_{ActiveDrugIngredient}$ **dosed as a** $\langle$**1.0 mg/kg**$\rangle_{Posology}$ $\langle$**subcutaneous injection**$\rangle_{IntakeRoute}$ **for** $\langle$**four doses**$\rangle_{Posology}$ $\langle$**did not alter the pharmacokinetics**$\rangle_{InteractionEffect}$ **of** $\langle$**eptifibatide**$\rangle_{ActiveDrugIngredient}$.

4.3 Experimental Setup

We measure and evaluate the performance of our model based on precision (P), recall (R) and F_1-measure (F_1) [18]. We report results in terms of overall and individual label performance. When dealing with multi-label classification and imbalanced labels, the performance on the individual labels can essentially be aggregated into overall performance results in two complementary ways: either we compute their arithmetic mean, giving equal weight to each of the labels (macro-averaged); or we compute the mean by weighting each label by the number of times it occurs in the data set (micro-averaged).

Table 1. Overall experimental results (in %) of CRF

Micro-average			Macro-average			Overall
Precision	Recall	F_1-measure	Precision	Recall	F_1-measure	accuracy
90.45	90.53	90.30	90.43	78.82	83.72	90.53

5 Results and Discussion

Table 1 presents a summary of the key performance. In general, our experiments show that the classifiers, with carefully designed features, can identify drug interactions related information with a resulting overall accuracy of around 90%. Although the data might contain noise inherent to manual annotation, the learning algorithms reach good performance. Expressing the problem of content extraction in the described machine learning approach is therefore promising.

The performance differences between the macro- and micro-averaged results suggest that some rare labels are often misclassified, as shown in their low recall in Table 2. Macro-averaged metrics, in fact, are often dominated by the performance on rare labels. Table 2 shows the evaluation results on the individual labels in terms of precision recall and F_1-measure. Overall, labels whose training examples are scarce suffer from relatively low performance. It is the labels *DiagnosticTest* and *OtherSubstance* that are hardest to extract. On the other hand, some other labels such as *AgeClass*, and *IntakeRoute*, although rare, perform better. Such labels, in fact, can rely on a more precise definition (i.e. they are often related to the same sequence of words), which is an important factor that contributes to the good performance. Although prior work is hardly comparable with our own, mainly due to the fact that the dataset are entirely different, we nevertheless report results from Segura-Bedmar et al [15]. They follow a similar machine learning based approach on the same task of drug-interaction extraction, yet use Support Vector Machine and rely on a corpus of documents from the DrugBank database. Their best method achieves a F_1-measure of 66.0%. Our experimental results compare favorably, since they have a F_1-measure of 90.30%.

Moreover, we investigate the influence of different feature groups (i.e. orthographical, neighboring word, prefix, punctuation and dictionary features) on the overall classification results. Table 3 looks at the performance when varying the employed set of features. Each features set differs only in the absence of a particular group that is specified in the first column of Table 3. For all evaluations, we tested numerous settings for the variance of the Gaussian regularizer and found the value to work best. This is because each feature is, in general, associated with a parameter. The more parameters the model has, the higher its degree of freedom and the more likely it is to overfit. This means that in comparing of different feature groups we should regularize differently. Particularly, the more features there are, the smaller the variance of the Gaussian prior needs to be. Regarding the results on the feature categories, not surprisingly, the neighboring word features have been shown to be the most beneficial ones when comparing the different feature sets, additionally because they represent the large majority of features. On the other hand, as expected, number, punctuation, prefixes and dictionary features don't have too great an impact on these results, especially because there are only few of them.

Table 2. Performance results (in %) of the classifier on individual labels

Label	N_{train}	N_{test}	Precision	Recall	F_1-measure
ActiveDrugIngredient	1196	894	97.39	87.70	92.29
AgeClass	16	8	100	75.00	85.71
ClinicalCondition	77	25	100	100	100
DiagnosticTest	77	51	100	56.86	72.50
DrugClass	1527	634	87.23	70.03	77.69
IntakeRoute	40	21	80.00	76.19	78.05
InteractionEffect	1698	1165	85.75	78.54	81.99
None	11378	7623	91.04	96.39	93.64
OtherSubstance	119	58	76.47	67.24	71.56
PharmaceuticalForm	1	-	-	-	-
PhysiologicalCondition	3	-	-	-	-
Posology	256	375	94.02	88.00	90.91
RecoveringAction	787	564	82.85	71.1	76.53

Table 3. Variation in performance (in %) for different features sets

Feature set	Variance	Micro-averaged			Macro-averaged		
		Precision	Recall	F_1-measure	Precision	Recall	F_1-measure
No Dictionary Features	100	89.73	89.81	89.58	89.95	79.71	84.26
No Number Features	100	90.48	90.53	90.31	90.57	78.28	83.48
No Prefix Features	200	90.25	90.32	90.08	89.98	77.85	82.86
No Punctuation Features	200	90.45	90.52	90.32	90.16	78.65	83.51
No Word Identity Features	1000	88.54	88.71	88.45	86.37	76.02	80.37
No Neighboring Features	10000	85.37	85.40	85.25	81.21	70.96	74.20

6 Conclusions

In short, we have presented a framework for simultaneously recognizing occurrences of multiple entity classes in textual drug fact sheets, using supervised machine learning techniques. Our empirical evaluation shows that the classifier achieves high overall accuracy. Although we have focused on drug interactions, the encouraging results and the ready adaptability of the approach we have adopted show that our system has significance for the extraction of detailed information about drugs (drug targets, contraindications, side effects, etc.) more generally.

References

1. Evans, D.A., Brownlowt, N.D., Hersh, W.R., Campbell, E.M.: Automating concept identification in the electronic medical record: An experiment in extracting dosage information. In: Proc. AMIA Annu. Fall Symp., pp. 388–392 (1996)
2. Friedman, C., Jonhson, S.B., Forman, B., Stanner, J.: Architectural requirements for a multipurpose natural language processor in the clinical environment. In: Proc. Annu. Symp. Comput. Appl. Med. Care, pp. 347–351 (1995)
3. Gold, S., Elhadad, N., Zhu, X., Cimino, J.J., Hripcsak, G.: Extracting structured medication event information from discharge summaries. In: Proc. AMIA Annu. Symp., pp. 237–241 (2008)
4. Haug, P.J., Ranum, D.L., Frederick, P.R.: Computerized extraction of coded findings from free-text radiologic reports. Radiology 174(2), 543–548 (1990)
5. Hripcsak, G., Kuperman, G.J., Friedman, C.: Extracting findings from narrative reports: software transferability and sources of physician disagreement. Methods Inf. Med., 1–7 (1998)
6. Lafferty, J.D., McCallum, A., Pereira, F.C.N.: Conditional random fields: Probabilistic models for segmenting and labeling sequence data. In: Proc. International Conference on Machine Learning, vol. 18, pp. 282–289 (2001)
7. Leape, L.L., Bates, D.W., Cullen, D.J., Cuper, J.: System analysis of adverse drug events. Journal of the American Medical Association 274(1), 35–43 (1995)
8. Levin, M.A., Krol, M., Doshi, A.M., Reich, D.L.: Extraction and mapping of drug names from free text to a standardized nomenclature. In: Proc. AMIA Annu. Symp., pp. 438–442 (2007)
9. McCallum, A.: Mallet: A machine learning for language toolkit. Tech. rep. (2002), `http://mallet.cs.umass.edu`
10. McCarry, A.T., Sponsler, J.L., Brylawski, B., Browne, A.C.: The role of a lexical knowledge in biomedical text understanding. In: Proc. SCAMC, pp. 103–104 (1987)
11. Meystre, S.M., Savova, G.K., Kipper-Schuler, K.C., Hurdle, J.F.: Extracting information from textual documents in the electronic health record: A review of recent research. In: IMIA Yearbook of Medical Informatics, pp. 128–144 (2008)
12. Pereira, S., Plaisantin, B., Korchia, M., Rozanes, N., Serrot, E., Joubert, M., Darmoni, S.J.: Automatic construction of dictionaries, application to product characteristics indexing. In: Proc Workshop on Advances in Bio Text Mining (2010)
13. Rubrichi, S., Leonardi, G., Quaglini, S.: A drug ontology as a basis for safe therapeutic decision. In: Proc. Second National Conference of Bioengineering, Patron (2010)

14. Sager, N., Friedman, C., Chi, E.: The analysis and processing of clinical narrative. In: Salamon, R., Blum, B., Jorgensen, M. (eds.) Proc. fifth Conference on Medical Informatics, pp. 1101–1105. Elsevier, Amsterdam (1986)
15. Segura-Bedmar, I., Martínez, P., de Pablo-Sánchez, C.: Extracting drug-drug interactions from biomedical texts. In: Workshop on Advances in Bio Text Mining (2010)
16. Shah, A.D., Martinez, C.: An algorithm to derive a numerical daily dose from unstructured text dosage instructions. Pharmacoepidemiology and Drug Safety 15, 161–166 (2006)
17. Sirohi, E., Peissig, P.: Study of effect of drug lexicons on medication extraction from electronic medical records. In: Proc. Pacific Symposium on Biocomputing, vol. 10, pp. 308–318 (2005)
18. Van Rijsbergen, C.J.: Information Retrieval. Department of Computer Science, University of Glasgow (1979)
19. Xu, H., Stenner, S.P., Doan, S., Johnson, K.B., Waitman, L.R., Denny, J.C.: Medex: a medication information extraction system for clinical narratives. Journal of the American Medical Informatics Association 17, 19–24 (2010)
20. Zanchetta, E., Baroni, M.: Morph-it!: a free corpus-based morphological resource for the italian language. In: Proc. Corpus Linguistics 2005 Conference (2005)

Automatic Verbalisation of SNOMED Classes Using OntoVerbal

Shao Fen Liang[1], Robert Stevens[1], Donia Scott[2], and Alan Rector[1]

[1] School of Computer Science, University of Manchester, Oxford Road, Manchester, UK M13 9PL
{Fennie.Liang,Robert.Stevens,Rector}@cs.man.ac.uk
[2] School of Informatics, University of Sussex, Falmer, Brighton, BN1 9QH, UK
D.R.Scott@sussex.ac.uk

Abstract. SNOMED is a large description logic based terminology for recording in electronic health records. Often, neither the labels nor the description logic definitions are easy for users to understand. Furthermore, information is increasingly being recorded not just using individual SNOMED concepts but also using complex expressions in the description logic ("post-coordinated" concepts). Such post-coordinated expressions are likely to be even more complex than other definitions, and therefore can have no pre-assigned labels. Automatic verbalisation will be useful both for understanding and quality assurance of SNOMED definitions, and for helping users to understand post-coordinated expressions. OntoVerbal is a system that presents a compositional terminology expressed in OWL as natural language. We describe the application of OntoVerbal to SNOMED-CT, whereby SNOMED classes are presented as textual paragraphs through the use of natural language generation technology.

Keywords: ontology verbalisation, natural language generation, describing ontologies.

1 Introduction

SNOMED-CT, managed by the International Health Terminology Standards Development Organisation (IHTSDO), is now mandated as a terminology for use in electronic health records in numerous countries including the USA, UK, Canada, Australia, several countries in continental Europe, and beyond. SNOMED describes diagnoses, procedures, and the necessary anatomy, biological processes (morphology) and the relevant organisms that cause disease. The goal is for terms from SNOMED to form a controlled vocabulary for filling electronic health records, with the controlled usage of terms, coupled with the hierarchy of SNOMED, enabling extensive querying to be made and statistics to be gathered.

SNOMED is developed using a Description Logic (DL) [2]. The DL structure allows compositional descriptions to be made of entities in a domain; that is, entities are described in terms of other entities, but this comes at the cost of cognitive complexity and unfamiliar notation. For example, the rendering of the concept heart disease in the Web Ontology Language (OWL) is:

M. Peleg, N. Lavrač, and C. Combi (Eds.): AIME 2011, LNAI 6747, pp. 338–342, 2011.

Class: Heart disease
EquivalentTo: Disorder of cardiovascular system
and RoleGroup some (Finding site some Heart structure)

While such descriptions are explicit, and can aid automated reasoners in building the terminology, they can be hard for humans to understand.

Other terminologies often include natural language definitions corresponding to the logical definitions. These should be easier to understand, especially when in a style of natural language used by the community in question. For instance, the above example could be verbalised as "*A heart disease is a disease that is found in a heart structure*". Such natural language definitions are, however, time-consuming to produce by hand. We have built a natural language verbaliser, *OntoVerbal*, to help automate the process of making OWL ontologies such as these more transparent. Automatic generation of natural language from knowledge representations such as OWL is known as "verbalisation" [3].

There is clearly an intuitive correlation between axioms and sentences, and between groups of related axioms and paragraphs. In generating such paragraphs we need to ensure that they are more than simply collections of individual sentences, each expressing a given axiom in the ontology; instead, they need to be structured, coherent and fluent. This can be achieved through four main operations: (a) grouping axioms together based on a shared topic; (b) aggregating axioms sharing a common pattern; (c) organising these as sentences according to theories of discourse structure, such as Rhetorical Structure Theory (RST) [7]; and (d) making use of linguistic devices designed to make the text hang together in a meaningful and organised manner — e.g., conjunctions [9], discourse markers [4] and punctuation.

2 The OntoVerbal System

OntoVerbal starts by grouping axioms relating to a designated class according to their relations to that class and the complexity of the grouped axioms' arguments. Axioms are defined as having *direct* relations to a class if the class is the first class that appears in its argument. For example an axiom like "A SubClassOf B" is in a *direct* relation to the class A, but is in an *indirect* relation to the class B. This example also represents a *simple* axiom, as only named classes appear in its argument. Axioms are classified as *complex* when they contain not only named classes, but also properties, cardinalities or value restrictions, or combinations of named classes in anonymous class expressions — e.g.: "A EquivalentTo B and hasRestriction some R" where R is the argument and contains another class expression.

Distinguishing between *direct* and *indirect* axioms allows all of the information about a given class to be brought together and presented in a rhetorically coherent way with a single topic; it also provides a framework for indicating to the reader when a topic has changed, by using linguistic devices for maintaining coherence of the text. We achieve this coherence through the application of RST, a theory of discourse coherence that addresses issues of semantics, communication and the nature of the coherence of texts, and which plays an important role in computational methods for generating natural language texts [10].

The *OntoVerbal* system has three main processes for axioms collected from a designated class.

The first process verbalises all *simple* axioms, where*by* axioms of the form "A SubClassOf B" are expressed as *"an* A *is a* B*"*. Where there are more subclass axioms, for example, "A SubClassOf C" and "A SubClassOf D" we treat this as a case requiring aggregation [6] to produce, for example, *"an* A *is a* B*, a* C *and a* D*"*. While SubClassOf relations are expressed through "is a" (and other semantically equivalent expressions), we treat EquivalentClass relations as definitions. So, for example, if the SubClassOf relation in the previous example were instead an EquivalentClass relation, the resulting text would be *"an* A *is defined as a* B*, a* C *and a* D*"*. In the cases mentioned so far, the relations are *direct* ones. Axioms in *indirect* relations will need to be inverted so as to be directed to the designated class. For example, in a context where the topic is B, the axiom we saw earlier, "A SubClassOf B", would be more properly expressed as *"a* B *includes an* A*"*, if the thread of discourse is to be maintained (i.e., for the text to "hang together"). In this context, the alternative, earlier, rendition would introduce a disfluency through the sudden shift of topic from B to A [11], and thus place an additional cognitive load on the reader [5].

The second process verbalises *complex*, but *direct* axioms. *Complex* axioms are necessarily longer than *simple* ones, and we ensure the maintenance of fluency and coherence between sentences through the use of relative clauses, discourse markers and punctuation. In our approach, *complex* SubClassOf axioms are expressed as *"an* A *is a* B *that* …" and *complex* EquivalentClass axioms are expressed as *"an* A *is defined as a* B *that* …". We use the discourse marker "additionally" to connect sentences from the outputs of the *simple* to the *complex* (*direct*) axioms process. This leads to results such as "*An* A *is a* B*, which includes a* C*, and both an* X *and a* Y *are an* A. *Additionally, an* A *is an* X *that …, and is defined as a* Y *that* …". However, if no sentence occurs from the *simple* axioms process then the discourse marker will be omitted.

The third process verbalises *complex*, but *indirect* axioms. In cases where *complex* axioms are in *indirect* relation to the designated class, this feature must be signalled in the generated text, since a change of topic (i.e., a new subject) is introduced. Without such signalling, the text will lack coherence and fluency and be harder to understand. We introduce these axioms through the use of key phrases, such as: *"Another relevant aspect of an* A *is that"* or *"Other relevant aspects of an* A *include the following:"*.

3 Discussion

Our attempts at verbalising SNOMED have so far focused on generating an appropriate rhetorical structure that conveys the basic meaning of the concept. There are obvious issues with articles and plurality in our verbalisations, and these will be addressed as *OntoVerbal* progresses. There are, however, several more substantial issues in verbalisation to tackle, some of which are generic to DL ontologies and some of which are peculiar to SNOMED.

For example, many SNOMED expressions are, in fact, redundant, and so *OntoVerbal*'s near-literal verbalisations can also seem redundant. Consider, for example, the generated paragraph:

> *A* Heart disease *includes a* Disorder of cardiac function*, and both an* Acute disease of cardiovascular system *and a* Heart disease *are an* Acute heart disease*. Additionally, a* Heart disease *is defined as a* Disorder of cardiovascular system *that has a* Finding site *some* Heart structure*. Other relevant aspects of a* Heart disease *include the following:* Hypertensive heart disease *is a* Heart disease *that has a* Finding site *some* Heart structure *and is* Associated with *some* Hypertensive disorder*; a* Chronic heart disease *is defined as a* Chronic disease of cardiovascular system *that is a* Heart disease *and has a* Clinical course *some* Chronic*; a* Structural disorder of heart *is defined as a* Heart disease *that has an* Associated morphology *some* Morphologically abnormal structure *and a* Finding site *some* Heart structure*; a* Disorder of cardiac ventricle *is defined as a* Heart disease *that has a* Finding site *some* Cardiac ventricular structure.

where the underlined sentence is clearly redundant in its multiple references to "chronic". This is a problem that combines issues for both the description logic representation and the verbalisation.

Similarly, because SNOMED's representation lacks a disjunction operator, it makes awkward use of complex intersections and this leads to infelicities of the sort seen here:

> *A* Lower body part structure *is a* Lower body structure*, which includes a* Pelvis and lower extremities. *An* Abdominal structure *is a* Chest and abdomen*, an* Abdomen and pelvis*, a* Structure of subregion of trunk *and a* Lower body part structure.

which should more properly read as the following, with the inclusion of the underlined words:

> *A* Lower body part structure *is a* Lower body structure*, which includes a* Pelvis and lower extremities *and an* Abdominal structure. *An* Abdominal structure *is a* Chest and abdomen*, an* Abdomen and pelvis*, a* Structure of subregion of trunk *and a* Lower body part structure.

We will be addressing these problems, refining our currently rudimentary treatment of plurals and articles, and exploring the use of layout (e.g., bulleted lists) [8] in future versions of the system.

There are two aspects of SNOMED that lead us to exceptionally depart for our stated goal of faithfulness of the generated output to the SNOMED input. The first involves the RoleGroup construct that is supposed to group aspects together. In reality, however, most of them appear to have only one role group, and therefore the RoleGroup is redundant in these cases. Our approach to this in *OntoVerbal* is to simply ignore such constructs.

The second aspect relates to multiple terms for class IDs. Most SNOMED class IDs have several associated terms, such as "preferred term" (that is expected to be used most commonly in medical records and interfaces), and "fully specified term" (that is intended to be completely unique and self explanatory) [1]. Given that there are thus many synonyms referring to a single concept, we have decided to let *OntoVerbal* in all cases use the stated "preferred term" to express SNOMED concepts.

4 Conclusions

OntoVerbal currently produces near-literal verbalisation of SNOMED concepts in well structured natural language. This addresses the problems of comprehension of complex logical descriptions of medical concepts in terminologies such as SNOMED, but also other DL based terminologies and ontologies. The need for automatically-generated verbalisations is especially important when post co-ordination is used, as without it there is no possibility of the provision of natural language versions of the concepts. Such verbalisations can provide much-needed documentation for artifacts like SNOMED, thereby making their content more accessible to users.

OntoVerbal's output currently lacks some linguistic polish, but having addressed the basic issues of grouping, aggregation and rhetorical structure in the verbalisations, other features of the output can be addressed. Then the role of automatic verbalisation of complex axiomatic descriptions in error detection, facilitation of users' comprehension, and creation of innovative presentations for artefacts such as SNOMED, can be explored.

Acknowledgments. This work is part of the Semantic Web Authoring Tool (SWAT) project (see www.swatproject.org), which is supported by the UK Engineering and Physical Sciences Research Council (EPSRC) grant EP/G032459/1, to the University of Manchester, the University of Sussex, and the Open University.

References

1. SNOMED-CT User Guide, http://www.ihtsdo.org/fileadmin/user_upload/Docs_01/SNOMED_CT/About_SNOMED_CT/Use_of_SNOMED_CT/SNOMED_CT_User_Guide_20090731.pdf
2. Baader, F., Horrocks, I., Sattler, U.: Description logics as ontology languages for the semantic web. In: Hutter, D., Stephan, W. (eds.) Mechanizing Mathematical Reasoning. LNCS (LNAI), vol. 2605, pp. 228–248. Springer, Heidelberg (2005)
3. Baud, R.H., Rodrigues, J.-M., Wagner, J.C., et al.: Validation of concept representation using natural language generation. Journal of the American Medical Informatics Association 841 (1997)
4. Callaway, C.B.: Integrating discourse markers into a pipelined natural language generation architecture. In: 41st Annual Meeting on Association for Computational Linguistics, vol. 1, pp. 264–271 (2003)
5. Clark, H.H.: Psycholinguistics. MIT Press, Cambridge (1999)
6. Dalianis, H.: Aggregation as a subtask of text and sentence planning. In: Stewman, J.H. (ed.) Florida AI Research Symposium, FLAIRS 1996, pp. 1–5 (1996)
7. Mann, W.C., Thompson, S.A.: Rhetorical Structure Theory: toward a functional theory of text organisation. Text 8, 243–281 (1988)
8. Power, R., Scott, D., Bouanyad-Agha, N.: Document structure. Computational Linguistics 29, 211–260 (2003)
9. Reape, M., Mellish, C.: Just what is aggregation, anyway? In: European Workshop on Natural Language Generation (1999)
10. Scott, D., Souza, C.S.: d.: Getting the message across in RST-based text generation. In: Mellish, C., Dale, R., Zock, M. (eds.) Current Research in Natural Language Generation, pp. 31–56. Academic Press, London (1990)
11. Walker, M.A., Joshi, A.K., Prince, E.F.: Centering Theory in Discourse. Oxford University Press, Oxford (1998)

Evaluating Outliers for Cross-Context Link Discovery

Borut Sluban[1], Matjaž Juršič[1], Bojan Cestnik[1,2], and Nada Lavrač[1,3]

[1] Jožef Stefan Institute, Ljubljana, Slovenia
[2] Temida d.o.o., Ljubljana, Slovenia
[3] University of Nova Gorica, Nova Gorica, Slovenia
{borut.sluban,matjaz.jursic,bojan.cestnik,nada.lavrac}@ijs.si

Abstract. In literature-based creative knowledge discovery the goal is to identify interesting terms or concepts which relate different domains. We propose to support this cross-context link discovery process by inspecting outlier documents which are not in the mainstream domain literature. We have explored the utility of outlier documents, discovered by combining three classification-based outlier detection methods, in terms of their potential for bridging concept discovery in the migraine-magnesium cross-domain discovery problem and in the autism-calcineurin domain pair. Experimental results prove that outlier documents present a small fraction of a domain pair dataset that is rich on concept bridging terms. Therefore, by exploring only a small subset of documents, where a great majority of bridging terms are present and more frequent, the effort needed for finding cross-domain links can be substantially reduced.

Keywords: text mining, creative knowledge discovery, outlier detection.

1 Introduction

In literature-based creative knowledge discovery one of the interesting goals is to identify terms or concepts which relate different domains, as these terms may represent germs of new scientific discoveries. The aim of this research is to support scientists in this creative knowledge discovery process, when analyzing scientific papers of their interest. A simplified cross-domain literature mining setting is addressed, where a scientist has identified two domains of interest (two different scientific areas or two different contexts) and tries to find concepts that represent potential links between the two different contexts. This simplified cross-context link discovery setting is usually referred to as a *closed discovery* setting [13]. Like Swanson [10] and Weeber et al. [13], we address the problem of literature mining, where papers from two different scientific areas are available, and the task is to support the scientist in cross-context literature mining.

This research investigates the role of *outlier documents* in literature mining, and explores the utility of outliers in this non-standard *cross-domain link discovery* task. This work provides evidence that outlier detection methods can contribute to cross-domain scientific discovery since outlier documents prove to be a rich source of cross-domain linking/bridging terms.

M. Peleg, N. Lavrač, and C. Combi (Eds.): AIME 2011, LNAI 6747, pp. 343–347, 2011.

2 Related Work

The motivation for new scientific discoveries from disparate literatures grounds in Mednick's *associative creativity theory* [4] and in the literature on domain-crossing associations, called bisociations, introduced by Koestler [3].

In the *closed discovery process*[1] defined by Weeber et al. [13] two domains of interest are identified by the expert prior to starting the knowledge discovery process. Weeber et al. have followed the work of creative literature-based discovery in medical domains by Swanson [10] who designed the *ABC model* approach that investigates whether an agent A is connected with a phenomenon C by discovering complementary structures via interconnecting phenomena B. In a *closed discovery process*, both A and C are known and the goal is to search for b-terms, i.e., bridging concepts (terms) b in B, in order to support the validation of the hypothesis about the hypothesized connection between A and C.

Smalheiser and Swanson [8] developed an online system ARROWSMITH, which takes as input two sets of titles from disjoint domains A and C and lists b-terms that are common to literature A and C; the resulting bridging terms are used to generate novel scientific hypotheses. As stated by Swanson et al. [11], the major focus in literature-based discovery has been on the closed discovery process, where both A and C are specified in advance.

Srinivasan and Libbus [9] developed an algorithm for bridging concept identification that is claimed to require the least amount of manual work in comparison with other studies. However, it still needs substantial time and human effort for collecting evidence relevant to the hypothesized connections.

In a closely related approach, rarity of terms as means for knowledge discovery has been explored in the RaJoLink system [6,12], which can be used to find interesting scientific articles in the PubMed database, to compute different statistics, and to analyze the articles with the aim to discover new knowledge. Recently, we have studied and improved the RaJoLink methodology by inspecting outlier documents[2] as potential source for speeding up the b-term detection process [5]. The methodology focuses on the search for b-terms in outlier documents identified by Ontogen, a semi-automated tool for topic ontology construction [2].

Classification noise filters and their ensembles, that were recently investigated by the authors [7], are used for outlier document detection in this work. Instances of a domain pair dataset that are misclassified by a classifier can be considered as domain outliers, since these instances tend to be more similar to regular instances of the opposite domain than to instances of their own domain. The utility of domain outliers as relevant sources of domain bridging terms is the topic of study of this paper.

---

[1] In contrast to closed discovery, *open discovery* leads the creative knowledge discovery process from a given starting domain towards a yet unknown second domain which at the end of this process turns out to be connected with the first one.

[2] In statistics, an outlier is an observation that is numerically distant from the rest of the data, or more formally, it is an observation that lies outside the overall pattern of a distribution.

3 Detecting Outlier Documents

This research aims at supporting the search for cross-domain links between concepts from two disparate literature sources by exploring outliers in the articles of the two domains.

The novelty of our work is to use noise detection approaches for finding domain outlier documents containing cross-domain links (bridging terms or *b*-terms) between different domains. When exploring a domain pair we search for a set of outlier documents with different classification noise filtering approaches [1], implemented and adapted for this purpose.

Classification noise filtering is based on the idea of using a classifier as a tool for detecting noisy and outlier instances in data. The proposed outlier detection method works in a 10-fold cross-validation manner, where repeatedly nine folds are used for training the classifier and on the complementary fold the misclassified instances are denoted as noise/outliers. Instances of a domain pair dataset that are misclassified by a classifier can be considered as domain outliers, since these instances tend to be more similar to regular instances of the opposite domain than to instances of their own domain.

4 Experimental Evaluation

This section provides experimental evidence for the claim that inspecting outlier documents can speed-up the search for bridging concepts between different domains of expertise.

In our experiments we used two domain pairs retrieved from the *PubMed database*[3] using domain name keyword queries: '*migraine*' – '*magnesium*' (dataset name abbr. MM) and '*autism*' – '*calcineurin*' (abbr. AC).

We performed outlier detection by a classification noise filtering algorithm, implemented with three different classifiers: Naïve Bayes (abbr. Bayes), Random Forest (RF) and Support Vector Machine (SVM). In addition to the outlier sets obtained by these three classification filters we examined also the union of those outlier sets and the so called 'Majority' outlier set containing outlier documents that were detected by at least two out of three classification filters.

To measure the relevance of the detected outlier documents in terms of their potential for containing domain bridging terms, we inspected 43 terms known as *b*-terms appearing in the MM domain pair, identified by Swanson et al. [11], and 13 known *b*-terms in the AC domain pair, identified by Petrič et al. [6]. We recorded the size of all detected outlier sets, the amount of *b*-terms present in these sets and the amount of *b*-terms present in randomly sampled document sets of same size as the outlier sets. A comparison of these recorded values relative to the whole datasets MM and AC can be found in Figures 1 and 2, respectively.

The results show two interesting points. Firstly, in all five outlier sets 70% to over 90% (for the 'Union' set) of all *b*-terms are present, which is on average in less than 10% of all documents from the MM dataset and in less than 5%

[3] PubMed: `http://www.ncbi.nlm.nih.gov/pubmed`

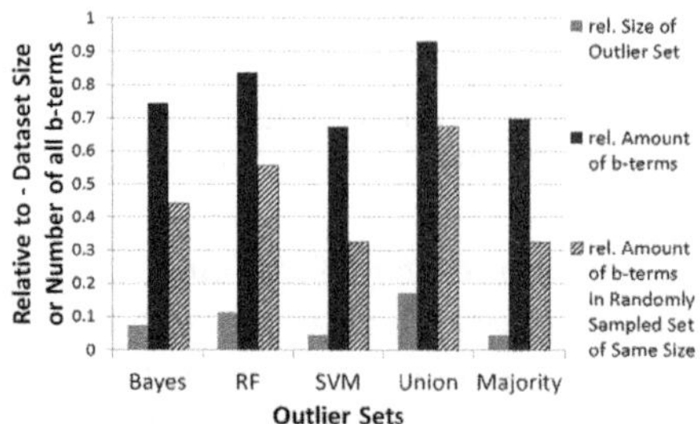

Fig. 1. Relative size of outlier sets and amount of *b*-terms for the MM dataset.

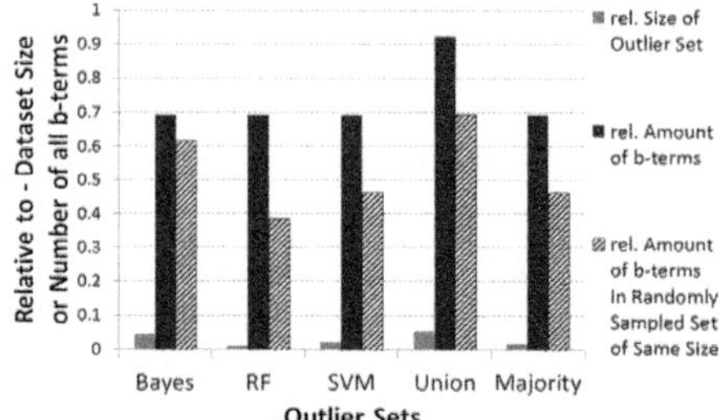

Fig. 2. Relative size of outlier sets and amount of *b*-terms for the AC dataset.

of all documents from the AC dataset. Secondly, more than 30% more of all *b*-terms from the MM dataset and more than 20% more of all *b*-terms from the AC dataset are present in outlier sets than in same-sized randomly sampled sets.

Additionally, we compared *relative frequencies of b-terms* in the detected outlier sets to those in the whole dataset, i.e. the fraction of documents containing a certain *b*-term among the documents of a chosen set. Figure 3 presents the increase of relative frequencies of *b*-terms in the 'Majority' outlier set detected in the MM and AC datasets.

We present the results of the majority voting based outlier detection approach because it is more likely to give high quality outliers on various datasets, since it reduces the danger of overfitting or bias of a single outlier detection approach to a certain domain by requiring the agreement of at least two outlier detection approaches for a document to declare it as an domain outlier.

Furthermore, the 'Majority' outlier sets achieve an overall most favorable ratio among the proportion of the size of the outlier set and the proportion of *b*-terms which are present in that outlier set (see Figures 1 and 2).

Finally, the relative frequency of all *b*-terms present in the 'Majority' outlier sets, except one in the AC dataset, is higher compared to the whole datasets, as can be clearly seen from Figure 3.

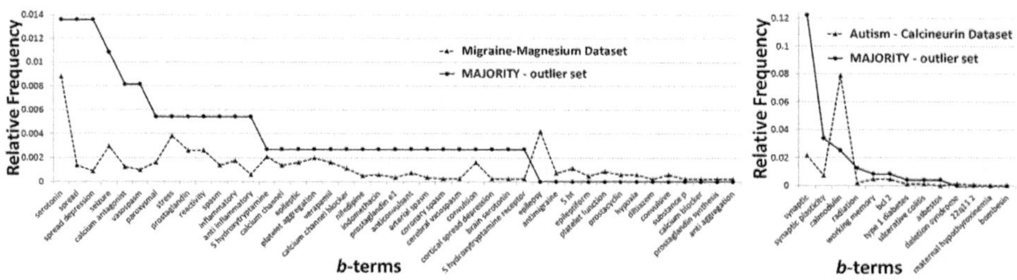

Fig. 3. Comparison of relative frequencies of bridging terms in the whole dataset and in the 'Majority' set of outlier documents detected by three different outlier detection methods in the MM dataset (left) and in the AC dataset (right[7]).

[7] Note that the scale of the chart on the right (AC dataset) is different from the scale of the chart on the left (MM dataset).

5 Conclusions

In our research we investigate the potential of outlier detection methods in literature mining for supporting the discovery of bridging concepts between two disparate domains. In our experiments we obtain five sets of outlier documents for each examined domain pair by three different outlier detection methods, their union and a majority voting approach, which proves to have the greatest potential for bridging concept detection. Experimental results prove that inspecting outlier documents considerably contributes to the bridging concept discovery process, since it enables the expert to focus only on a small fraction of documents that is rich on b-terms. Thus, the effort needed for finding cross-domain links is substantially reduced, as it requires to explore a much smaller subset of documents, where a great majority of b-terms are present and more frequent.

In further work we will examine other outlier detection methods in the context of cross-domain link discovery and use outlier documents as a focus in the search for potential b-terms on yet unexplored domain-pairs.

This work was supported by the European Commission under the 7th Framework Programme FP7-ICT-2007-C FET-Open, contract no. BISON-211898.

References

1. Brodley, C.E., Friedl, M.A.: Identifying mislabeled training data. Journal of Artificial Intelligence Research 11, 131–167 (1999)
2. Fortuna, B., Grobelnik, M., Mladenić, D.: Semi-automatic data-driven ontology construction system. In: Proc. of the Information Society Conf., pp. 223–226 (2006)
3. Koestler, A.: The act of creation. MacMillan Company, New York (1964)
4. Mednick, S.A.: The associative basis of the creative process. Psychological Review 69, 219–227 (1962)
5. Petrič, I., Cestnik, B., Lavrač, N., Urbančič, T.: Outlier detection in cross-context link discovery for creative literature mining. The Computer Journal (2010)
6. Petrič, I., Urbančič, T., Cestnik, B., Macedoni-Lukšič, M.: Literature mining method RaJoLink for uncovering relations between biomedical concepts. Journal of Biomedical Informatics 42(2), 220–232 (2009)
7. Sluban, B., Gamberger, D., Lavrač, N.: Performance analysis of class noise detection algorithms. In: Proceedings of STAIRS 2010, pp. 303–314 (2011)
8. Smalheiser, N.R., Swanson, D.R.: Using ARROWSMITH: a computer-assisted approach to formulating and assessing scientific hypotheses. Comput. Methods Programs Biomed. 57(3), 149–153 (1998)
9. Srinivasan, P., Libbus, B., Sehgal, A.K.: Mining MEDLINE: Postulating a beneficial role for curcumin longa in retinal diseases. In: BioLINK, pp. 33–40 (2004)
10. Swanson, D.R.: Undiscovered public knowledge. Libr. Quar. 56(2), 103–118 (1986)
11. Swanson, D.R., Smalheiser, N.R., Torvik, V.I.: Ranking indirect connections in literature-based discovery: The role of medical subject headings (MeSH). Jour. Am. Soc. Inf. Sci. Tec. 57(11), 1427–1439 (2006)
12. Urbančič, T., Petrič, I., Cestnik, B., Macedoni-Lukšič, M.: Literature mining: towards better understanding of autism. In: Bellazzi, R., Abu-Hanna, A., Hunter, J. (eds.) AIME 2007. LNCS (LNAI), vol. 4594, pp. 217–226. Springer, Heidelberg (2007)
13. Weeber, M., Vos, R., Klein, H., de Jong-van den Berg, L.T.W.: Using concepts in literature-based discovery: Simulating Swanson's Raynaud–fish oil and migraine–magnesium discoveries. Jour. Am. Soc. Inf. Sci. Tec. 52, 548–557 (2001)

Diagnosis Code Assignment Support Using Random Indexing of Patient Records – A Qualitative Feasibility Study

Aron Henriksson[1], Martin Hassel[1], and Maria Kvist[1,2]

[1] Department of Computer and System Sciences (DSV), Stockholm University
Forum 100, 164 40 Kista, Sweden

[2] Department of Clinical Immunology and Transfusion Medicine, Karolinska University Hospital, 171 76 Stockholm, Sweden

Abstract. The prediction of diagnosis codes is typically based on free-text entries in clinical documents. Previous attempts to tackle this problem range from strictly rule-based systems to utilizing various classification algorithms, resulting in varying degrees of success. A novel approach is to build a word space model based on a corpus of coded patient records, associating co-occurrences of words and ICD-10 codes. Random Indexing is a computationally efficient implementation of the word space model and may prove an effective means of providing support for the assignment of diagnosis codes. The method is here qualitatively evaluated for its feasibility by a physician on clinical records from two Swedish clinics. The assigned codes were in this initial experiment found among the top 10 generated suggestions in 20% of the cases, but a partial match in 77% demonstrates the potential of the method.

Keywords: ICD-10 Assignment, Random Indexing, Electronic Patient Records, Qualitative Evaluation.

1 Introduction

1.1 Diagnosis Code Assignment Support

Patient records comprise a combination of structured information and free-text fields. Free-text fields allow healthcare personnel to record observations and to reason about possible diagnoses and actions in a flexible manner. Fixed fields, i.e. closed classes, are on the other hand often desirable as they can easily be aggregated to produce meaningful statistics. The 10th revision of the *International Classification of Diseases and Related Health Problems* (ICD-10) is a classification system that is used to record medical activity. Its main purpose is to enable classification and quantification of diseases and other health-related issues [1].

Assigning ICD-10 codes is a necessary yet time-consuming task that keeps healthcare personnel away from their core responsibility: tending to patients. To facilitate the selection of diagnosis codes among a myriad of options, computer-aided coding support has been an active research area for the past twenty years or so (see [2] for a literature review).

M. Peleg, N. Lavrač, and C. Combi (Eds.): AIME 2011, LNAI 6747, pp. 348–352, 2011.

The most common approach is to base coding support on natural language processing of clinical documents. This study is to all intents and purposes similar to that of Larkey and Croft [3]. They assign ICD-9 codes to discharge summaries using three classifiers trained on a prelabeled corpus. By giving extra weight to words, phrases and structures that provide the most diagnostic evidence, results are shown to improve. A combination of classifiers yields a precision of 87.9%, where the principal code is included in a list of ten recommendations.

A large number of related studies were sparked by the Computational Medicine Center's 2007 Medical NLP Challenge[1], where a limited set of 45 ICD-9-CM codes were to be assigned to free-text radiology reports. Many of the solutions are hand-crafted rule-based systems, giving at best an 89.1% average F-score.

1.2 Word Space Models

A common trait of the aforementioned methods is that they in some way attempt to represent features of the classified text passage. Word space models constitute a family of models that capture meaning through statistics on word co-occurrences. Since its introduction, *Latent Semantic Analysis* (LSA) [4] has more or less spawned an entire research field with a wide range of word space models as a result. Numerous publications report exceptional results in many different applications, such as information retrieval, various semantic knowledge tests (e.g. TOEFL), text categorization and word sense disambiguation.

The idea behind word space models is to use statistics on word distributions in order to generate a high-dimensional vector space. Words are here represented by context vectors whose relative directions are assumed to indicate semantic similarity. The basis of this is the *distributional hypothesis*, according to which words that occur in similar contexts tend to have similar properties (meanings/functions). If we repeatedly observe two words in the same contexts, it is not too far-fetched to assume that they also refer to similar concepts [5].

2 Method

We employ the *Random Indexing* word space approach [5], [6], which presents an efficient, scalable and inherently incremental alternative to LSA-like word space models. The construction of context vectors using Random Indexing can be viewed as a two-step process.

First, each context—defined as the document or paragraph in which a word occurs, or as a (sliding) window of a number of surrounding words—is assigned a unique and (usually) randomly generated label. These labels are sparse, high-dimensional and ternary vectors. Their dimensionality d is usually in the range of a couple of hundred to several thousands, depending on the size and redundancy of the data, and they consist of a very small number (usually about 1-2%) of randomly distributed +1s and -1s, with the rest of the elements in the vectors set to 0. Next, the actual context vectors are produced by scanning the text: each

[1] `http://www.computationalmedicine.org/challenge/2007/index.php`

time a token w occurs in a particular context, the d-dimensional random label of that context is added to the context vector of w. Thus, each context that a token w appears in has an effect, through its random label, on the context vector of w. Words are in this way effectively represented by d-dimensional context vectors, which are the sum of the random labels of the co-occurring contexts.

In our experiments, we set the context to an entire document, as there exists no sequential dependency between the diagnosis code and the words. A document contains all free-text entries concerning an individual patient made on consecutive days at a single clinic, as well as the associated ICD-10 codes. The data used for training and testing the model is a part of the *Stockholm EPR* corpus [7] and contains 273,888 documents written in Swedish, 12,396 distinct ICD-10 codes and 838 clinical units[2]. A document contains an average of 96 words and 1.7 ICD-10 codes. All documents are first pre-processed. In addition to lemmatization, which is done using the *Granska Tagger* [8], punctuation, digits and stop words[3] are removed. The data is then split 90:10 between training and testing, where the training documents include the associated codes, while, in the testing data, they are retained separately for evaluation.

In the testing phase, a document is input: for each word, a ranked list of semantically correlated words is produced by the model. As our interest lies in assigning ICD-10 codes only, the result set is restricted to such tokens. The lists for each of the words in the document are combined to yield a single ranked list of ten ICD-10 codes. The results are manually evaluated by a physician on a total of 30 documents: 15 from an emergency ward and 15 from a rheumatology clinic. The recommended codes are evaluated for their relevance compared to the clinical text and matched with the codes assigned by the physicians.

3 Evaluation

We found the assigned code among the ten suggestions in 20% of the cases (Table 1). It should be noted that, although this number seems low, matching the assigned code exactly is difficult, given the structure of ICD-10. The codes contain four levels, going from general categories to more specific descriptions, with codes typically assigned at the two most specific levels. As a result, the model will sometimes generate suggestions that are either more or less specific than the assigned code(s), even if they are otherwise similar. For partial matches[4], however, there was at least one match in 77% of the cases. Another complicating factor is that some closely related diagnoses belong to different categories altogether, resulting in a reasonable suggestion not even yielding a partial match.

We therefore also evaluated to what extent the recommended codes were reasonable. On average, 23% of the suggestions were reasonable in the sense that they were deemed possible diagnoses by a physician based on the clinical

[2] This research has been approved by the Regional Ethical Review Board in Stockholm (Etikprövningsnämnden i Stockholm), permission number 2009/1742-31/5.

[3] Frequently occurring words that have a low discriminatory value.

[4] A partial match is defined as matching the assigned code on any of the levels.

text. Some of these—with occurrences in more than half of the documents—were diagnoses that were not assigned a code, either because they could not yet be confirmed or due to their lesser degree of relevance in relation to the problem at hand. We also measured the proportion of the suggested diagnoses which had a palpable connection—in the form of clinically significant words—to the text. We found such a word-based connection in 45% of the recommended codes.

Table 1. Evaluation of recommended codes in relation to input document and assigned code. Word connections and reasonable suggestions are calculated for all recommended codes (10/doc), while full and partial matches are calculated on a document level.

	Word connection	Reasonable suggestion	Assigned code in top 10	
			Full match	Partial match
Rheumatology	43% (±25)	23% (±18)	33%	87%
Emergency	47% (±16)	23% (±13)	6.7%	67%
Overall	45% (±21)	23% (±16)	20%	77%

The results between the two clinics are fairly similar when it comes to word connections and reasonable suggestions, which indicates that the method is equally applicable to two very different types of clinics. The difficulty of the task is not necessarily identical, however, as the results of the full and partial matches demonstrate. A possible explanation for this could be that a rheumatology clinic consists of a more homogenous group of specialists using a limited set of well-known diagnosis codes, whereas the number of possible codes is likely to be larger in an emergency ward, where the specificity of the code may also depend on the specialty of the coder.

4 Discussion

Even if ICD-10 codes may sometimes be used in a complementary manner to the free-text fields in patient records, in our evaluation there was almost always a connection between the text and the assigned code(s). This is encouraging, as it constitutes a prerequisite for the application of Random Indexing—or any other implementation of the word space model—to be successful in recommending diagnosis codes. There are, however, a number of limitations to the method, especially in its current mold.

In addition to the difficulties mentioned earlier, a big challenge is posed by the present inability to capture the function of negations. This is particularly problematic when applying the method to the clinical domain, where ruling out possible diseases, symptoms and findings is inherent in the operations of clinical practice. The consequence is, of course, that diagnosis codes will be associated with symptoms and findings that are negated in the text.

In this rather naive implementation, all words have an equal say in "voting" for the most appropriate diagnosis code. A means of countering this is to incorporate some form of weighting. We plan initially to employ the well-established *tf-idf* (term frequency-inverse document frequency) weighting scheme, which is based on the prominence of tokens (*tf*) and their discriminatory value (*idf*). Giving more weight to words in the ICD-10 descriptions and to certain sections of the patient record may also yield improved results.

Given the large amount of possible diagnosis codes, domain-specific models trained on a single type of clinic may possibly perform better. Taking advantage of structured information, such as age and gender, is also likely to limit the classification problem by ruling out, or giving less weight to, unlikely correlations. Finally, building word space models based on bigrams, which have a higher discriminatory value than unigrams, is also something we plan to investigate.

Once we have implemented some of these features, we will also conduct a quantitative study, in which all the test data will be evaluated in relation to the assigned diagnosis codes.

5 Conclusion

We have introduced Random Indexing of patient records as a new approach to the problem of diagnosis code assignment support. The outcome of the qualitative evaluation is fairly encouraging—particularly as it is here applied in a rather elementary fashion—with 20% full matches and 77% partial matches against a list of ten recommended ICD-10 codes. With further room for improvement, it may prove an efficient and effective solution.

References

1. World Health Organization: International Classification of Diseases (ICD) (Internet). WHO, Geneva (2010), `http://www.who.int/classifications/icd/en/` (accessed February 2010)
2. Stanfill, M.H., Williams, M., Fenton, S., Jenders, R.A., Hersh, W.R.: A systematic literature review of automated clinical coding and classification systems. J. Am. Med. Inform. Assoc. 17, 646–651 (2010)
3. Larkey, L.S., Croft, W.B.: Automatic Assignment of ICD9 Codes to Discharge Summaries. In: PhD thesis University of Massachusetts at Amherst, Amherst, MA (1995)
4. Landauer, T.K., Foltz, W., Laham, D.: Introduction to Latent Semantic Analysis. Discourse Processes 25, 259–284 (1998)
5. Sahlgren, M.: The Word-Space Model: Using distributional analysis to represent syntagmatic and paradigmatic relations between words in high-dimensional vector spaces. In: PhD thesis Stockholm University, Stockholm, Sweden (2006)
6. Sahlgren, M.: Vector-Based Semantic Analysis: Representing Word Meanings Based on Random Labels. In: Proceedings of Semantic Knowledge Acquisition and Categorization Workshop at ESSLLI 2001 (2001)
7. Dalianis, H., Hassel, M., Velupillai, S.: The Stockholm EPR Corpus: Characteristics and Some Initial Findings. In: Proceedings of ISHIMR 2009, pp. 243–249 (2009)
8. Knutsson, O., Bigert, J., Kann, V.: A Robust Shallow Parser for Swedish. In: Proceedings of Nodalida (2003)

Author Index

<u>GPSR Compliance</u>

The European Union's (EU) General Product Safety Regulation (GPSR) is a set of rules that requires consumer products to be safe and our obligations to ensure this.

If you have any concerns about our products, you can contact us on ProductSafety@springernature.com

In case Publisher is established outside the EU, the EU authorized representative is:

Springer Nature Customer Service Center GmbH
Europaplatz 3
69115 Heidelberg, Germany

Batch number: 09496765

Printed by Printforce, the Netherlands